Skin Care:
Beyond the Basics

Skin Care:
Beyond the Basics

Mark Lees, Ph.D.

MILADY

THOMSON LEARNING

Australia • Canada • Mexico • Singapore • Spain • United Kingdom • United States

Skin Care: Beyond the Basics
by Mark Lees

MILADY STAFF:

President:
Susan Simpfenderfer

Publisher:
Marlene McHugh Pratt

Acquisitions Editor:
Pamela Lappies

Development Editor:
Judy Roberts

Executive Production Manager:
Wendy A. Troeger

Production Editor:
Eileen M. Clawson

Executive Marketing Manager:
Donna J. Lewis

Channel Manager:
Nigar Hale

Cover Design:
Dutton and Sherman Design

For permission to use material from this text or product, contact us by
Tel   (800) 730-2214
Fax   (800) 730-2215
www.thomsonrights.com

Library of Congress Cataloging-in-Publication Data

Lees, Mark.
   Skin care: beyond the basics / Mark Lees.
      p. cm.
   Includes bibliographical references and index.
   ISBN 1-56253-625-7 (softcover)
   1. Skin--Care and hygiene. 2. Self-care, Health. I. Title.
RA776.5 .L43 2000
646.7'26--dc21

                                                   00-052551

NOTICE TO THE READER

Dedication

This book is dedicated to my parents, Richard and Virginia Lees.
Thank you for your lifelong encouragement.

Contents

Acknowledgments

Very special thanks to the following people and organizations for contributing in many ways to this book. The author very much appreciates their efforts.

Editors and staff of Milady/Thomas Learning.

Reviewers: Carroll Pierson, Crystal Gutshall, Billie Smith, Laurol Boik, Martin Dow, Barbara Spencer, Kim Fullen, Sally Deitz, Virginia Burge, Judith Culp, Ellen Thorpe.

Erica Miller, Correlations, Inc., Dallas, Texas.

Rube Pardo, M.D., Ph.D., Dept. of Dermatology, University of Miami.

Samuel J. LaMonte, M.D., Facial Plastic Surgeon, Pensacola, Florida.

Kirk Smith, M.D., Plastic Surgeon, Pensacola, Florida.

David Wanetik, Skin Culture Institute, New York, New York.

Howard Murad, M.D., Murad Skin Research Laboratories, Los Angeles, California.

Rebecca James, Cosmetic Chemistry Instructor, UCLA.

Thibiant International/Guinot-Paris, Beverly Hills, California.

My wonderful staff, family, and friends for putting up with me while I was writing this book.

Timothy Berger, M.D., Dermatologist, San Francisco, California.

Michael Bond, M.D., Dermatologist, Memphis, Tennessee.

Melvin Elson, M.D., Dermatologist, Nashville, Tennessee.

George Fisher, M.D., Dermatologist, Pensacola, Florida.

Figures 12–2, 12–3, 12–5, 12–6, 12–8 are reprinted from *Acne Morphogenesis and Treatment* by Gerd Plewig, M.D., and Albert M. Kligman, M.D., Ph.D.; permission of publishers, Springer-Verlafg, New York, U.S.A., Heidelberg, Berlin, Germany.

National Rosacea Society

Charles Mizelle, Los Angeles, California

Marta Martine, Martine Business Development, Santa Barbara, California

Sothys USA, Miami, Florida

St. Tropez, Inc., Santa Clarita, California

Dermascope Magazine, Sunnyvale, Texas

Les Nouvelles Esthetiques—American Edition, Coral Gables, Florida

Skin Inc., Carol Stream, Illinois

About the Author

Dr. Mark Lees is recognized as one of the world's renowned skin-care specialists, having been quoted and interviewed by *Glamour, Teen, Self,* the *Miami Herald,* the Associated Press, Discovery Channel, and NBC News, to name a few. His professional awards are numerous and include *American Salon Magazine* Esthetician of the Year, the *Les Nouvelles Esthetiques* Crystal Award, the Dermascope Legends Award, the Rocco Bellino Award for outstanding education from the Chicago Cosmetology Association, and Best Educational Skin Care Classroom from the Long Beach International Beauty Expo.

Dr. Lees holds a Ph.D. in Health Sciences, a Master of Science in Health, and the prestigious CIDESCO International Diploma, and also serves as an International CIDESCO Examiner. He has been in practice in Northwest Florida for almost twenty years at his CIDESCO-Accredited Dayspa and Salon.

Dr. Lees is president of the Esthetics Manufacturers and Distributors Alliance (EMDA), a division of the American Beauty Association. He is former chairperson of EstheticsAmerica, the skin-care division of the National Cosmetology Association, former vice president of CIDESCO, USA, and is a member of the Society of Cosmetic Chemists.

His company, Mark Lees Skin Care, Inc., specializes in the development of science-based skin-care products and cosmetics for acne-prone, sensitive, and sun-damaged skin. The product line is now used and sold in salons and dermatology clinics all over America, and is also distributed in other countries.

Dr. Lees is an accomplished writer, having published dozens of skin-care, technical, and business articles for almost every major beauty and esthetics trade publication. He serves on the editorial advisory board of *Les Nouvelles Esthetiques—American Edition.* He authored a chapter on esthetics for the dental textbook *Esthetic Dentistry.*

An extremely popular and award-winning speaker, Dr. Lees is constantly in demand for his classes at professional beauty and medical conventions, as well as consumers and women's groups, and major universities including UCLA, Purdue, and Columbia. He has also made appearances in both Australia and Europe.

Letter to the Reader

It is amazing to me how much science can change in just a few years. I am excited to have had the opportunity to expand—and literally rewrite—much of this book. Whether you are currently practicing professional skin care, are just entering the field as a student, or just want more practical information about scientific care of the skin, I hope you will find this real-world book helpful. I have tried to keep this book as user-friendly and as helpful in day-to-day practice as the first edition.

We understand more than ever about the treatment of aging skin. It is now accepted by the scientific community that the corneum of the skin is dead, yet very chemically and biologically active.

AIDS, fortunately, is now being managed more successfully, and rosacea is being diagnosed more frequently. Many more people seem to have sensitive skin, and laser skin resurfacing is a routine cosmetic surgery procedure. Hence, there is new and expanded information about these and other topics.

I am thrilled with the response to the first edition of this book, and have tried to add and develop subjects for which I have had many requests, including the addition of color picture inserts.

I am so flattered when estheticians tell me that they always keep my book within reach. I hope you find this second edition—*Skin Care: Beyond the Basics*—even more help in your understanding and treatment of the skin.

Mark Lees, Ph.D.
CIDESCO Diplomate
Pensacola, Florida

Chapter 1

Advanced Anatomy and Physiology of the Skin

Objectives

In this chapter you will learn about the anatomy and functions of cells. You will also recognize different types of tissues and their functions. You will learn, in detail, about the different layers of the skin and functions of various reactions that take place in the different layers of the skin. Skin penetration will be studied, as well as some techniques for better penetrating, moisturizing, and conditioning treatments for the skin.

Before we can fully understand how to treat cosmetic disorders of the skin, we must first fully understand the functions and activities of the body, more specifically, the **cell**. The cell is almost a self-contained factory of life. Cells are the building blocks of the human body. Within each cell, many chemical and physical processes constantly take place. To simplify, let's think of the cell as a very, very small living body. This is, of course, an oversimplification, but it will help us understand the many miraculous functions that happen inside each cell of the human body.

1

THE STRUCTURE OF THE CELL

Cell is a very small, self-contained unit of life. Within the human body, cells specialize in individual functions.

Cell membrane gives the cell structure and shape and contains the many internal parts of the cell.

Selective permeability means that the cell membrane can let substances into the cell, such as food, water, and oxygen. It can also let substances out of the cell, such as waste and carbon dioxide.

Receptor sites are small structures on the cell membrane that are "docking stations" for hormones and other chemicals. Receptor sites receive chemical messages from other cells or organs that cause the cell to behave in a certain way.

Cytoplasm is a fluid inside cells that is made of water and other substances.

Organelles are small structures within the cell that have their own function.

Endoplasmic reticulum is a structure inside cells that is formed like a maze. This network of material forms little canals within the cytoplasm that allows substances and other organelles to move around.

Mitochrondria are the "lungs" and "digestive system" of the cell.

Much like the skin that covers our bodies, the cell is protected by an outer shell known as the **cell membrane** (Figure 1–1). The cell membrane gives the cell structure and shape and contains the many internal parts of the cell. The cell membrane is made of a network of lipids (fatty matter) and protein. The cell membrane possesses a function known as **selective permeability**. Selective permeability means that the cell membrane can let substances into the cell, such as food, water, and oxygen. It can also let substances out of the cell, such as waste and carbon dioxide. The cell is furnished food, water, and oxygen by the blood. Blood is also the vehicle that carries waste materials and carbon dioxide away from the cell membrane and eventually out of the body. Blood itself is made up of cells.

Located on the cell membrane are special structures called **receptor sites**. Receptors are the communication system between different cells, tissues, organs, and different parts of the body. Each tissue has cells with unique receptor sites that carry out the activity of a particular type of cell. Receptors receive messages from hormones and other chemical messengers made by other cells. Receptor sites work with these chemical messengers like a "lock and key" system. The receptor site is the "lock," and the chemical it comes in contact with is the "key." When a chemical comes in contact with its specific special receptor, a message is sent to the cell, which carries out specific functions. A good example of this is sebaceous gland activity. Production of sebum in the sebaceous gland is stimulated by male hormones that are received by the receptor sites in the cells of the sebaceous gland. The sites are like "switches" that are "turned on" when a male hormone stimulates the receptor site.

Inside the cell is a fluid called **cytoplasm**. Cytoplasm is made of water and other substances. It has a gel-like consistency. Cytoplasm allows other structures to move around inside the cell. If you think of the cell as a human body, the cytoplasm would play the part of the blood, allowing transportation within the cell.

Organelles

Organelles are small structures within the cell that each have their own function. You can think of organelles as being miniature body organs in the cell. For many years, scientists did not know about the existence of organelles. But as science progressed, these super-small structures were discovered.

Inside the cell cytoplasm, there is a structure that is formed like a maze, sort of like a house of mirrors at a carnival. This maze is called the **endoplasmic reticulum**. This network of material forms little canals within the cytoplasm that allow substances and other organelles to move around. Think of the endoplasmic reticulum as blood vessels within the body.

The **mitochondria** are the "lungs" and the "digestive system" of the cell. The mitochondria can be thought of as the cell's nutritionist. They convert oxygen and nutrients so that they can be used as energy by the cell. The mitochondria are also responsible for converting oxygen to carbon dioxide, which is an essential part of the oxygen usage system within the body. The mitochondria have "departments" that also control the amount of water and other substances that are allowed into the cytoplasm at particular

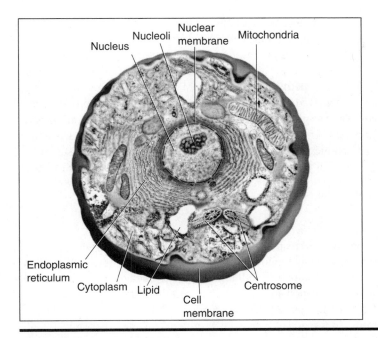

Figure 1–1 Structure of the cell

times. As a "digestive factory" they help to break down simple sugars, fats, and parts of proteins called **amino acids**. These are broken into smaller units that can more easily be used by the cell for energy. The **Golgi apparatus** is a storage mechanism that helps store proteins for later conversion to manufacture other necessary chemicals when the cell needs them. Think of the Golgi apparatus as a tiny "silo" storing fuels for a future date.

    Ribosomes are very small organelles that help build protein structures that the cell needs. They are the protein "construction division" of the cell.

    Lysosomes are the "demolition crew" of the cell. They manufacture enzymes that help break apart large molecules entering the cell so that they can be more easily converted to other necessary chemicals and substances. Lysosomes also are the "self-destruct" mechanism for the cell. When a cell dies, the lysosome releases enzymes that help destroy the cell membrane.

    Vacuoles are often one of the biggest organelles. They are the "storage vats" for waste and excess food supplies.

A DAY IN THE LIFE OF A CELL

Let's go through an oversimplified yet representative "day in the life of a cell." The blood cells deliver foods for the cell that have already been substantially broken down by the digestive system, absorbed through the intestinal wall, and absorbed by the blood. The blood also delivers fresh oxygen from the lungs. First the cell membrane

Amino acids are proteins that help break down simple sugars, fats, and parts of proteins.

Golgi apparatus is a storage mechanism that helps store proteins for later conversion to manufacture other necessary chemicals when the cell needs them.

Ribosomes are very small organelles that help build protein structures that the cell needs.

Lysosomes manufacture enzymes that help break apart large molecules entering the cell so that they can be more easily converted to other necessary chemicals and substances.

Vacuoles are the "storage vats" for waste and excess food supplies.

acts as a "guard," allowing certain substances into the cytoplasm. Once inside, they may be guided to their destination by the canals of the endoplasmic reticulum. The lysosomes start breaking down the large protein molecules. The ribosomes are building or "rebuilding" the proteins that the cell needs at the time. The mitochondria serve as a "power plant" making usable energy for the cell from the variety of proteins, sugars, oxygen, and fats that have arrived. Excess food product and waste from production are stored in the vacuoles. The Golgi apparatus stores proteins to use later for manufacturing enzymes and hormones. After production is over, waste materials and carbon dioxide are released by the cell membranes to the blood. The blood takes the waste away to the lungs, where the carbon dioxide is breathed out, and to the kidneys, which filter out the other waste.

THE NUCLEUS

We have discussed some of the respiratory, digestive, and synthesis functions of the cell. But what controls these many functions? Where is the "brain" of the cell? Centered in the cytoplasm is a large structure called the **nucleus**. The nucleus of the cell is made largely of protein and is also responsible for building certain proteins. It contains fibers called **chromatin**. Chromatin is largely responsible for cell division, which will be discussed later. The chromatin is made of a mixture of protein and special chemicals called **nucleic acids**. The most important of these acids is deoxyribonucleic acid, better known as DNA. DNA is a long, spiral-shaped molecule, which looks like a twisted ladder. The DNA has the power to duplicate itself, and within it are the "directions" for running the cell operations. Therefore, it may pass on instructions to new cells as it duplicates, ensuring that each type of cell will know the "blueprint" for life.

Cells divide and reproduce by a process known as mitotic division, or **mitosis**. Hereditary traits for the cell are found in small structures in the DNA called **genes**. When the cell divides, the chromatin fibers line up and are seen as **chromosomes**. The entire "blueprint" is duplicated in the DNA, and the cell splits into two separate cells, both containing the exact same DNA, and genes (Figure 1–2). By this process cells are constantly reproducing themselves, carrying out the same functions.

CELL SPECIALIZATION

Many types of cells are found within the human body. Groups of cells that perform the same function are called **tissues**. There are many different types of tissue.

Muscular tissue is of three types, which include visceral muscle, skeletal muscle, and cardiac muscle.

Visceral muscle is responsible for involuntary muscle actions. Involuntary muscle actions are movements that happen subconsciously. Movement of the lungs expanding and contracting, muscles of the intestines, and muscles of the digestive system are involuntary muscles. In other words, these muscle structures operate on "automatic pilot." Involuntary muscles are also known as smooth muscle tissue.

Nucleus of the cell is made largely of protein and is also responsible for building certain proteins.

Chromatin is largely responsible for cell division.

Nucleic acids are a mixture of protein and special chemicals that make up chromatin.

Mitosis is the division and reproduction of cells.

Genes are small structures that contain hereditary traits.

Chromosomes are chromatin fibers.

Tissues are groups of cells that perform the same function.

Muscular tissue is of three types, which include visceral muscle, skeletal muscle, and cardiac muscle.

Visceral muscle is responsible for involuntary muscle actions.

Skeletal muscles are responsible for the movement of the bones and the body's physical motion.

Striations are stripes on skeletal muscles that control body movement. These muscles are known as striated muscles.

First Phase

Second Phase

Third Phase

Fourth Phase

Fifth Phase

One cell has divided to create two cells.

Figure 1–2 Indirect division of the human cell

Skeletal muscles are responsible for the movement of the bones and the body's physical motion. Because these muscle cells have stripes, or **striations**, they are also known as striated muscles. Skeletal muscles are responsible for voluntary movement and therefore are known as voluntary muscles. These muscles are controlled by the conscious brain, which means the brain directly controls their movement. Walking across a room to pick up an object is a motion in which the brain has complete control and is an example of a voluntary muscle action.

Cardiac muscle tissue used to be considered an involuntary smooth muscle, but it has since been established that this tissue is also striated, so it is classified in a separate category. Cardiac muscle is both striated and involuntary.

Connective tissue is a group of cells that specialize in providing support and cushioning for the body. **Cartilage** and **ligaments** are examples of connective tissue. They help to connect bones to each other, and bones to muscle. The ear and nose are made of cartilage.

Skeletal tissue makes up the bones in the body.

Cardiac muscle tissue is both striated and involuntary.

Connective tissue is a group of cells that specialize in providing support and cushioning for the body.

Cartilage is a type of tough connective tissue that helps form structures in the body.

Ligaments are connective tissues that connect the bones of the body.

Skeletal tissue makes up the bones of the body.

Nerve tissue is a group of cells that control the brain and nerves.

Liquid tissue includes blood and lymph.

Plasma makes up the liquid part of the blood.

Red corpuscles complete oxygen–carbon dioxide transport to and from the cells.

White corpuscles are responsible for defending the body against bacterial invasion.

Lymph nodes are filters in the lymph system.

Adipose tissue is fat tissue.

Endothelial tissue refers to inner tissues that line the walls of the intestines, lungs, and other internal organs.

Epithelial tissue refers to outer tissues that line the outer and exposed body surfaces.

Subcutaneous layer is the most internal layer of the skin.

Lamellated corpuscles are nerve endings in the subcutaneous skin layer.

Dermis, often called the "live layer of the skin," lies next to the subcutaneous skin layer.

Papillary layer is the upper part of the dermis.

Dermal papillae attach to the epidermis.

Epidermis is the outermost layer of the skin and is made up of five layers.

Meissner's corpuscles are nerves located in the papillary layer that are sensitive to firm touch.

Nerve tissue are cells that control the brain and the nerves. Nerve cells transmit messages to all parts of the body. There are many types of nerve cells in the skin, which will be discussed later in this chapter. Think of the nerves as a long line of dominoes that possess the ability to transmit messages by touching one another. This "domino effect" enables the nerves to transport commands from the brain and information to the brain. Let's pretend that you accidentally touch a hot stove. The heat and pain nerve cells in the skin transmit the feeling up the body to the brain in a split second. The brain, in turn, sends a response in another split second, telling your arm muscles to immediately remove your hand from the hot stove.

Liquid tissue includes blood and lymph. The blood is responsible for carrying oxygen and food to all the cells in the body, and for carrying waste and carbon dioxide away from the cells. Blood is mostly made of a substance called **plasma**. Plasma makes up the liquid part of the blood. Floating in the plasma are red blood cells, or **red corpuscles**, whose function is to complete oxygen-carbon dioxide transport to and from all the cells. The other main type of blood cells are white blood cells, or **white corpuscles**, which are largely responsible for defending the body against bacterial invasion. Much more about the white blood cells will be discussed in Chapter 2, The Immune System.

Lymph is a liquid that bathes all the tissues of the body and helps filter wastes from the bloodstream and the body. Filters in the lymph system are present in many areas of the body such as the armpits, groin, and neck. These filters are called **lymph nodes**. When you are sick, sometimes you will have swollen areas in your neck or other areas. This is because the lymph is filtering debris and dead bacteria from the body, attempting to rid the body of these wastes. The lymph nodes swell when they are filtering lots of debris.

Adipose tissue is fat tissue. Fat, although it has a bad reputation, contributes to many functions within the body. It helps cushion all the other types of tissue. Imagine sitting on a sofa that had no cushions. It would be very hard and would break more easily if it was dropped or damaged. Fat helps the body in the same way, helping to soften injuries and protect the organs. Fat also is needed to produce hormones and other chemicals necessary for life.

Endothelial tissue refers to inner tissues that line the walls of the intestines, lungs, and other internal organs.

Epithelial tissue refers to outer tissues that line the outer and exposed body surfaces. The skin is an example of epithelial tissue.

PHYSIOLOGY OF THE SKIN

The skin is comprised of three major layers (Figure 1–3). The **subcutaneous layer** is the most internal layer of the skin. It contains large layers of fat to provide cushion for the internal organs, as previously discussed. Winding through the subcutaneous layer are blood vessels and lymph vessels, again insulated by fat tissue. The subcutaneous layer also contains nerve endings called **lamellated corpuscles**, which are responsive to pressure.

The **dermis** is the next layer toward the skin surface. The dermis is often called the "live" layer of the skin. The upper part of the dermis is called the **papillary layer**, con-

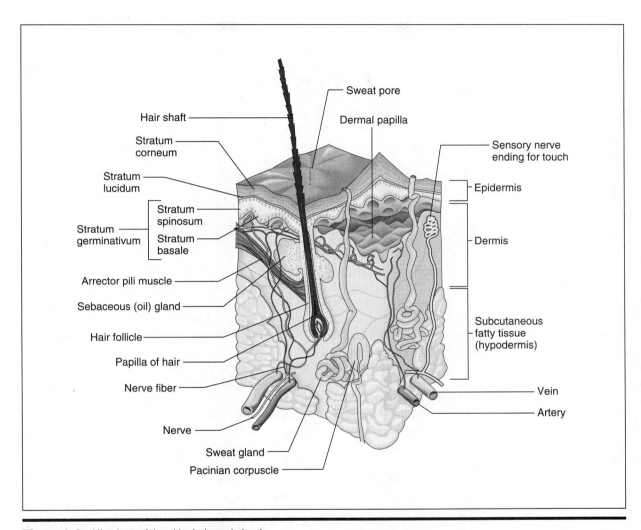

Figure 1–3 Histology of the skin, hair, and glands

taining the **dermal papillae**. Think of the dermal papilla as a "handlike" structure that attaches to the **epidermis**, the outermost of the three layers. The dermal papillae look like fingers "holding" the two layers together. Inside the papillae are many small blood vessels called capillaries, spiraling through the papillae. Also found in the papillary layer are some nerves sensitive to firm touch, called **Meissner's corpuscles**. These nerves sense deep touch. As an experiment, gently touch your hand. Next, exert more pressure on your hand. Doesn't it have a completely different feeling? This is because deeper nerves are stimulated when the skin is touched or pushed in a firmer manner.

The lower, more internal area of the dermis is called the **reticular layer**. The reticular layer contains a multitude of structures and activity. **Collagen** and **elastin fibrils**

Reticular layer is the lower, more internal area of the dermis.

Collagen are large, long-chain molecular proteins that lie on the top of the skin and bind water, also helping to prevent water loss.

Elastin fibrils intertwine throughout the reticular layer and give the skin firmness and elasticity.

intertwine throughout the reticular layer. Both of these fibers are made of protein and are examples of connective tissue. They give the skin firmness and elasticity. Collagen is not flexible and gives skin its firmness and inability to stretch very much. Elastin is the fibrous structure that gives skin elasticity and the ability to "bounce back." Fat globules are also in this layer, as well as numerous blood vessels (arteries and veins), lymph vessels, and nerve endings that are sensitive to pain, heat, cold, and pressure. The base or bottom part of the hair follicle is also found in the reticular layer, as well as the **sudoriferous glands**, or sweat glands, and the **sebaceous (oil) glands**.

The sebaceous glands secrete an oily mixture of fatty materials known as **sebum**. Sebum's main functions are to protect the surface of the corneum against dehydration, and to provide an acid barrier against outside bacterial invasion.

The **intercellular cement** or **interstitial fluid** is the substance found between the cells in the epidermis. The epidermis has been compared to a brick wall by many scientists. This intercellular material is the "mortar" between the "bricks," and is also often referred to as the **barrier function** of the skin. The barrier function is largely responsible for binding water between the cells of the epidermis, helping the skin look smooth and firm. This also prevents **transepidermal water loss (TEWL)**, which dehydrates the skin surface, interferes with proper functioning of epidermal cells, and can lead to irritation. The barrier function also helps the skin resist invasion by foreign objects or substances such as certain chemicals. Keeping the barrier function intact is a major factor in preserving healthy and attractive skin.

The sudoriferous glands produce sweat. There are two kinds of sweat glands: the **apocrine glands** and the **eccrine glands**. The apocrine glands are present in the groin area and the armpits. They produce a thicker form of sweat and are basically responsible for producing the substance that, when in contact with bacteria, produces body odor.

The eccrine glands are abundant on the face and other parts of the body. They are present in extremely large numbers in the palms of the hands and the soles of the feet.

Sweat is a mixture of water, salt, urea, uric acid, ammonia, broken-down proteins (amino acids), simple sugars, and vitamins. Sweat is a function of the body that controls temperature. As sweat evaporates, it helps to cool the surface of the skin. Some wastes are excreted by sweat, but body temperature regulation is its major function. When looking through a microscope, eccrine glands take the form of a spiral tube, much like the inside of a refrigerator. Apocrine glands are branched, appearing more like blood vessels off a major artery.

The epidermis, which is the major part of the skin that the esthetician treats, is made up of five basic layers.

The basal layer is the innermost layer of the epidermis. Within it are **melanocytes**, the cells that are "pigment factories" for the skin. Different color skin types have the same number of melanocytes, but people of certain races and ethnic backgrounds simply carry genes that make the melanocytes produce more **melanin** or pigment. Sunlight, injuries to the skin, and hormones can also stimulate melanin production. This is what causes an individual to become tan after a day at the beach. The primary function of melanin is to shield and protect the skin from damaging sun rays or injury. It is the body putting up a "parasol" to deflect ultraviolet rays. So, essentially a "healthy looking" tan is

Sudoriferous glands, or sweat glands, are found in the reticular layer.

Sebaceous (oil) glands are found in the reticular layer.

Sebum is an oily substance secreted onto the skin surface by the sebaceous gland in the dermis that helps prevent dehydration of the corneum cells.

Intercellular cement is the cushion of lipid substance between the cells of the corneum that keeps the skin from dehydrating and helps protect the skin from irritative substances.

Interstitial fluid is the fluid between the cells.

Barrier function refers to the protective barrier furnished by the corneum and intercellular cement. This protects against dehydration of the epidermis and exposure to irritative substances.

Transepidermal water loss (TEWL) is the evaporation of excess intercellular water.

Apocrine glands are present in the groin area and armpits. They produce a thicker form of sweat and are responsible for producing the substance that, when in contact with bacteria, produces body odor.

Eccrine glands are sweat glands found in the face and other parts of the body.

Melanocytes are cells that are "pigment factories" for the skin.

Melanin is the pigment of the skin.

actually the body defending itself from something unhealthy. The melanocytes "inject" melanin into the cells at the basal layer, and as they drift upward toward the surface, the cells are eventually shed from the surface. This is what causes the "loss" of a tan.

The basal cells are constantly dividing through mitosis, constantly pushing upwards to the outside of the skin. As they divide and move toward the surface, the intercellular structures discussed earlier begin to change. They produce a protein called **keratin**, which is the "magic" that helps protect the skin against invasion. As the cells change they also produce a variety of fats, or lipids, which help hold the keratinized cells together, much the way mortar holds a brick wall together.

> **Keratin** is a protein that helps protect the skin against invasion.

Protein keratin synthesis begins in the basal layer, where fibrils of keratin begin to form out of the cytoplasm in the cell. As the cells move up from the basal layer, they start to form the next cellular layer, or **stratum**. The spiny layer, or **stratum spinosum**, is so called because the cells appear to have little spines or thorns on the outside of the cell membranes. In this layer, the cells change shape from cubelike to multisided.

> **Stratum** is a layer of the skin or epidermis.
>
> **Stratum spinosum** is so called because the cells appear to have little spines or thorns on the outside of the membrane.

The next layer is the **stratum granulosum**, or granular layer. The granular looking cells are filled with a substance called **keratohyalin**, which helps to form keratin from the microtubule structures first formed in the basal cell layer. Keratohyalin is produced by the endoplasmic reticulum, as previously discussed. The nuclei of the dying cells are breaking down, and the cell is dying. In the granular stage new lipids are formed, which will again help to serve as a medium or "mortar" for the outer cell layer.

> **Stratum granulosum** is the layer where cells are filled with keratohyalin, which helps form keratin.
>
> **Keratohyalin** helps form keratin.

It is this group of lipid substances that forms the barrier function of the epidermis. They include triglycerides, sphingolipids, and glycolipids, also known as ceramides, cholesterol, phospholipids, waxes, and fatty acids.

The next layer of the skin is the **stratum lucidum**, or clear layer, so called because it appears lucid or clear on microscopic examination. It is filled with a substance called **eleidin**, which is produced from keratohyalin, and will eventually form keratin.

> **Stratum lucidum**, or clear layer, is filled with a substance called eleidin.
>
> **Eleidin** is a substance produced from keratohyalin, and will eventually form keratin.

The outermost layer of the epidermis is called the **stratum corneum**, or "horny" layer, so called because the cells are piled up on top of one another in layers and have a horny appearance on the microscopic surface. Cells in this layer are referred to as **corneocytes**. In the "mortar" of the "bricks" in this layer are small structures called **lamellar bodies**. Lamellar bodies are thought to be produced during the stage of keratinization in the granular layer of the skin. Their function is to produce more lipids, which will serve to permit certain substances in and out of the corneum. In other words they will permit certain substances into the "mortar" of the cell layer and will allow certain gases and toxins produced by the skin to escape through the same pathway. The fats formed by the lamellar bodies serve almost the same purpose as the cell membrane discussed earlier. They possess the characteristic of selective permeability.

> **Stratum corneum** is the outermost layer of the epidermis.
>
> **Corneocytes** are cells of the stratum corneum.
>
> **Lamellar bodies** are thought to be produced during the stage of keratinization in the granular layer of the skin. Their function is to produce lipids.

Let's take a minute to review the process of keratinization. The epidermis is divided into five layers:

1. The basal layer, which is a live layer, where the cells are dividing and constantly pushing upward. The melanocytes are also present in this layer. As cells drift upwards through the five layers, they die. In the process of dying, they form keratin, a resilient protein that will eventually serve to protect the skin from invasion.

2. The spiny layer, where the shapes of the cells have changed.
3. The granular layer, where keratin continues to form, and where fats that will make up the "mortar" begin to form.
4. The clear layer, where the process of keratinization continues.
5. Ultimately, the cells reach the top of the skin in the horny layer or stratum corneum, where they become the "bricks" in the outer, protective layer of skin. The cells are filled with keratin protein. The lamellar bodies are small "fat factories" and help produce "mortar" to seal between the cellular "bricks," but have the unique ability to allow certain substances in and out of the skin.

SKIN PENETRATION

Not long ago, scientists and physicians believed that the skin was a barrier to almost everything. Now we know that a number of substances could indeed penetrate the skin. Drugs were developed that were absorbed **transdermally**, which means that these drugs penetrate the epidermis and the dermis, and then are absorbed into the bloodstream. This discovery opened new pathways for many treatments, including treatment of heart irregularities and motion sickness, and now include nicotine and even hormone patches.

Transdermally means to penetrate the epidermis and the dermis, and then be absorbed in the bloodstream.

One of the first signs that the skin is more penetrable than first thought was an incident in which hexachlorophene, an antimicrobial, which, at the time, was available in an over-the-counter cleanser, was found to penetrate the skin readily, and hence was taken off the over-the-counter market, and is now only available by prescription.

A variety of tests have been developed to measure skin penetration of substances, using techniques involving dyes and substances that have been "labeled" with radioactive compounds. These radioactive substances can be measured in the tissue or the blood to determine the amount and level of penetration.

Routes of Penetration

The investigation of skin penetration is still largely theoretical. Although we know that many substances can penetrate the skin to varying degrees, we know that many cannot. The issue of drug claims versus cosmetic claims influences the following few paragraphs. Please be careful with the claims you make for cosmetics. For more information on this issue, please read Chapter 11, Claims in Cosmetics.

It is generally accepted that there are four means of penetrating the skin (Figure 1–4). Certain substances can penetrate the skin through the following routes:

1. The hair follicle, which is essentially a hollow tube that begins with its opening at the epidermis and ends with its root in the dermis. It is theoretically possible that small enough substances could go into the hair follicle and end up a lot closer to the blood vessels, because the hair follicle extends into the dermis. The inner walls of the follicle are lined with epidermal cells. The layers of the epidermis basically dip into the follicle. The problem here is that the space is relatively limited, because the hair follicles occupy a relatively small proportion of the entire epidermis.

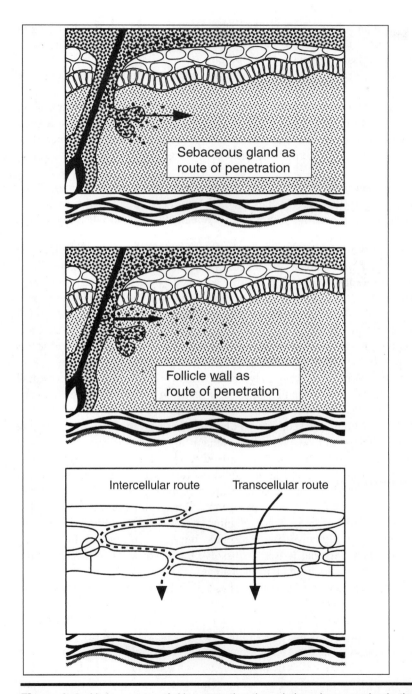

Figure 1–4 Various routes of skin penetration: through the sebaceous glands, the follicle wall, and intercellular and transcellular routes. (*Courtesy Thibiant International/Guinot-Paris.*)

2. The sebaceous glands may also provide a pathway for certain substances. Many of these glands empty directly into the hair follicle; however, some of the apocrine glands may not be associated with a hair follicle.
3. The sudoriferous duct, which is relatively small compared to the size of a follicle (pore) opening.
4. The intercellular ("mortar") fluids are probably the best vehicle for penetration of the epidermis. Its surface area is large. But how do we penetrate the stacks of keratinized corneocytes, which are impermeable to many substances? The fatty fluid holding the cells together is actually permeable by certain substances.

Remember that earlier in the chapter we discussed how cells migrate from the basal layer to the corneum. In this process they die and form keratin, but also manufacture new lipids, along with the lamellar bodies that secrete more lipids into the intercellular cement.

These lipids in the intercellular cement will accept similar substances. In other words, theoretically, if we can make substances that are similar to the lipids in the intercellular cement, these substances may be readily accepted by the intercellular cement.

Other factors that affect skin penetration include the specific area where penetration is attempted. The order of permeability of various areas of the body are, in descending order: the genitals, head, trunk, and finally the arms and legs. So the face is generally more accepting of skin penetration than the back, and so forth. The forehead seems to be the most penetrable area of the skin on the face.

The size of the corneocytes may play an important role in penetration potential. The forehead's corneocytes are smaller than other areas on the face. The thickness of the stratum corneum may also be a factor. Another issue is the condition of the skin being treated. Torn or injured tissue, or skin that has a rash or abrasion, may be more easily penetrated. This is simply explained. Skin that is injured or suffering from a rash, eczema, or abrasion is said to have a **compromised** barrier function, which means that the barrier function is not working like it should because of the injury or disorder. A compromised barrier function will enable the skin to be more permeable by sometimes nondesirable materials such as allergens and irritants. Barrier function can be injured or decreased by exposure to detergents, acids, alkaline substances, keratolytics, or injuries. Even overexposure to an alphahydroxy acid could interfere with barrier function by exposing lipids to chemicals that loosen or dissolve the lipids within the intercellular fluids. The corneocytes are not as thick in such areas.

The size of the molecule being penetrated has a big effect on its permeability. Large proteins like collagen are not permeable. They are simply too big to go between the cells. However, smaller molecules with more affinity for lipids like sodium PCA (a humectant), retinoids, squalane, and fat-soluble vitamins such as vitamins A, D, and E seem to have good permeability. Some large molecules such as collagen do not need to penetrate the skin to be useful cosmetically. Collagen is a substantive, which means that it adheres readily to the surface of the corneum, helping to bind water and reduce water loss from within the epidermis. Cleansers, sunscreens, and makeup foundations are other examples of substances that should not be penetrated. They totally lose their cos-

Compromised is to be impaired or injured, not completely functional.

metic effectiveness at lower levels, assuming they could be penetrated at all. Keratolytics like salicylic acid need to stay on the surface because they work solely on the corneum; we do not want to dissolve other layers. However, for medicinal purposes, we would obviously want to penetrate the full epidermis in many cases. Cosmetically, moisturizers will work better and hold moisture for longer periods of time if they are able to penetrate deeper into the corneum.

Other Factors That Influence Penetration

The thickness of the stratum corneum will obviously have an effect on skin permeability. If there is a large buildup of dead cells on the surface, penetration is hindered. When applying a moisturizer, for example, an excessively thick corneum will not absorb the moisturizer as well. The buildup of cells is usually dry and brittle, due to the large amount of keratin present within each cell, and will "grab" the moisture from the moisturizer. Therefore, the lower corneum is less likely to benefit from the moisture treatment.

Excessive oily skin will have a layer of excess sebum on the surface, further slowing penetration. Doctors often apply an strong solvent such as acetone before applying chemical peel solutions. This is to cut the excess sebum on the surface, so that the chemical peeling solution can better adhere to and affect the desired area. This, of course, is for a medical procedure, and not recommended for salon services.

Temperature of the skin also influences its acceptance of preparations. Warm skin is generally more accepting. Heat causes activity within molecules, kind of "stirring up" the molecules in the intercellular cement and the cell activity itself. On the other hand, certain substances such as hydrocortisone are known to absorb better when cold compresses are applied to the area.

Salon Application Techniques for Good Absorption of Topical Preparations

Because some routes of penetration are more effective than others, some techniques can be used in the salon to get products to penetrate better. Moisturizing and conditioning treatments will be more effective if they can get deeper into the corneum.

Preparing the Skin for Treatment

Cleansing the skin helps rid the surface of dirt, dust, pollutants, makeup, and excess secretions such as sweat and sebum. Some dead keratinocytes (corneal cells) are removed during basic cleansing.

Using toners, fresheners, and astringents helps to remove more excess sebum on the surface. Using these products both in the salon and at home will help to better prepare the surface for penetration of appropriate cosmetic treatment preparations.

The amount of alcohol, propylene glycol, and other solvents will have a direct effect on the amount of sebum removed. The oilier the skin is, the more solvent should be present in the toner. This process can work against us as well. For example, if you use a strong astringent on dry, dehydrated, thin, sensitive skin, and then apply a treatment that is too strong, it can irritate the skin instead of helping it. In this type of incidence, the chemicals will dissolve part of the lipid barrier, reducing the barrier function. A toner for oily skin is often not appropriate for dry skin. Be careful to choose the appropriate cleanser and toner for the skin type you are treating.

Removing cellular buildup—for skin types with excess corneum the use of mechanical, enzyme, or cosmetic peeling or other exfoliating treatments will help remove excess corneocytes. Removing these dead cells will help improve the appearance of the skin in four ways.

1. Removing these dead keratinized cells will immediately improve the skin's surface appearance, making it look smoother and clearer. Removing the cells that surround wrinkles will make wrinkles look less apparent. If you think of a wrinkle as a ditch, a mound of dead cells on either side of the ditch will make the ditch look deeper. Removing the mounds will reduce the space between the bottom of the wrinkle and the skin surface, making it look less obvious.
2. Makeup will apply more evenly to a more even surface. Clients report that makeup applies much easier for up to two weeks after a good exfoliation.
3. Removal of the cells increases the cell turnover rate, stimulating the division of cells and the production of intercellular lipids, therefore improving the barrier function. The improved barrier function and increased intercellular lipids make the skin look healthier and smoother, with improved circulation and glow.
4. Removing the cells increases physical penetration of moisture treatments or other preparations applied after the exfoliation.

We must remember that too much exfoliation disturbs the barrier function, causing skin irritation and making the skin more susceptible to inflammation and irritation from topical substances, allergens, and the environment. It can also cause redness and scaling, and cause skin to look less smooth and less firm.

Types of Exfoliation

Mechanical exfoliation means that the cells are mechanically removed by physically removing them from the skin. They are actually being "bumped" from the surface of the skin. Good examples of mechanical exfoliation are the use of a brushing machine or granulated scrub. "Peel-off" masks and drying preparations that are rubbed off are also good examples of mechanical exfoliation.

Proteolytic means protein dissolving.

Enzyme treatment uses **proteolytic**, or protein dissolving, enzymes that actually dissolve the excess corneocyte buildup. Enzyme "peeling" is a common salon treatment that will be discussed in more detail in Chapter 18, Chemical Peeling and Exfoliation Procedures.

Chemical solvents and light chemical peeling are used to reduce excess corneocytes on the surface. Glycolic acid, resorcinol, salicylic acid, and lactic acid are chemicals used in this type of procedure, which will be discussed in more detail in Chapter 18.

Microdermabrasion uses a pump-driven machine to exfoliate the skin by propelling small particles onto the skin surface.

Corundum is an aluminum oxide crystal powder often used in microdermabrasion.

Another relatively new mechanical exfoliation technique is **microdermabrasion**. This procedure uses **corundum**, or aluminum oxide crystals, to "sandblast" the skin. This procedure will be further discussed in Chapter 18.

Increasing Physical Absorption of Moisture Treatments

Besides improving the surface permeability by the skin preparation techniques we have just discussed, using various techniques or tools to increase absorption can make penetration of treatment preparations more likely.

Massage stimulates the skin both physically and thermostatically, meaning that the heat generated by friction with the skin actually warms the surface, as well as warming the preparation you are using. A good but gentle massage with the appropriate moisturizer will increase its penetration and effectiveness.

Use the knowledge you obtain in this book to help select the right preparation. Manufacturers now develop preparations that are more readily accepted by the lipids in the intercellular cement. Examples are lipid-containing moisture products and liposome treatments. Creams that are very heavy or greasy may be less permeable due to the large size of the molecules in their base formulations. Classic "massage creams," usually based with petrolatum or mineral oil, are good examples of nonpermeable creams.

Use of heat and cold will increase cream penetration. Infrared lamps and infrared "skin irons" release heat, which aids absorption. Heat masks and paraffin treatments produce similar results. Warning! Do not use direct heat on sensitive skin; red, irritated skin; or skin with enlarged or distended capillaries!

Cold penetration with cold "globes" may be more appropriate for sensitive skin. Globes are glass or plastic balls that contain cryogenic (extremely cold) liquids. You can cut irritation from globes by placing a large piece of gauze over the face after applying the treatment and before using the cold therapy. Cold globes are also very helpful in reducing redness and irritation.

High-frequency treatment releases heat deeper into the skin layers, helping to stimulate the skin and increase product absorption.

Iontophoresis or **ionization** uses electrical current to polarize preparations into the skin (Figure 1–5). Ions are repelled into the skin by use of galvanic current. See Gerson, *Milady's Standard Textbook for Professional Estheticians* for further instructions on machine usage.

Use of masks over creams restricts evaporation of the creams, therefore increasing penetration.

Warning! Some types of treatments should not be used with these penetration techniques and certain individuals are not good candidates for some of these techniques. Use common sense and follow manufacturers' instructions for all treatments, preparations, and devices.

High-frequency treatment releases heat deeper into the skin layers, helping to stimulate the skin and increase product absorption.

Iontophoresis uses electrical current to polarize preparations into the skin.

Ionization uses electrical current to polarize preparations into the skin.

Topics for Discussion

1. What is the function of the cell membrane?
2. What is selective permeability?
3. Why is the nucleus of the cell so important?

Figure 1–5   The electrode on the client's face is the positive pole. The current flows to the negative pole in the client's hand. Positively charged, water-based materials are repelled by the positive pole and attracted to the negative pole, increasing absorption of material into the skin surface. Desincrustation, using negatively charged alkaline liquids, is performed by switching the electrodes—using negative on the face while the client holds the positive electrode. (*Courtesy Mark Lees Skin Care, Inc.*)

4. What is the difference between involuntary and voluntary muscles?
5. Discuss the three major layers of skin and the structures contained in each.
6. Discuss in detail methods for helping creams penetrate the skin better in the salon.
7. What is a receptor site?
8. What is barrier function and why is it important?
9. Why should estheticians be careful with exfoliation procedures?

Chapter

2

The Immune System

The body's immune system is a very complex system. It is the body's defense mechanism against disease and other invaders. This chapter describes how the immune system functions and some of the many reactions that take place in the body's fight against disease. You will learn the many immune functions of the skin and why the skin is one of the most important parts of the immune system.

The **immune system** is the body's mechanism for fighting disease. The immune system involves a complex series of specialized cells, the blood, the nervous system, organs, hormones, and many complex chemical reactions. When a person possesses the necessary substances and characteristics to avoid getting a disease, that person is said to be **immune** to that disease.

Let's suppose that your body is invaded by a pathogenic organism. A **pathogenic organism** is a type of bacteria, virus, or other one-celled organism that causes disease. This kind of bacteria is, of course, foreign material to the body. An **antigen** is a foreign substance that the body recognizes as foreign, and therefore attempts to defend against. The body will produce a special kind of protein called an **antibody** that helps to neutralize foreign organisms entering the body. When you have already had chickenpox,

Immune system is the body's mechanism for fighting diseases.

Immune describes the body's defense against disease and inability to contract an illness due to excellent function of the immune system.

Pathogenic organism is a type of bacteria, virus, or other one-celled organism that causes disease.

Antigen refers to a foreign substance recognized by the immune system as an invader.

Antibody is a protein that helps to neutralize foreign organisms entering the body.

Acquired immunity antibodies the body builds to disease when you are sick.

Natural immunity is immunity to certain diseases that you have had since you were born.

Polymorphonuclear leucocytes are white blood cells that attack bacteria and other pathogenic organisms.

Polymorphs are white blood cells that attack bacteria and other pathogenic organisms.

Phagocytosis is the process in which polymorphs attack bacteria and other pathogenic organisms.

Necrotic tissue is dead tissue.

Macrophage is a large type of white blood cells that act as a guard, constantly patrolling the body looking for foreign invaders.

Lymphocyte is produced in the lymph nodes, the spleen, and the thymus gland.

B cells, also called B lymphocytes, make antibodies that are proteins that help to prevent further infection or reoccurrence.

T cells, also called T lymphocytes, help alert the immune system.

you cannot get chickenpox again. This is because your body produced antibodies the first time you had the illness. When your body builds antibodies to diseases when you are sick, the process is called **acquired immunity**. In other words, you acquired immunity to a future illness of the same type that you did not have before you were ill.

Natural immunity is immunity to certain diseases that you have had since you were born. You obtain the antibodies for natural immunity from your mother's blood and your parents' genes before you are born. In Chapter 1, we mentioned white blood cells. White blood cells are largely responsible for fighting disease in the immune system. White blood cells are produced by the bone marrow, but also by the spleen, liver, and lymph nodes. There are 8,000 white blood cells per milliliter of blood. When the body has an infection, there may be up to 50,000 white blood cells per milliliter!

COMPONENTS OF THE IMMUNE SYSTEM

There are two kinds of white blood cells. **Polymorphonuclear leucocytes** are referred to as **polymorphs**. Polymorphs are divided into three types: esoinophils, basophils, and neutrophils. Polymorphs attack bacteria and other pathogenic organisms in a process called **phagocytosis**. They surround foreign bodies and destroy them. They also help in disposing of **necrotic** (dead) tissue. Pus is largely comprised of defeated, dead polymorphs. You can understand this better if you think about a pimple. When acne bacteria take over a pore, polymorphs rush to the rescue. Some are killed by the bacteria and some die during the struggle. Their bodies are the main component of pus in the pustule.

A very large variety of white blood cells is called a **macrophage**. Macrophage means "large phagocyte." It acts as a guard, constantly patrolling the body looking for foreign invaders (Figure 2–1). Its cell membrane will surround and "swallow" bacteria. It is large enough to swallow and destroy even a hundred bacteria at a time. Macrophages can identify foreign bodies and determine that they are invaders, and not part of the body's cells. In other words, they can tell the difference between the body's own cells and foreign invading organisms.

The other type of white blood cell is called the **lymphocyte**. Lymphocytes are produced by the lymph nodes, the spleen, and the thymus gland. The thymus gland is located under the breastbone in the chest. It secretes hormones and helps to trigger synthesis of more lymph tissue.

There are two types of lymphocytes. They are called B lymphocytes and T lymphocytes, also known as **B cells** and **T cells**. T cells are of three types. T-helper cells help alert the immune system. Think of T-helper cells as messengers. When a macrophage identifies a foreign organism, the T-helper cell runs to the lymph nodes, where another type of T cell, the T-killer cell, is waiting. T-killer cells are activated and rush to the invasion site of the foreign organism. The T-killer cells work to kill the organisms. After the battle is won, another type of T cell called T-suppressor cells stop the T-killer cells from fighting and signal them that the battle is over.

The T-helper cell also plays another role in the immune system. It signals the B cells, which are in the lymph nodes. The B cells make antibodies that are, as we dis-

Figure 2-1   A macrophage guarding the epidermis

cussed previously, proteins that help to prevent further infection or reoccurrence. Antibodies are also called **immunoglobulins**, called Igs by scientists. Igs float through the bloodstream and help protect against invasion by organisms they recognize.

Let's put all this information in perspective. Think of the body as a community. The immune system is the "fire department" (Figure 2–2). The macrophage is the fire patrol unit, constantly looking for "fires" (foreign organisms). If it spots a "fire," it holds it and checks it out, making sure it is not a "false alarm." Once the macrophage has established that the organism is real, it signals the T-helper cells, who rush to the "fire station" to alert the T-killer cells, who are waiting to "slide down the pole!" The T-killer cells rush to the scene, fiercely battling the "blaze" of foreign organisms, killing all the organisms. Watching the battle is the T-suppressor cell—sort of a lookout. When the "fire is out," the T-suppressor cells blow the whistle to let the T-killer cells know that the fire is under control. The T-helper cells have also alerted the B cells in the lymph nodes. The B cells start producing "fireproofing materials" (antibodies, Igs). The Igs serve as safety officers to make sure that this type of "fire" never starts again.

Immunoglobulins, or Igs, are antibodies that protect against specific invaders.

HOW THE IMMUNE SYSTEM COMMUNICATES WITH ITSELF

In Chapter 1 we discussed how DNA replicates itself in cell division and how each cell is a self-contained life system connected to other cells, specialized into the different tissues.

The information contained in the DNA of each cell allows the cell to duplicate an exact copy of itself, passing on the instructions from one cell generation to the next. This is a unique code in each individual person.

Just as the DNA is coded, so is the surface of the cell membrane. Each cell membrane has on its surface special codes called **receptors**. Receptors are basically how cells communicate. Receptors can receive messages from other cells or other tissues. Hormones often communicate to cells via their receptors. Receptors inform T cells of what type of cell it is and that it is an "official" cell of the body and not an antigen (foreign body). The receptors on the cell membranes are made of special proteins. These proteins

Receptors inform T cells of what type of cell it is and that it is an "official" cell of the body and not an antigen.

1. The macrophage spots a "fire" and signals the T-helper cells.

2. The T-helper cells run to the "fire department."

3. The T-killer cells rush to the scene of the "fire."

4. The T-killer cells kill invading organisms.

5. Y-suppressor cell "blows whistle" to let T-killer cells know that everything is under control.

6. B cells manufacture antibodies ("fireproofing"), helping to prevent another invasion.

Figure 2–2 The Immune Fire Department

specifically fit similar protein structures on the surface of immune system cells, such as macrophages. It works like a lock and key (Figure 2–3). As long as the macrophage's "key" fits a cell's "lock," the macrophage recognizes the cell as part of the body's tissue. When the key does not fit, the macrophage starts the process of investigating the unidentified body.

The T cells communicate with each other by releasing a hormone-type substance called **interleukin**. Interleukin is present in the cytoplasm of T cells and is released as an alarm system when the T cell is alerted to a foreign body. It is sort of like a skunk spraying when it is disturbed! The other T cells receive a similar alarming message from the interleukin.

Interleukin is present in the cytoplasm of T cells and is released as an alarm system when the T cell is alerted to a foreign body.

ABOUT CANCER

Cancer is one of the most intriguing and destructive diseases. Cancer starts in one cell. The cell becomes deformed and then duplicates through mitosis, but the process of mitosis does not stop. The abnormal cell keeps dividing, creating more and more cancerous cells.

With the thousands of cell duplications happening constantly in our bodies, some cells become **mutated**, or changed, from time to time. They become deformed and are recognized as deformed by the immune system. The immune system will kill these cells. So it is theoretically probable that cancerous cells develop periodically, but that these cells are usually killed by the immune system. However, when the immune system does not function properly, or when the cancerous cells divide too fast to be killed by the immune system, cancer, as we know it, develops.

Mutated means changed.

Cancer cells can also "disguise" themselves. The T cells are trained to react to receptors on the cell membrane that help them distinguish body cells from foreign bodies. In a cancerous cells, the cell membrane is actually the same as the membrane of a

Figure 2–3   Lock and key of the membrane

normal body cell. The T cells cannot tell that the cell is cancerous. The T cell treats the cell as a normal cell, ignores it, and does not attack. Cancerous cells that have abnormalities in their cell membrane may be recognized as unusual, but normal cell membranes will indicate no problem to the immune system. Cancer is abnormal cells duplicating out of control. This is how cancer can spread so quickly. Spreading of cancer is called **metastasis;** the cancer is said to be metastasizing.

Metastasis is the spreading of cancer.

T cells, as we have already discussed, are produced by the thymus gland in the chest. The thymus gland is very productive early in life and then significantly reduces production. T cells, unlike other body cells, live for about 60 years, then start to die. This may explain why older people are more likely to get cancer and illnesses of any kind.

Onco- means "tumor," and *-ology* means "the study of." **Oncology** is the study of cancer. Physicians who specialize in the treatment of cancer are called **oncologists**.

Oncology is the study of cancer.

Oncologists are physicians who specialize in the treatment of cancer.

Let's review for a moment some things we learned in Chapter 1. In the nucleus of cells in our body lies the DNA. DNA contains instructions for running the cell. In the DNA are the genes, which determine our hereditary traits.

Among the genes are the **oncogenes**. Oncogenes play an important part in cell duplication. They help trigger the replication process. Everything is fine unless they get out of control. Scientists believe that oncogenes out of control may initiate the beginning of that one cancerous cell.

Oncogenes are specialized genes that regulate and trigger cell duplication.

Cancer Causes

What specifically causes oncogenes to go out of control is not known. However, some substances are **carcinogenic**. Carcinogenic means "cancer-causing." Substances that are carcinogenic are called **carcinogens**. There are many well-known carcinogens. Let's start with the one discussed the most—smoking!

Carcinogenic means cancer-causing.

Carcinogens are substances that cause cancer.

Smoke insults the body like almost no other substance. Smoke is, of course, foreign to the body. So the body tries to get rid of it like any other foreign substance. The chemicals within smoke kill cells and contain more free radicals (defined later in this chapter) and poisons than almost any other substance. Exposure of the cells to these substances severely damages cells. The cells have to work hard to repair the tissue damaged by the chemicals. This hurried process to repair the cells in the tissues, along with possible aggravation of the oncogenes by the chemicals, may cause abnormal cell replication and therefore cancerous cells. Because the body is stressed by the repair process, the immune system is overworked during this rebuilding process. The "tired" immune system is less likely to react well to invaders. So one effect of smoking is that it decreases immune functions in the body.

Many other substances can contribute to "slowing" of the immune system. Excessive alcohol, illegal drug use, stress, improper diet, too much fat, lack of exercise, and many other factors can contribute to malfunctions of the immune system. Let's think about these factors individually.

Alcohol in excessive amounts can cause a tremendous stress on all body systems. It is in fact a poison in significant quantities. Continual, repetitive damage is done day after day to the body of an alcoholic. Alcoholics also tend not to eat correctly, not to get enough sleep, and cause themselves stress by creating problems for those around them.

Illegal drug use also damages the body. The effects are similar to that of alcohol. High stress levels, poor diet, and irritation to the tissues are all effects of drug use. Drug users also risk the danger of overdose, which often kills.

Stress insults every function of the body. Scientists and physicians are learning more and more about stress and its influence on disease. It is generally accepted that stress can be a factor in almost every disease. When the body is under stress, the immune system is overworked. **Immunosuppression** refers to the slowing of the immune system by any of the factors mentioned in this section.

> **Immunosuppression** refers to the slowing of the immune system.

Improper diet robs the body of its fuel—the fuel it needs to carry out all the chemical reactions that take place in every single cell in the body. Imagine how you would feel if you were not able to eat for several days. The cells cannot function properly without proper nutrition. And the immune system is made of cells!

Too much fat in the diet causes a buildup of cholesterol and triglycerides in the blood vessels. This **plaque** obstructs blood flow. How do cells receive their food and oxygen? From the blood! If the "road" is blocked, the supplies cannot get through. And the cells of the immune system are on the delivery route.

> **Plaque** is a buildup of cholesterol and triglycerides in the blood vessels.

Regular aerobic exercise such as walking, biking, aerobics, or swimming improve the oxygen transport system of the body. This means that the body gets more oxygen. Exercising regularly also can lower blood pressure, reduce cholesterol and triglycerides, and reduce stress. All of these factors we have just discussed involve one thing—common sense! Treat your body with respect and it will treat you with respect.

FREE RADICALS

Anyone who reads health magazines has heard of free radicals. **Free radicals** are wild, unstable atoms or molecules. Often they are unstable oxygen atoms. Oxygen occurs in the atmosphere as O_2, or two oxygen atoms linked together. They are stable because they have a stable number of electrons in their outer orbit. (See Chapter 7, Essential Knowledge of Chemistry.) When a cell or a chemical reaction within the body needs an atom of oxygen, it takes one of the two atoms, leaving one unstable atom that no longer has the right number of electrons to be stable. This is a free radical, which, in this case, is also referred to as **singlet oxygen**.

> **Free radicals** are oxygen atoms that are unstable because they have lost an electron in their outer orbit. They are attracted to fats and lipids, which have extra electrons available to stabilize these oxygen atoms.

It is the sole mission of every atom to become stable by obtaining enough electrons in their outer energy levels. (See Chapter 7.) So the unstable oxygen atom desperately looks for electrons to fill its outer energy orbital. One great source for electrons is fat. Fatty materials tend to have electrons that are easy to steal. Lipids and, more specifically, lipids within a cell membrane are easy targets. Singlet oxygen steals electrons from these fats to stabilize itself, but creates another free radical called **lipid peroxide**. Lipid peroxide can create yet another free radical called **hydroxyl radical**, one of the most aggressive and destructive free radicals. Different kinds of free radicals are known as **reactive oxygen species (ROS)**.

> **Singlet oxygen** describes a very reactive single oxygenation, lacking the proper electrons for stability.
>
> **Lipid peroxide** is a fat that has been attacked by singlet oxygen.
>
> **Hydroxyl radical** is a very destructive form of free radical.
>
> **Reactive oxygen species (ROS)** defines any type of molecule that is a free radical and contains a form of oxygen.

So what's the big deal about losing an electron, or forming a new substance? Chemical reactions are very dependent on electron transfer, or trading electrons to form new compounds and reactions. So, if a substance or atom has the wrong number of electrons, this can easily interfere with proper chemical reactions, and therefore, proper body and cellular functioning.

Let's pretend there are three estheticians who work in the same salon: Deborah, Joanne, and Lisa. Each has her own room and her own equipment.

Deborah arrives at work at 8:45, and discovers that her steamer is broken. She looks into Joanne's room and sees that she is not there yet. So Deborah borrows Joanne's steamer for her 9:00 client.

Joanne arrives around 9:00 for her 9:20 appointment, and discovers that her steamer has been taken. She looks into Lisa's room and sees that Lisa is not there yet, and so she borrows Lisa's steamer.

Lisa arrives at 9:15 for her 9:30 appointment and discovers her steamer is missing. She looks into Deborah's room, whose client is now under a mask, and sneaks Deborah's (really Joanne's!) steamer out of the room.

And so goes the day! We have all known days like this, whether it is a broken steamer, or a series of clients late for their appointments. The point of this story is that the estheticians taking the steamers from each other's rooms work like free radicals stealing electrons from various other atoms. What would that day be like in the salon? Chaotic? Irritating? Free radicals do create havoc and chaos, and often real irritation, even it is not clearly visible. Irritation that does not have physical objective symptoms is called **subclinical irritation**.

Subclinical irritation is an irritation with no obvious physical symptoms.

DNA damage from free radicals can occur and is possibly a factor in skin cancer. It has also been suggested that hyperpigmentation is linked to free radicals. One of the biggest causes of free radicals is sun exposure.

Although free radical oxygen atoms are a by-product of many normal chemical reactions within the body, free radicals are also formed readily from smoking, alcohol, stress, and pollution. Whereas free radicals can affect all the body cells, and are probably significantly responsible for the aging of the entire body, free radicals have a particularly strong effect on the skin. We will discuss treating and preventing free radical formation in Chapter 9, Active Agents and Performance Ingredients.

HOW MEDICINE HELPS THE IMMUNE SYSTEM

Vaccines

Vaccines are an artificial way of tricking the immune system into making antibodies, or Igs.

Vaccines are an artificial way of tricking the immune system into making antibodies, or Igs. Vaccines introduce very small amounts of antigen (foreign organisms) into the body. Not enough of the organism is introduced to cause the body to become ill, but enough that it triggers the B cells to make immunoglobulins to protect against whatever organism is being used in the vaccination process.

Sometimes the vaccination process will produce minor symptoms of the illness. You have probably heard of people getting slightly ill after receiving a flu vaccine. In cases where small amounts of the organisms are enough to trigger disease, doctors sometimes use dead viruses or irradiated organisms in vaccines. Irradiated organisms used in vaccines have been treated with some form of radiation before being used. They are still alive, but the radiation treatment renders the organisms unable to reproduce. These are sometimes called **modified live vaccines**.

Vaccines are available against a large variety of diseases, including polio, smallpox, measles, mumps, certain types of influenza (flu), and many other diseases.

Modified live vaccines are still alive, but radiation treatment renders the organisms unable to reproduce.

Antibiotics

Antibiotics are drugs that are made from extracts obtained from living organisms. Penicillin is probably the best known form of antibiotic. It is derived from a type of mold. Antibiotics do not produce long-term, or active, immunity. They simply kill the bacteria.

Antibiotics are drugs that are made from extracts obtained from living organisms that fight bacterial infections.

Science has yet to develop much effective treatment for viruses. Viruses are different from bacteria in that they do not have the same characteristics as one-celled organisms. Viruses are particles instead of cells. They do not have the same structure as a cell. They invade the body by "injecting" themselves into healthy cells. They reproduce in great numbers inside the body cell, eventually killing the cell. When the cell dies, the many viruses are released to invade other cells.

The immune system is our best protection against viruses. Scientists have developed immune system stimulants and synthetic immunoglobulins that may help the body's own immune system fight viruses. However, no drugs to kill viruses are yet available that are as effective as antibiotics are against bacterial infections.

Sometimes antibiotics kill the wrong bacteria as well as the ones they were intended to kill. It is not unusual for someone taking antibiotics to have gastrointestinal disturbances while they are taking antibiotics. This is because the antibiotics also kill "good guy" bacteria while they are attacking the pathogenic organisms. Many bacteria present in our bodies help with necessary chemical reactions that happen within the body constantly. When these bacteria are killed by an antibiotic, normal body functioning may be affected.

THE IMMUNITY ROLE OF THE SKIN

The fact that the skin is the outer shield of the body makes it an immune barrier. Keratin in the corneocytes helps to protect the body against invasion by foreign bodies and organisms. The fact that the skin will resist being punctured by a needle illustrates this point. If you press your finger against the point of a needle, the skin will not be pierced unless pressure is applied to the needle.

Microorganisms are found all over the surface of the skin at all times. These organisms generally do not penetrate the skin because of the layers of corneocytes preventing absorption. The **acid mantle**, or the layer of lipids and sweat secretions on top of the skin, help kill many bacteria. What if we tear the skin or puncture it with that needle? When we puncture the skin, we break the barrier of the corneocytes and expose the broken

Acid mantle is the layer of lipids and sweat secretions on top of the skin that help kill bacteria.

skin and blood to the many microorganisms that are on the needle, as well as those on the surface of the skin.

Diseases that cause breaks in the skin surface, such as eczema, acne, and dermatitis, make the skin more susceptible to invasion by microorganisms. Dermatitis is often accompanied by a secondary infection such as a fungus or bacteria.

The second possibility for passing the barrier of the corneum is through the routes of skin penetration we discussed earlier. It is physically possible for a microorganism to penetrate the skin through the intercellular fluids or cement that we discussed in Chapter 1. But this organism would have to penetrate the corneum, its layers of keratinized cells, the acid mantle, and the intercellular cement.

Let's suppose that a microorganism gets through the outer layer. The microorganism is first noticed by the **Langerhans cell**. Langerhans cells are "guard" cells that constantly patrol the epidermis. Langerhans cells look like spiders, because one end has many tentacle-like structures called **dendrites**. On the other end of the Langerhans cell is a pseudopod. **Pseudopod** means "false foot." The Langerhans cell is able to extend this oval-shaped foot to help it move.

When the Langerhans cell is stimulated by a foreign body, it breaks off a sample piece of the antigen. The Langerhans cell then presents the sample piece to the macrophage, which is present in the epidermis just under the Langerhans cell. The macrophage then identifies the antigen, and if it is indeed a pathogenic organism, it signals the T cells to the rescue.

The Langerhans cells are particularly sensitive to sun exposure. A moderate amount of sun exposure will knock them out of commission for a few days. Repeated sun exposure may knock them out of commission long enough for skin cancer cells to get a good start. With the Langerhans cells "on sick leave" from the sun exposure, the skin is left vulnerable to other microorganisms. This explains why many people get flares of herpes simplex (fever blisters) when they are exposed to the sun. This lack of immune protection may also have a domino effect on other parts of the immune system within other parts of the body.

For many years scientists thought that the epidermis was dead and had no chemical processes. Whereas keratinocytes are technically dead or dying, we now know that there are numerous functions and vital chemical reactions that are carried out in the epidermis.

The keratinocytes in the epidermis also help to secrete a number of important immune substances. The keratinocytes secrete a protein substance called apolipoprotein-E, apo-E for short. Apo-E helps transport cholesterol, which makes up a part of the intercellular cement. Keratinocytes also help to neutralize potential carcinogens and produce two different forms of interleukin, the hormone-like substance that helps immune cells communicate. The keratinocytes also produce another substance called granulocyte-macrophage colony-stimulating factor (GM-CSF), which helps promote replication of the macrophages in the granular layer of the epidermis. Last but not least, the keratinocytes produce a substance very similar to that produced by the thymus gland. These hormones help cause T cells to mature.

Langerhans cells are "guard" cells that constantly patrol the epidermis.

Dendrites are tentacle-like structures on the end of some cells including nerves, melanocytes, and Langerhans cells.

Pseudopod means false foot.

Also present in the epidermis are the Granstein cells, which are believed to play a part in suppressing immune function. It is theorized that the Granstein cells act similarly to T-suppressor cells in discontinuing actions of the immune system.

Cosmetic and medical scientists are now learning more and more about the function of the epidermal cells, and how they may be manipulated by topical agents. It is now possible to stimulate lipid synthesis, speed up epidermal cell turnover, and send signals to the cells to perform other functions. Research of this type may be important to both the cosmetic and medical worlds, as this type of treatment might help a number of problems ranging from wrinkles to wound healing.

AUTOIMMUNE DISEASES

Autoimmunity is a condition in which the immune system cannot distinguish the difference between antigens and its own body cells. The immune system essentially starts attacking the body cells. A good example of an autoimmune response is what happens sometimes after an organ transplant. We have all heard about a kidney transplant patient who "rejected" the new kidney. The immune system sees the new kidney as a foreign body and works to attack and reject the new kidney.

Autoimmune diseases also cause rejection, but the person's own body cells are being rejected.

Probably the most frequent condition that estheticians see involving autoimmunity is **lupus erythematosus**, usually called lupus. Lupus patients have developed antibodies to their own cells.

The body is constantly cleaning itself of dead body cells. In lupus, the lymphocytes also produce antibodies to these dead cells. While the lymphatic and blood systems are still trying to rid the body of these dead cells, the antibodies produced by the malfunctioning immune system bind themselves to the dead cells, creating "traffic jams" in the blood vessels. Damage to the blood vessels results.

Lupus mostly affects the skin, the joints, the nervous system, and the kidneys. The skin is marked by a butterfly-shaped rash on the cheeks. Sun exposure can cause sudden attacks of the disease.

Lupus is managed by medical specialists called rheumatologists or immunologists. They control the symptoms of lupus with steroids and other symptom-relieving drugs. These drugs may cause additional medical as well as esthetic problems. If you have a lupus patient in your skin-care practice, consult with the physician before beginning esthetic treatment. Let the doctor know what treatment you are planning to use and what topical preparations you will use. Most lupus patients can greatly benefit from esthetic treatment.

Autoimmunity is a condition in which the immune system cannot distinguish the difference between antigens and its own body cells.

Lupus erythematosus, commonly known as **lupus,** is an autoimmune disease that primarily affects the skin, the joints, the nervous system, and the kidneys.

Topics for Discussion

1. What is the function of the immune system?
2. What is the difference between acquired and natural immunity?

3. Describe the process of the immune system functioning on a foreign body.
4. What are some factors that suppress the immune system?
5. Discuss the skin's immune function.
6. What is an autoimmune disease? What is one of the most prevalent autoimmune diseases the esthetician sees?
7. Explain why free radicals are bad for cells.

Chapter 3

AIDS

Objectives

AIDS (acquired immune deficiency syndrome) is a devastating disease that has already affected millions of people, and continues to affect millions more. In this chapter you will learn how the AIDS virus affects the immune system and the body. We will discuss how AIDS is transmitted and what can be done to prevent further spread of AIDS. We will discuss AIDS symptoms in the body, including many symptoms that may appear in the skin. Management of the AIDS patient will be reviewed so that you will be knowledgeable about the medical treatment of AIDS and AIDS-related conditions.

AIDS is a syndrome caused by a virus known as the human immunodeficiency virus (HIV), which is capable of destroying the immune system in persons infected with it. The immune system is the vital natural defense system against diseases. Without a properly functioning immune system, the body is unable to fight off infections that threaten it.

As we learned in Chapter 2, viruses work by "injecting" themselves into healthy cells. Once they are inside the healthy cells, they reproduce in great numbers, eventually killing the cell. The cell ruptures, releasing millions of new viruses. Each of these new viruses can "inject" other cells, repeating the process and duplicating even more viruses.

When the body is infected with HIV, the virus invades certain types of white blood cells known as T cells or CD4 cells, and the genetic material of the virus becomes a part of the blood cell. The virus tricks the blood cell into duplicating its genetic material, eventually overtaking the cell while breeding new virus capsules. It essentially uses the cell to duplicate itself, and the new viruses attack other T cells. Eventually, the number of T cells dwindles to the point where there are not enough to defend the body against invasion by disease-causing organisms. These organisms, normally kept in check by a properly functioning immune system, begin attacking the body. Such diseases are called **opportunistic infections**, which means they are diseases that rarely affect a normal, healthy body, and cannot be eradicated as they normally would be by a properly functioning immune system.

Opportunistic infections are sicknesses that the immune system normally has no trouble fighting off.

When persons die of AIDS, it is because the body simply can no longer defend itself against disease. No one actually dies of AIDS; they die of infections or diseases that infest the body owing to failure of the immune function.

HOW PEOPLE GET INFECTED WITH AIDS

HIV has been linked to a similar virus in African green monkeys. The monkeys carry this similar virus but are not always affected by it. When viruses or other organisms duplicate many times, the DNA in the organism sometimes changes slightly. This change is called a **mutation**. Many scientists believe that the AIDS virus mutated in a human after the human was bitten by a monkey in Africa. The virus was then probably spread sexually. There are many, many cases of AIDS in Africa, mostly in heterosexuals. Because HIV attacks white blood cells, it can spread very rapidly in the body. Blood, as you know, flows through the body. There are some blood cells in every body fluid. Body fluids are blood, semen, urine, vaginal secretions, spinal fluid, tears, and saliva, and amniotic fluids in pregnant women. Semen and blood appear to be the only real sources of infections. No infection from tears or saliva has ever been documented.

Mutation means change.

Intravenous drug users are infected by the AIDS virus by using dirty hypodermic needles that contain small amounts of blood from another person. When they inject their illegal drugs, they also inject the other person's HIV-infected blood.

Many patients who received blood transfusions before blood was being checked for HIV contamination became infected. Organ donors infected with HIV donated organs that were also contaminated, causing AIDS to develop in some people. However, now that there are tests to screen blood and tissue donations, infection through blood transfusions or organ transplants is highly unlikely.

The number one risk source for HIV infection is sexual intercourse. Sexual intercourse involves direct transmission of body fluids from one individual to another. The vagina, the penis, and the rectum all have many small blood vessels that can break during intercourse, causing direct exposure. When HIV-infected blood enters the body, infection can occur. Once the virus enters the body, it can spread very quickly. However, symptoms caused by the breakdown of the immune system may not be noticed for months or years.

Anyone who has been infected by HIV can transmit the virus to others through sexual contact, whether or not that person has symptoms. During the early stages of the disease, it is virtually impossible to tell if an individual is infected by simply looking at that individual.

TESTING FOR THE AIDS VIRUS

When the body is infected with HIV, the B cells produce antibodies to the virus. These antibodies can be identified by blood tests, which are able to isolate the antibody.

The first test done for the HIV antibody is called the ELISA test. This test is a screening test for the HIV antibody. If the test is positive, this indicates that the patient has antibodies to the virus. Confirmation of a positive ELISA test is completed by a second blood test called a western blot test. If the second test is also positive, the patient definitely has HIV antibodies. Doctors refer to these patients as HIV positive. Persons who do not have the virus or antibodies are called HIV negative. HIV-positive individuals, as we said before, may not show symptoms of AIDS for months or for as long as ten years or more. Medical scientists believe, however, that without antiviral treatment, all HIV-positive individuals will eventually develop AIDS symptoms.

Sometimes a person with HIV infection will not test positive for the virus immediately. Let's suppose an individual was exposed through sexual contact but did not test positive when he was tested for HIV two months later. However, several months later he tested positive for the virus. This delayed reaction occurs because the B cells have not yet produced antibodies to the virus. The B cells eventually produced antibodies, and they were identified during the later test. The period of time between exposure to HIV and the time antibodies are made is called a **window phase**. Individuals will not test positive if there are no antibodies, because the test identifies the antibodies, not the virus. For high-risk individuals, several tests should be performed at intervals over a period of a year to eighteen months. During that time the individual must abstain from contact to prevent the possibility of another window phase from occurring.

Window phase is the period of time between exposure to HIV and the time antibodies are made.

There have been over 500,000 cases of AIDS diagnosed in the United States. Over a million individuals are HIV positive, a few of whom have not shown symptoms in 15 years, and most of whom developed AIDS in the first ten years. That is about 1 in 250 Americans. Persons who are HIV positive may infect an uninfected person through sexual contact or exchange of blood, semen, or other body fluids. The test for HIV is now available through private physicians, state and local health departments, and other health care facilities. There is currently an at-home mail-in test available that can be purchased at pharmacies.

THE SYMPTOMS OF HIV INFECTION

Many small infections can occur in an HIV-positive person before strong symptoms develop. Strange skin rashes and lesions, repeated infections such as frequent flu-like symptoms, chronic tiredness, and other symptoms may be caused by HIV infection. Of course many other diseases can have these same symptoms. Because a person has symptoms like these does not necessarily mean the person is infected with HIV. The beginning of immune system breakdown, however, may result in multiple minor infections.

In order to call HIV infection AIDS, a person must both be HIV positive and show signs of advanced immune system breakdown, identified by the presence of a definite opportunistic disease or extremely low T cell counts. We will discuss these diseases shortly. Doctors often refer to patients with these symptoms as having "full-blown" AIDS.

Common AIDS Symptoms

Pneumocystis carinii pneumonia (PCP) affects AIDS patients. This form of pneumonia produces high fever, a horrible hacking cough owing to fluid in the lungs, and almost always results in hospitalization.

Other forms of lung infection are also prevalent in AIDS patients. Fungal and yeast infections of the lungs are common, as well as fungal and yeast infections of the esophagus. Other forms of bacterial infection may also occur in the lungs. Some of these infections may occur simultaneously.

Swollen lymph nodes are also common in HIV-infected individuals. The immune system is trying to fight off infection, but is losing the battle. Swollen lymph nodes may indicate the presence of a large number of dead T cells killed by HIV.

Dementia is an infection of the brain or cerebrospinal tissues. This may result in personality disorders or mental illnesses. Various forms of cancer are much more likely to occur in AIDS patients. Again, the immune system no longer can protect the body. **Chronic wasting syndrome** refers to rapid, unexplained weight loss. Any sort of recurrent infection may be a symptom. A simple infection may be treated with antibiotics, but reoccurs in a short period of time. These are only a very few general symptomatic diseases of AIDS. Again, it must be stressed that all of these diseases may occur in healthy, HIV-negative persons. But, they are most likely to occur when the immune system is not functioning well, as is the case with HIV infection. These diseases are sometimes called AIDS-indicator diseases. Doctors know that if an HIV-infected person has these diseases, AIDS is often indicated.

Dementia is an infection of the brain or cerebrospinal tissues resulting in abnormal thought processes.

Chronic wasting syndrome refers to rapid, unexplained weight loss.

TREATMENT OF AIDS AND HIV INFECTION

Although there is still no cure for AIDS, there has been much progress made in understanding the biochemistry and physical aspects of the virus and its physiology in relation to the immune system.

Great strides have been made in the management of the HIV-infected patient. It is important that patients with HIV receive testing regularly to monitor their immune systems. Constant monitoring can help doctors slow the progress of the disease. New tests have been developed that measure **viral load**, which is an indication of how many viral particles are actually in the infected patient's blood. Other tests can now monitor CD4 cells, a specific type of T cell severely affected by HIV. A low CD4 is an indication of low resistance to diseases.

Viral load is a measurement of how many viral particles are in a patient's blood.

The immune system must be in good shape to fight off disease and infections. To help restore or partially restore the immune system in HIV patients, scientists have developed drugs known as **enzyme inhibitors**, which interfere with the normal activity of the HIV virus. AZT is an example of this type of drug. This drug therapy results in reduction of the virus replicating process, and therefore reduces the amount of HIV in the body, allowing the body to restore immune function, or at least partially restore it. Combinations of drugs, known as **"drug cocktails,"** interfere with various biochemical reactions the virus needs to complete its replication.

Enzyme inhibitors are chemicals that interfere with enzyme activity. In the case of HIV infection, they interfere with enzymes that cause viral replication.

Drug cocktails are mixtures of several different drugs that work well together.

By combining antiviral drugs, doctors can now lower and keep viral loads in check, thus keeping CD4 counts higher. These drug groups are already keeping HIV-positive patients healthy, enabling them to live much longer, productive lives as well as have a higher quality of life. There are some indications, although it is very early to tell, that HIV patients will be able to live out normal lifespans, if they are properly monitored.

Some of these drugs have side effects in some people, and not all patients are able to take them. Side effects include intestinal symptoms, such as diarrhea, and tiredness. Many of these drugs are also very expensive, placing financial burdens on the patient, on the patient's family, as well as on society.

Unfortunately, in some cases, the drugs stop working or stop working as effectively. This may mean that the virus has adapted to the drugs. At this point the virus could spread again and immune suppression take place, leaving the patient susceptible to many infections. Fortunately, there are several types of drug cocktails, and doctors can sometimes adjust the combination of drugs to try a new approach.

There also has been progress in the preparation of a vaccine against AIDS. Although tests are not complete as of this writing, scientists have prepared a vaccine that has proved successful in monkeys for a period of one year. This, however, does not mean that the vaccine will necessary work in humans, nor does it mean that it will work for longer periods of time. It is significant progress, though, and it does mean that there is hope for more long-range treatment. Even if a cure is not found, perhaps someday it can be managed like diabetes or thyroid disease.

One of the problems with the virus is that it mutates frequently, and there are several types or **strains** of HIV. This means that the virus can change and adapt itself to the drug therapy. In fact, 20 percent of persons with AIDS today have now been infected with viruses mutated from the cocktails, indicating that they probably had sexual intercourse with persons being treated with the enzyme inhibitors.

Strains are slightly genetically different forms of the same virus.

PREVENTION OF AIDS

Prevention is still the best treatment for AIDS. Prevention means taking steps to stop people from getting a disease. In this case, it means stopping people from becoming infected with HIV. The best way to prevent the spread of the virus is through education. This is where the esthetician can play a very important part. If you are knowledgeable about AIDS you can help your clients understand the syndrome as well as answer questions about preventing the spread of AIDS. It is, therefore, very important that all estheticians, and in fact all health and personal care professionals, be aware of prevention techniques.

Prevention Techniques

There are basically only two ways to get HIV infection or AIDS through contact with infected individuals. Both ways involve the exchange of blood, blood products, or body fluids contaminated with HIV between individuals.

Because sexual contact is the number one cause of the spread of AIDS, "safe sex" practices must be implemented. Any exchange of blood, semen, or vaginal fluids during sexual contact may cause HIV infection if one person is infected. Precautions must be carefully carried out to prevent exchange of these fluids. The absolute safest prevention technique is abstinence. **Abstinence** means that the persons do not engage in sexual intercourse at all. If sexual partners choose to have sexual intercourse, using a condom (rubber) is important. A latex condom is the only type that is safe to use. Some condoms are made of skin taken from lambs. Skin, as we discussed in Chapter 1, can be permeable. It is possible that a condom made of lambskin will leak semen and cause infection. Condoms must be worn throughout sexual relations, from start to finish.

Avoiding body penetration is also helpful in preventing AIDS. When the penis enters any body orifice, such as the vagina, rectum, or mouth, the disease transmission possibility is greatly increased.

Monogamy means that two persons who engage in sex are faithful to one another and never have sex with any person other than their spouse or partner. Persons who are in a monogamous relationship where both persons have tested negative for HIV and have received medical counseling regarding proper HIV testing need not worry about HIV infection, as long as there are no other risk factors. Other risk factors include use of intravenous drugs.

The use of intravenous drugs (illegal drugs that are injected by a hypodermic needle into the body) is terrible for the health of any individual. Besides the many health risks that illegal drug use causes, HIV infection is also very possible. People who are addicted to intravenous drugs are often careless about health and hygiene. They use other addicts' needles or share needles that are dirty and contaminated with HIV or many other diseases. Direct injection of HIV-infected blood almost certainly leads to HIV infection.

One of the newest concerns is complacency due to the news of successful drug therapy. Some people are being careless about safe sex and needles, thinking AIDS is controllable. It isn't.

HIV infection among homosexual males has declined, but the infection rate has increased among women and teenagers and is increasing among African-Americans and Hispanics.

ABOUT HEPATITIS

Hepatitis is an inflammation of the liver that is caused by a viral infection. There are five known viruses that cause hepatitis: hepatitis A, B, C, D, and E.

Abstinence means that the persons do not engage in sexual intercourse at all.

Hepatitis is an inflammation of the liver.

The liver is an extremely important organ in the body. It helps break down fats and helps store energy. It helps with food digestion, and also acts as a disposal system for toxins and blood wastes. A person cannot survive without a functioning liver.

Hepatitis interferes with the liver's ability to function properly. Severe viral infection can cause liver failure, which is often fatal. Hepatitis viruses are extremely infectious, and the odds of becoming infected with a hepatitis virus are much higher than with HIV. This is a result of the virus being present in much higher numbers. Symptoms of hepatitis include **jaundice**, which is a yellowing of the skin and eyes, abdominal pain, fever, and constant fatigue. Hepatitis can result in permanent damage to the liver. The hepatitis virus can also live quietly in the liver after symptoms have gone away. If the virus lives after the initial disease, the person can still infect other people and is known as a **carrier**.

Jaundice is a yellowing of the skin and eyes.

Carrier refers to a person who is infected with an illness and able to transmit it to another person. A carrier may or may not show symptoms of the disease.

Types of Hepatitis

Hepatitis A is caused by eating food contaminated with the virus, usually through fecal material and poor sanitation. This is the type of hepatitis associated with eating raw oysters and other raw shellfish. Oysters eat by filtering water, and bay water can be contaminated with human waste from sewage. Hepatitis A is the least dangerous of the hepatitis viruses, and most people recover completely.

Hepatitis B is a much more serious type of infection, and is most often spread by sexual contact or body fluids, similar to HIV. Unlike HIV, however, hepatitis B can be contracted by kissing. Hepatitis B symptoms may last for months. Although most people recover fully from it, a few develop permanent liver damage, and about 10 percent become carriers. Liver cancer is known to often occur in long-term carriers after 30 or more years.

Hepatitis C was identified only a few years ago. The symptoms are similar to hepatitis B, and it is sometimes associated with HIV infection.

Hepatitis D affects those already infected with hepatitis B. This is a serious infection and permanent damage is much more likely to occur.

Hepatitis E, which is similar to hepatitis A, occurs mainly in underdeveloped countries.

Vaccines and Prevention of Hepatitis

Hepatitis B and C can be prevented or avoided by the same precautionary measures as for HIV. Hepatitis A can be prevented by proper sanitation, proper hand washing, and by following general cleanliness guidelines.

There are now vaccinations available for hepatitis A and B. They are administered in a series of injections, which slowly builds the body's immunity to the virus. Hepatitis vaccinations are highly advisable for estheticians, because they are periodically exposed to blood and body fluids.

Hepatitis and the Salon

Proper sterilization of implements, proper disposal of contaminated materials, the use of one-use implements, and the use of hospital-grade disinfectants as discussed in

Chapter 4, Hygiene and Sterilization Techniques, are the best methods for preventing accidental exposure to hepatitis viruses in the salon.

Technically, hepatitis viruses are harder to kill than HIV and are much more numerous in body fluids. It is much more likely for someone to contract hepatitis rather than HIV from an improperly sanitized or contaminated implement. Risk can be reduced greatly by use of proper sanitation and sterilization procedures.

For much more information on these subjects, read *HIV/AIDS and Hepatitis* by Doug Schoon, available from Milady Publishing.

PERSONAL PRECAUTIONS

HIV infection and AIDS are preventable. Following are some general tips for prevention:

1. Do not have unprotected sex. Use a latex condom from start to finish.
2. Sex with multiple partners is extremely risky. Promiscuous sex is also very risky. Any sexually active persons with multiple sexual partners, regardless of sexual preference, expose themselves to blood or semen.
3. Do not use intravenous drugs or have sex with anyone who does. AIDS is rampant among IV drug users, many of whom are also prostitutes.
4. HIV infection is on the rise in teenagers, heterosexuals, and females.
5. Never assume that anyone is not HIV positive. Persons may have HIV and appear perfectly healthy.
6. Even if a potential sexual partner tells you that he or she has tested negative for HIV, there is a "window phase" in which a person being tested may not have developed antibodies to the virus yet. All HIV tests detect antibodies in the blood. Someone who is in a window phase may test negative, yet still have the virus. Always use a condom.

DISPELLING MYTHS ABOUT AIDS

When people do not fully understand something that is life-threatening like AIDS, they tend to be afraid. Because they are afraid, rumors often get started about how the disease spreads. Let's stop some of those rumors. These are the facts about AIDS.

1. The only way to get AIDS is to exchange blood or body fluids contaminated with blood from an HIV-infected person.
2. You cannot get AIDS from casual contact. Sitting next to someone who is infected cannot transmit HIV.
3. You cannot get AIDS by drinking after someone or sharing eating utensils.
4. You cannot get AIDS by hugging, touching, social kissing (on the cheek), or by eating food prepared by someone who is infected.
5. You cannot get AIDS from mosquito or insect bites.
6. No cases of AIDS have ever been associated with French kissing.
7. AIDS is not a gay disease. Anyone can become infected if they engage in unsafe sex or share needles with an infected person.

AIDS AND THE ESTHETICIAN

Exposure to HIV in the cosmetology workplace has not been documented, but it is extremely important to use the hygiene and sterile techniques listed later in this chapter.

There have been some incidences where a health care worker became infected with HIV due to needle-stick injuries. This means that the health care worker was accidentally stuck with a used, dirty needle from an HIV-infected patient.

This, of course, can cause infection in the same way as intravenous drug users. It is very important that all health care workers and personal care workers take precautions to avoid such accidents.

We, of course, do not work with body fluids as health care workers do. However, certain procedures performed by estheticians may sometimes result in very small amounts of blood surfacing on the skin. Extraction, waxing, tweezing, and electrolysis are examples of such procedures. Clients may express concern about your salon's techniques for sterilizing equipment to prevent HIV infection. Because we work in a field that sometimes involves contact with small amounts of body fluids and blood, we must take special precautions when handling clients. We must make sure to follow strict sanitation guidelines and make sure that all our utensils and equipment are thoroughly disinfected at all times. We will discuss techniques to prevent transmission of AIDS and many other diseases in Chapter 4, Hygiene and Sterilization Techniques.

SKIN SYMPTOMS ASSOCIATED WITH AIDS

Fortunately, early detection of HIV now allows medical management of the HIV-positive patient. Skin problems as well as other problems that occur due to immune system dysfunction are therefore less likely to occur. Nevertheless, we should discuss the skin symptoms and problems that may be associated with HIV and AIDS.

There are many HIV-related symptoms that may occur in the skin. These include unusual or severe cases of common diseases such as shingles (herpes zoster), herpes simplex, venereal herpes, venereal warts, seborrheic dermatitis, unexplained rashes, warts, impetigo, fungal infections, folliculitis, athlete's foot, and other infections of the mouth and throat. Although these infections can occur in normal, HIV-negative persons, in HIV-positive persons they are often recurrent or extremely severe. They may also prove resistant to normal treatment. All of the preceding symptoms are medical conditions, regardless of patient type, and should be referred to a physician immediately.

The skin is a major organ of the immune system, where some of the first symptoms of HIV infection or AIDS show up. HIV and AIDS are often first diagnosed in a dermatologist's office. Although estheticians are not in the business of diagnosing or treating disease, it is important to be aware of these possible symptoms, and encourage clients who show signs of these illnesses to see a physician, regardless of HIV status.

Again, it is important to remember that these symptoms may all be present in normal, healthy, HIV-negative individuals. The esthetician should never mention the AIDS relationship of these symptoms to the client. The esthetician should only refer these problems to a doctor, as you should for any medical condition.

The symptoms, which affect many people anyway, tend to be much more severe and chronic in HIV-positive persons. The treatments for these symptoms administered by physicians are often more intensive to treat skin problems associated with AIDS patients. Many of these symptoms may also affect mucous membranes, such as the inside of the mouth, rectum, vagina, and eye.

Herpes

Herpes refers to a group of viruses.

Herpes is a virus that comes in many different forms. Most people think of genital herpes when they hear the word **herpes**. But, as we said before, there are many different herpes viruses and not all are transmitted by sexual contact (Plate 1).

Cold sores, for example, result from one form of the herpes virus. Genital herpes is another form. In patients with HIV, herpes flareups tend to be much more severe and happen more often. Physicians may give these patients antiviral medications to help the depressed immune system heal the lesions associated with a herpes infection.

Herpes zoster is the virus that causes both shingles and chickenpox.

Shingles, known also as herpes zoster, is caused by the same virus that causes chickenpox. The lesions of herpes zoster look like multiple red blisters.

Another form of herpes is called **herpes zoster**, better known as **shingles**. Shingles is actually an adult manifestation of chickenpox. It can be very painful. Shingles in HIV-positive patients is often much worse and widespread than in normal healthy individuals (Plate 2).

Warts

Warts are caused by a variety of viruses known as papovaviruses or verrucae.

Warts are often recurrent and more widespread in HIV-positive patients. They may occur in unusual places such as the beard area, mouth, and tongue. Plantar warts on the feet or hands may also be present. The physician may find that these warts are resistant to normal treatment. Venereal warts on the genitals, anus, and vagina are also often seen.

Molluscum contagiosum is a viral infection frequently seen on the faces of children, which appear as groups of small, flesh-colored papules.

Molluscum contagiosum is often seen in normal children. It often looks like a large group of warts and is frequently seen on the face.

Infections

Impetigo is a skin infection that is characterized by large, open, weeping lesions.

Impetigo is a bacterial infection, again often seen in small, normal children. In AIDS patients, the lesions can be much worse. Impetigo is characterized by multiple lesions, often in the mouth and chin area. They have a crusty top, but ooze transparent fluid. Impetigo is extremely contagious. Refer the patient to a physician immediately.

Mycosis are fungal infections.

Mycosis infections are fungal infections. Many fungal infections can affect both the skin and the internal organs of the AIDS patient. Skin infections from fungi may be indicative of internal fungal infections in AIDS patients. Fungal infections may show many different forms of symptomatic lesions.

Folliculitis is a bacterial infection of the hair follicle.

Folliculitis is an irritation of the hair follicle and is caused by a bacterial infection. The follicles appear inflamed, are in groups or patches, and often may appear as patches of very tiny pustules.

Seborrheic dermatitis, or seborrhea, is an inflammation of the sebaceous glands and follicles resulting in redness, flaking, and itching in oily areas of the face.

Severe **seborrheic dermatitis**, or seborrhea, may be seen in HIV-positive patients. Many clients may have a small area of seborrheic dermatitis, but in AIDS patients the seborrhea may be much worse. Red, scaly patches in all areas of the face, but especially the hairline and ears, are apparent. Severe seborrhea may cause cracks in the skin and bleeding. Oozing lesions may also be present. The scalp can be severely affected as well. Again, seborrhea affects many healthy individuals, but in AIDS patients it is much more widespread, inflamed, and chronic. Normal treatment may prove to be unresponsive. More potent topical steroids are often needed to control the disorder (Plate 3). Psoriasis may develop or worsen in AIDS patients.

Mouth Symptoms

One of the earliest symptoms of AIDS may be a yeast infection of the mouth called **oral thrush**. *Candida albicans* is the name of the yeast that causes thrush. Thrush symptoms include an abnormally thick, white paste covering mouth tissues. It often occurs in HIV-positive patients. It looks like cotton stuck to patches in the mouth. Thrush is often a problem for small children who do not have AIDS. It is not seen as often in normal, healthy adults.

Oral thrush is an infection of the mouth and throat caused by the yeast known as *candida albicans*.

Hairy leukoplakia is a tumor-like eruption that can occur on the tongue or the insides of the cheeks. It is hard and scaly looking. Herpes lesions, or "fever blisters," may also affect the inside of the mouth of AIDS patients.

Hairy leukoplakia is a tumor-like eruption that can occur on the tongue or the insides of the cheeks.

Other Skin Symptoms

Many unusual skin lesions plague HIV-positive patients. Strange skin bumps and lesions may be apparent. Because AIDS patients have lowered resistance to infection, physicians constantly see new and strange lesions on the skin of patients.

SKIN CANCERS ASSOCIATED WITH AIDS

Kaposi's sarcoma (KS) was, at one time, a frequent skin symptom of AIDS. It appears as purple-brown lesions. It is a rare form of skin cancer, but it can affect AIDS patients because the AIDS patient's body is immunosuppressed. Because progress has been made in antiviral treatment, HIV-positive patients are now much less likely to develop Kaposi's sarcoma (Plate 4).

Kaposi's sarcoma is a rare form of skin cancer characterized by purple-brown lesions.

Other skin cancers are also seen in AIDS patients. Although not as prevalent as Kaposi's sarcoma, basal and squamous cell carcinomas have been detected in AIDS patients and seem to spread much faster. Malignant melanoma may also be seen and also has a tendency to spread faster in immunosuppressed patients.

THE MENTAL AND EMOTIONAL STATE OF AIDS PATIENTS

It is possible for an AIDS patient to experience many different emotions concerning the illness. Because it is a relatively new disease, much is still to be learned about AIDS. Although we basically understand its transmission and its effect on the immune system and the body, we are still learning about management of the HIV-positive individual. Because of these uncertainties, AIDS patients may have great difficulty coping with their situations. There is no permanent cure for AIDS.

AIDS or HIV-positive patients may feel anger toward others or themselves about the disease. They may also deny having the disease. They experience many of the same emotional conflicts felt by cancer patients. The stigma originally attached to AIDS, a so-called "gay disease," is decreasing, but many people are still not educated about its transmission. This, again, is where the esthetician can play a part in helping to educate the public. If a client says something incorrect about AIDS, tactfully correct the client. Only by getting the right word out can the many misunderstandings about this illness be clarified.

HANDLING CLIENT QUESTIONS ABOUT AIDS

Clients may have questions regarding AIDS and the salon, specifically questions about sanitation and sterilization. It is acceptable for clients to ask these questions, and for you to answer. It is very important that you are knowledgeable about the salon's sterilization procedures, and to be familiar with the requirements of your state regarding proper sanitation in the salon.

The client may be completely misinformed about AIDS and HIV. Cosmetology professionals are in a unique position to educate the consumer about issues such as AIDS. Rumors about AIDS are rampant, and it is important for you to always remain well-informed to help dispel these rumors.

Following are some tips about handling questions:

1. Answer the questions factually and briefly, but do not dwell on the subject.
2. Reassure the client that everything you use is sterile or disposable, and that you have taken all the precautions possible. (Make sure that you do!) A poster or plaque listing your sterilization and sanitation practices is a good idea. There is one available from EMDA—the Esthetics Manufacturers and Distributors Alliance, 401 North Michigan Avenue, Chicago IL 60601.
3. Make sure that your salon is always spotless. Let your client observe you washing your hands and following aseptic procedures. The impact of an immaculately clean salon or clinic will squelch most doubts the client may have.
4. Make sure that all coworkers are equally informed with the facts about AIDS and aseptic and sterile procedures.
5. A client may confide in you, or come to you for advice concerning his or her exposure or sickness. Refer the client to a physician immediately. Use the same caring attitude you would with any client. These people will need lots of help and understanding.

AIDS AND THE FUTURE

At the time of this writing, 1 in 250 people in the United States is HIV positive. In your lifetime it is likely that you will know someone who is HIV positive or who has AIDS. Although great progress in treatment has been made, we all hope that a cure or a vaccine is on the horizon.

AIDS/HIV KNOWLEDGE QUIZ

True or False:

_____ 1. Any person can get AIDS.

_____ 2. To become infected with HIV, infected blood or body fluids must enter the body.

_____ 3. One in 250 Americans is now infected with HIV.

_____ 4. Prevention is still the best treatment for HIV and AIDS.

_____ 5. AIDS can be spread by mosquitoes.

_____ 6. Anyone who gets AIDS is a promiscuous individual.

_____ 7. There are other diseases more transmissible than AIDS.

_____ 8. You can easily spot an HIV-infected person.

_____ 9. It is against the law to discriminate against AIDS patients and HIV-infected persons.

_____10. If a person has a negative HIV test, the person absolutely does not carry the virus.

_____11. The best way to prevent diseases of any type in the salon is to assume that all your clients are HIV positive.

_____12. Persons with HIV may not show symptoms for years.

_____13. The biggest increase in AIDS is currently seen in teenagers, women, African Americans, and Hispanics.

Answers:

1. True.
2. True.
3. True.
4. True.
5. False. No cases of AIDS or HIV infection have ever been traced to mosquito bites, casual contact, kissing, swimming pools, toilet seats, contact through cosmetology, pets, drinking fountains, food handling, or donating blood. You can only get AIDS from exchange of blood, blood products, or body fluids.
6. False. Although promiscuous sex is risky, anyone can get HIV from unprotected sex with an infected person.
7. True. Hepatitis and many other diseases are much easier to catch than AIDS/HIV.
8. False. Symptoms of AIDS may not show up for years. It is often impossible to tell by sight if a person has HIV or AIDS.
9. True.

10. False. HIV tests may be false-negative if the person has yet to develop antibodies to the virus, which is what HIV tests detect. Persons should be tested several times, several months apart, without participating in any risky activity during that time.
11. True. The very best way to ensure proper hygiene is to assume that all clients are HIV positive.
12. True.
13. True.

Topics for Discussion

1. Why is it possible for an HIV-infected person to show no symptoms?
2. Discuss the medical management of the HIV-infected person.
3. What can be done to prevent the spread of AIDS?
4. Why is it important to know that AIDS often affects the skin?
5. Why are skin infections in AIDS patients so much more severe than in healthy individuals?
6. Discuss the future of the AIDS epidemic.
7. What progress has been made in the management of HIV-positive individuals?

Chapter

4

Hygiene and Sterilization Techniques

Objectives

Sterilization, aseptic techniques, good hygiene, and disinfection methods are essential for every health and personal care practice. Esthetics is no exception. You will learn techniques for disinfecting many salon implements, as well as the importance of aseptic techniques. You will learn to protect yourself and your clients from exposure to pathogenic organisms.

Germs are microorganisms that literally cover almost every surface, including the skin of the human body. Because this is true, it is important that we learn how to control microorganisms through proper sanitation and sterilization.

Let's take a minute to review some of the various types of microorganisms. Bacteria are one-celled microorganisms. There are both pathogenic (disease-causing) and non-pathogenic (non-disease-producing) bacteria. In fact, our bodies need certain types of bacteria to help process foods. However, this chapter will not focus on "good guy" bacteria. We are concerned here about disease-producing, pathogenic bacteria (Figure 4–1).

Figure 4–1   Bacterial shapes

There are basically three types of bacteria:

Bacilli are rod-shaped bacteria that cause a variety of diseases, including tuberculosis and tetanus.

Cocci are round bacteria that often occur in groups.

Spirilla are spiral in shape. Syphilis is the best known disease caused by spirilla.

1. **Bacilli** are rod-shaped bacteria that cause a variety of diseases. Among these diseases are tuberculosis and tetanus.
2. **Cocci** are round bacteria that often occur in groups. There are three types of cocci. Staphylococci grow in small groups. Pustules are an example of an infection caused by staphylococci. Staphylococci can produce various systemic infections, which are those that affect the entire body. Localized infections are confined to one area. A pustule is an example of a localized infection. If an infection spreads into the bloodstream, then it is said to be systemic. Staphylococci infections are sometimes called staph ("staff") infections. Streptococci infections cause strep throat. They are another form of cocci. Diplococci, still another form of cocci, cause pneumonia.
3. **Spirilla** are a third form of bacteria. Spirilla are also called spirochetes. They are spiral in shape. Syphilis is probably the best known disease caused by spirilla.

Bacteria can be active or inactive. In their inactive stage, they form cocoon-like shells called spores. Spores are much harder to kill than active bacteria. This is important to know when we discuss sterilization later in the chapter.

Viruses are another form of microorganism. As we discussed in Chapter 2, viruses are not really cells, in that they do not have membranes. They are more like pieces of DNA proteins and are very small.

There are various types of fungi. Mold and mildew are examples of fungi. Fungal infections in humans are known as **mycoses**. Many, many illnesses are caused by microorganisms. The variety of bacteria, viruses, and fungi, and the various diseases they can cause, is much too extensive to discuss in this book. We touch on the basics in order to understand the importance of hygiene and sterilization.

Mycoses are fungal infections.

Sterilization is the process of killing all microorganisms, including good and bad ones. Sterilization also kills spores—bacteria that are in their inactive phase.

Autoclave is a machine that sterilizes equipment, utensils, and other materials through a combination of steam heat and pressure.

STERILIZATION

Sterilization is the process of killing all microorganisms, including good and bad ones. Sterilization also kills spores—bacteria that are in their inactive stage.

True sterilization is performed by a process called autoclaving. An **autoclave** is a machine that sterilizes equipment, utensils, and other materials through a combination of steam heat and pressure. It works similarly to a pressure cooker. Microorganisms cannot survive in an autoclave (Figure 4–2).

Autoclaves have a large metal chamber in which can be placed metal surgical instruments, sponges, gauze, and other materials. After the chamber is filled with the materials to be sterilized, a heavy-duty door is shut, locking and forming an air-tight seal. The autoclave then heats up, at the same time building pressure inside the chamber. The temperature of the heat goes above the boiling point of 212 degrees Fahrenheit. Articles are sterile when they have been exposed to very high heat (usually about 260 degrees), and sufficient pressure has built up inside the autoclave. Once the autoclave has reached a sufficient temperature and pressure, materials are left to sterilize for about 20 minutes. The autoclave is then vented, allowing the pressure and temperature to drop. The pressure is so high that it is impossible to open an autoclave during the sterilization cycle.

Items placed in the autoclave are placed in sealed special plastic or paper envelopes so they remain sterile once the autoclave has completed sterilizing. It is important to read the manufacturer's instructions well before operating an autoclave, because different manufacturers will have different instructions for sterilizing procedures.

Some materials cannot be autoclaved. Glass, for example, cannot withstand the high pressure. Check manufacturers' instructions to see what items cannot be autoclaved.

An autoclave is a very important tool for the esthetician as well as any other personal care or health care professional. In this age of AIDS, it is very important to protect your clients and yourself from exposure to any pathogenic microorganisms. The AIDS epidemic brought great attention to sterilization procedures. However, the AIDS virus is relatively easy to kill through sterilization. Hepatitis viruses, tuberculosis bacteria, and other microorganisms actually pose a much greater health risk in terms of sterilization procedures.

Disinfection is the process of killing the majority of pathogenic microorganisms. Disinfection is the general procedure that is usually followed in the cosmetology industry. Because we do not perform **invasive procedures**, or procedures that enter the body, we do not have to concern ourselves with the types of sterilization that are used in

Disinfection is the process of killing the majority of pathogenic microorganisms.

Invasive procedures are procedures that enter the body.

Figure 4–2 Example of an autoclave

hospitals. However, we do perform procedures such as extraction, waxing, and tweezing that sometimes expose blood on the surface of the skin. Because of this exposure to blood, we must be very careful to use excellent hygiene and sterile or disinfected materials.

Disinfectants are chemicals that kill pathogenic microorganisms. The most popular disinfectant chemical used in the cosmetology industry is quaternary ammonia. Seventy percent isopropyl alcohol is another commonly used disinfectant for surface disinfecting.

Disinfectants are also used in maintenance, such as disinfectant floor detergents and aerosol sprays, to kill bacteria in the air and control the odors they cause.

Antiseptics are a weaker form of disinfectant. They are usually mild enough to use on the skin. Hydrogen peroxide and other first-aid chemicals are examples of antiseptics.

Aseptic procedure is the term scientists use to describe proper handling techniques of sterilized and disinfected equipment. Placing a sterile comedone extractor on a dirty towel is a violation of aseptic procedure. Handling sterile equipment with other sterile materials is good aseptic procedure.

Theoretically, nothing is completely sterile once a seal has been broken on an envelope of an autoclaved utensil. Because bacteria, viruses, and other microorganisms are in the air, they land on the sterile equipment. But we cannot sterilize a building or a room, so we must do the next best thing in handling disinfected and sterile equipment with the best hygienic techniques possible.

Some hospital disinfectants are somewhat stronger than quaternary ammonia and are being used more frequently in salons, particularly in esthetics and electrolysis practices.

Popular stronger disinfectants are glutaraldehyde, formaldehyde solutions, benzalkonium chloride, and sodium hypochlorite (household bleach). These types of disinfectants are very strong. If they are not thoroughly removed by lots of rinsing, the residue can cause allergic and irritating reactions to the skin.

Glutaraldehyde solutions are excellent for disinfecting mask brushes, metal instruments such as tweezers, and other implements that cannot be autoclaved. Glutaraldehyde is available from medical and esthetic supply houses under a variety of trade names.

Glutaraldehyde often comes in concentrated form. It is mixed with water to form a solution that is potent in killing many microorganisms for three weeks. Read the label well and follow all manufacturer's instructions. Household bleach can be diluted 1:10 with water and serves as a good disinfectant for many articles. Besides being used for laundry, bleach can also be used to disinfect sponges and other linens. Do not use bleach to disinfect metal instruments. Chlorine is extremely corrosive to metals!

DISPOSABLE MATERIALS

The best way to ensure aseptic procedure is to use disposable materials. These materials should be used once and discarded. There is no way to transfer microorganisms from one client to another if you are using disposable materials.

Popular disposable items include:

Disinfectants are chemicals that kill pathogenic microorganisms.

Antiseptics are a weaker form of disinfectant. They are usually mild enough to use on the skin.

Aseptic procedure is the term scientists use to describe proper handling techniques of sterilized and disinfected equipment.

- cleansing pads made of sheet (roll) cotton
- disposable one-use lip brushes
- one-use mascara wands
- disposable eyeshadow sponges
- inexpensive cellulose sponges
- cotton swabs
- facial tissue
- wax strips
- disposable spatulas for wax or junior size tongue depressors
- paper towels and sheets

Lancets should always be presterilized for one use and disposable. Never use a lancet more than once! Electrolysis needles and filaments are also available in disposable types.

Disposables should be discarded in sealed plastic bags. Sharp items such as lancets and electrolysis needles should be disposed of in a "sharps box." A sharps box is a plastic box with a hole in the top in which you place used lancets and needles. The plastic box helps to prevent you or any other persons handling the refuse from accidentally injuring themselves with used lancets or needles. Even though blood is a rarity, it is best to protect everyone by using these precautions.

NONDISPOSABLE ITEMS

Some items must be used more than once. Because of expense and practicality, items such as brush attachments, high-frequency electrodes, mask brushes, suction apparatuses, comedone extractors, and other items must be either sterilized or disinfected.

When cleaning utensils you must be careful not to cross-contaminate the utensils. Cross-contamination means that utensils are accidentally re-exposed to microorganisms during handling. Examples of cross-contamination are rinsing utensils in a non-disinfected bowl, handling clean brushes with dirty towels, and re-dipping used spatulas into the same jar of cream.

You must use extreme care not to ever contaminate any item used in treatment by touching it with something that is dirty or has been used on a client. The following are instructions for properly disinfecting implements, utensils, or equipment pieces.

Always wear disposable gloves when practicing disinfectant procedures.

Disinfection of Brushes

Mask brushes should be autoclaved, if possible, but most brushes do not hold up well in the autoclave. The high temperature melts the glue that holds the brush together. In at least one state, the use of reusable mask brushes is against the sanitary code. Masks can also be applied with gloved hands or disposable spatulas. Soak brushes well in a disinfectant soap solution. The soak will help loosen mask materials from the brush. After soaking the brushes, put on a pair of gloves and rinse them well in a bowl. After they are thoroughly rinsed, place them in a solution of glutaraldehyde or other medical disinfectant. Let brushes soak for 20 minutes in the disinfectant. Remove them, rinsing well in a different rinsing bowl. It is best to label your rinsing bowls so that you don't rinse disinfected brushes in the soap-rinsing bowl. Remember to rinse very well so that you do not have disinfectant residue on the brushes. Store the disinfected brushes in a large jar until dry. After they are dry, they should be kept in a clean, closed container, a clean drawer, or a UV sanitizer.

UV sanitizers are good for storing clean, disinfected items. They kill some types of microorganisms with ultraviolet light. They do **not** sterilize. Utensils still must be disinfected before they are stored in a UV sanitizer.

Machine brushes should be washed well or soaked in a soap solution to remove all debris. They should then be soaked in a disinfectant solution, similar to mask brushes. Rinse machine brushes well and store in a clean, dry place.

High-frequency electrodes should be carefully cleaned with 70 percent isopropyl alcohol. After initial cleaning immerse the bulb part of the electrode (not the metal part) in a disinfectant solution for 20 minutes. Rinse the glass well with cool water, being very careful not to get the metal part of the electrode wet. Gently dry with a clean towel. Because high frequency is performed after extraction, it is possible that small amounts of blood or bacteria may be present on a used electrode. You should have more than one electrode so that one may be used while another is being disinfected. Do not attempt to autoclave electrodes! Galvanic desincrustation attachments should be thoroughly cleaned with 70 percent isopropyl alcohol after each use. Using cotton covers over desincrustation attachments will also help to reduce contamination.

Iontophoresis rollers should be thoroughly cleaned with 70 percent isopropyl alcohol. The metal rollers can be detached and soaked in a disinfectant solution for 20 minutes. Follow manufacturer's directions for cleaning, because attachments may differ. Be careful not to immerse any electrical parts of the machine. Again, it is advisable to have additional machine attachments so that one can be used while another is being disinfected.

Suction attachments should be thoroughly cleaned with 70 percent isopropyl alcohol, then allowed to soak in a disinfectant solution for 20 minutes. Store in alcohol or in a clean, dry place.

Comedone extractors are very likely to contain small amounts of blood or debris after use. Clean them well with 70 percent alcohol. It is important to autoclave comedone extractors! If an autoclave is unavailable, soak the clean comedone extractor in a glutaraldehyde solution for 20 to 25 minutes. Rinse thoroughly. Never use an extractor on more than one person without sterilizing!

Tweezers should be cleaned well with 70 percent isopropyl alcohol after each use. Metal tweezers can be autoclaved or disinfected. Store tweezers in a bowl or jar with quaternary ammonia and rinse well before each use.

It cannot be stressed enough that it is important to have additional implements of all types available. It is also very important to be extremely systematic about cleansing and disinfecting all materials at all times. Your entire staff should be aware of salon sterilization procedures so that all staff members follow the same techniques and cross-contamination does not occur (Figure 4–3).

Cleaning Sponges

Ideally, cleansing sponges should be used once and discarded. Many salons include the price of the sponges in the service and then give the used sponges to the client so that they may be used at home between salon treatments.

If disposable sponges are not a possibility, sponges should be washed in the washing machine with chlorine bleach. After washing they should be removed from the washing machine and autoclaved. If an autoclave is not available, the following disinfecting procedure is recommended. Collect several dozen sponges after they have been washed in the washing machine. Place the sponges in a garment washing bag (the kind used for hosiery). Place the bag in the washing machine. Fill the washer with cold water and mix in about a gallon of household bleach. Allow the sponges to soak for 15 to 20 minutes in the bleach solution. Depending on the size of your washing machine, more or less bleach may be added. The bleach solution should be 1 part bleach to 10 parts cold water. After allowing sponges to soak for 15 to 20 minutes, put the washing machine on the rinse cycle. It may be necessary to run the sponges through two rinse cycles to remove all the bleach solution. The spin cycle will remove most of the water. Allow the sponges to dry in a clean place. It is best to store sponges in a UV sanitizer.

GENERAL CLEANING

The facial room should be cleaned between clients. Utensils and equipment should be thoroughly disinfected. All towels and linens should be replaced between clients.

At the end of each day, the room should be very thoroughly cleaned.

The following are instructions for room "shut-down" procedures at the end of each day:

1. Put on a pair of latex gloves.
2. Remove all dirty laundry from the hamper. Spray the hamper with a disinfectant aerosol spray or wipe down with disinfectant. Mildew grows easily in hampers.
3. Remove all dirty spatulas, used brushes, and other utensils. Most of these should have been removed between clients during the day. Thoroughly disinfect all materials.
4. Wipe down all counters, the facial chair, machines, and other furniture with 70 percent isopropyl alcohol or other disinfectant. The magnifying lamp should be cleaned on both sides in the same manner.
5. Replenish the room with fresh linens, spatulas, utensils, and other supplies so it is ready for the next day.
6. Change disinfecting solution as necessary.
7. Maintain vaporizer as necessary.
8. Check the room for dirt or smudges on the walls, baseboards, or dust in corners or on air vents.

COMMONLY USED DISINFECTANTS

Name	Form	Strength	How to Use
Quaternary Ammonium Compounds (Quats)	Liquid or tablet	1:1000 solution	Immerse implements in solution for 20 or more minutes.
Formalin	Liquid	25% solution	Immerse implements in solution for 10 or more minutes.
Formalin	Liquid	10% solution	Immerse implements in solution for 20 or more minutes.
Alcohol	Liquid	70% solution	Immerse implements or sanitize electrodes and sharp cutting edges 10 or more minutes.

COMMONLY USED ANTISEPTICS

Name	Form	Strength	Use
Boric Acid	White crystals	2–5% solution	Cleanse the eyes.
Tincture of Iodine	Liquid	2% solution	Cleanse cuts and wounds.
Hydrogen Peroxide	Liquid	3–5% solution	Cleanse skin and minor cuts.
Ethyl or Grain Alcohol	Liquid	60% solution	Cleanse hands, skin, and minute cuts. Not to be used if irritation is present.
Formalin	Liquid	5% solution	Cleanse shampoo bowl, cabinet, etc.
Chloramine-T (Chlorazene; Chlorozol)	White crystals	½% solution	Cleanse skin and hands, and for general use.
Sodium Hypochlorite (Javelle water; Zonite)	White crystals	½% solution	Rinse the hands.

Other approved disinfectants and antiseptics are being used in beauty salons. Consult your state board of cosmetology or your health department.

Figure 4–3   Commonly used disinfectants and antiseptics

9. Vacuum and mop the room with a disinfectant.
10. Spray the air in the room with a disinfectant aerosol spray.
11. Replenish any empty jars. If you are reusing jars for dispensing creams from a bulk container, always use up the entire content of the small jar before replenishing. Never add cream to a partially used jar. Rinse the empty jar well with hot water and then disinfect with alcohol, rinsing thoroughly. Allow to dry before refilling the jar.

Following these procedures on a daily basis will serve three purposes:

- Your room will always be ready the next morning.
- Cleaning at night cuts down on the number of microorganisms that can breed overnight.
- Your room will always be spotless, making your clients confident and reassured that they are being treated in a hygienic environment.

Laundry

Anyone handling dirty laundry should always wear thick rubber or latex gloves during the entire laundry procedure. Dirty lancets, sponges, and gauze may be contaminated and can accidentally get mixed in with the laundry. Sheets and towels should be washed well with chlorine bleach and immediately dried in the dryer. Headbands, turbans, smocks, and labcoats should also be washed in the same manner.

Linen service is an alternative to washing. Linen services are familiar with hospital sanitation procedures and are a good choice if you have little space in your salon.

ABOUT OSHA

The **Occupational Safety and Health Administration (OSHA)**, is a federal government agency, part of the Department of Labor, formed to help ensure that places of employment maintain a safe and healthy environment for employees.

Salons are expected to have a program in place to educate employees about possible hazards in the workplace. In the skin-care profession, we must educate employees about safe practices in sanitation and precautions to avoid possible exposure to chemicals, as well as precautions to avoid exposure to bodily fluids. Universal precautions for blood-borne pathogens include the use of protective equipment such as gloves, labcoats, and the proper disposal of used or contaminated tools such as lancets, waxing supplies, and other soiled or used implements.

Manufacturers of skin-care products are required to furnish **Material Safety Data Sheets (MSDS)**, which are special instruction sheets that describe safe concerns of products used in the skin-care practice. Data include how to safely clean up accidental spills and any special instructions regarding eye contact or accidental ingestion. Because skin-care products are designed to be applied to the skin, there are often very few, if any, precautions listed. Nevertheless, product manufacturers are required to furnish you with MSDS when requested.

MSDS are only necessary for professional products used in the salon. They are not necessary or required for retail products intended for home use.

Occupational Safety and Health Administration (OSHA) is a federal government agency, part of the Department of Labor, formed to help ensure that places of employment maintain a safe and healthy environment for employees.

Material Safety Data Sheets (MSDS) are special instruction sheets that describe safety concerns of products used in the skin-care practice.

In the skin-care salon, MSDS for antiseptics, germicides, disinfectants, and nail chemicals are probably the most important. Many of these types of chemicals are more dangerous if mishandled or accidentally spilled.

For more information on OSHA rules and precautions, contact the U.S. Department of Labor, Occupational Safety and Health Administration, 200 Constitution Ave. N.W., Washington, DC 20210. More information on this subject can also be found in *The Esthetician's Guide to Working with Physicians* by Susanne Warfield, available from Milady Publishing.

PROTECTING YOU AND YOUR CLIENTS FROM DISEASE

Besides the many sanitation, disinfection, and sterilization procedures already discussed, it is important that you personally carry out personal sanitation procedures on a routine basis. You must be careful not to reuse disposable items or to contaminate your products by using a spatula more than once. To avoid cross contamination while removing creams from jars, there are several good techniques to use:

1. Always remove creams from jars with a disinfected spatula. Use spatulas only once before discarding or disinfecting.
2. When removing creams from jars, remove enough for the entire service. It is better to remove too much product than to have to re-dip into a jar. If you need more cream, use a fresh spatula. Place used spatulas in a soaking bowl for later cleaning and disinfecting. You should have at least six spatulas for each client you see per day.
3. It is a good idea to use small, disposable paper cups for dispensing creams. You may prepare measured portions of various products early in the day before clients arrive. Because you have measured the correct amount, this procedure eliminates all chances of contamination because you never touch a client's skin during preparation. Store cream portions wrapped in plastic wrap, or use small portion cups with plastic lids, like the kind used in restaurants for ketchup or sauces.
4. Pumps are another great idea, because they prevent contamination. Cleansers, fluids, and moisturizers can easily be dispensed from pumps. Squeeze bottles with flip-tops are another good type of dispenser. Using these types of dispensers also saves time in the treatment room.
5. Tubes or pumps are by far the most sanitary method for retail client use products. Your clients should also be instructed to use spatulas for jars at home. Using tubes or pumps eliminates this problem.
6. Wax, should also be dispensed using one spatula per dip. Again, a larger amount of wax may be removed and placed in a paper cup for application.

Use of Antiseptic Washes

Always wash your hands between clients with a good antiseptic soap or wash. Dispensers are the most sanitary method of accomplishing this. Bar soap is not appropriate because you touch and retouch the bar each time you wash your hands.

Gloves

You absolutely must use latex gloves when performing waxing, or any service that might involve exposure to blood or body fluids. It is strongly suggested to use gloves from start to finish of all facial treatments, electrolysis, and waxing (Figure 4–4).

Gloves will protect your hands from exposure to many microorganisms. If you don't use gloves for the entire facial treatment, at least wear them during and after extraction, through the remainder of the treatment. If you have any cuts, abrasions, or irritations on your hands, you must use gloves at all times!

The best type of glove to use is latex examination gloves. They conform much better to the hands than vinyl or plastic gloves and are much more comfortable for both the esthetician and the client. Many estheticians think that gloves take away the "personal touch" from the client. The truth is that most clients think that gloves feel smoother than hands for massage, and they appreciate your efforts to use sanitary procedures.

Some people, however, are allergic to latex. It is important to have vinyl gloves on hand in case you have a client who is allergic to latex.

Some gloves are powdered with talc or cornstarch for ease in putting on the gloves. Unfortunately, health care workers, including estheticians, often become allergic or develop contact dermatitis from glove powders. There are gloves available now that are completely powderless. Also be sure to purchase gloves that are the right size. Gloves that are too tight can rub and irritate the skin.

Gloves need not be sterile. Nonsterile, disposable, latex gloves usually are available in small, medium, and large sizes from a medical, dental, or esthetic supply house.

Techniques for Avoiding Blood Exposure During Treatment

Always begin extractions from the chin and work upward on the face. If you should encounter blood, gravity will pull the blood down the face and away from areas you will be extracting from next. While wearing gloves, try to avoid touching anything but the client's skin. Prepackaged, portioned products discussed earlier will help to prevent you from touching any bottles, jars, or other utensils while extracting.

Using a magnifying lamp during extraction helps protect your eyes from exposure to debris. Although masks and eye goggles are necessary for many health care workers, they are not necessary for estheticians. If you work with an assistant, the person should also wear gloves. Blood may accumulate under a mask in an acne treatment, for example. Wear gloves when removing masks or finishing the treatment. It is generally not necessary to wear gloves during makeup application unless you are working with a patient with acne or performing paramedical makeup on a client with open abrasions or incisions. Makeup brushes should also be washed and disinfected between uses. Makeup brushes are damaged much more easily during disinfection than are mask brushes. Be careful to use a mild disinfectant for makeup brushes.

When applying gloves, carefully slip your hand into the glove and then check the glove for any small tears or holes. Gloves with holes should be immediately discarded. To remove soiled gloves, grab a section of the cuff (the wrist part of the glove), and

Figure 4–4 It is important for estheticians to wear gloves during many procedures including facial treatments, extraction, waxing, and electrolysis.

remove the glove, turning the glove inside out. Repeat with the other glove. Turning the gloves inside out will prevent accidental contact with the soiled part of the glove. Discard used gloves immediately.

Other Diseases

Most states have cosmetology laws that prevent cosmetology professionals from working on clients with infectious diseases or on clients who have open sores suggestive of infectious disease. Taking a good client history on all new clients will help inform you of diseases that the client may have. Clients with infectious diseases such as conjunctivitis (pinkeye), impetigo, herpes infection, or other infectious diseases should not be worked on until a doctor certifies that they are well.

IN CONCLUSION

The esthetician is at relatively little risk of infection with most microorganisms. However, it is important to take precautions to always avoid contact with blood or other body fluids. Always wear gloves and use the disinfection and sterilization procedures outlined in this chapter. Laws vary slightly from state to state. Make sure you are thoroughly acquainted with your state sanitation rules and laws regarding the practice of esthetics. Most important, use common sense. Always be aware of your professional hygiene techniques. Constantly practicing good techniques will become a habit.

Topics for Discussion

1. What is the difference between disinfection and sterilization?
2. What is an invasive procedure?
3. What is aseptic procedure?
4. Discuss various methods for disinfecting equipment and materials.
5. Discuss general cleaning procedures.
6. Why are gloves important?
7. Discuss the correct ways to put on and take off latex gloves.
8. Why is it important to have both latex and vinyl gloves?
9. What is OSHA and why is it important?
10. What is an MSDS?

Chapter

5

Hormones

Objectives

Every esthetician needs to be familiar with the endocrine system and hormones. Hormones have very definite effects on the skin, and their functioning is directly related to many skin problems. This chapter will familiarize the esthetician with the major glands of the endocrine system and their function. You will also learn about the menstrual cycle, pregnancy, menopause, and diseases and disorders of the endocrine system. How hormones affect the skin will be discussed in depth.

Hormones are basically chemical messengers that are manufactured or **secreted** by glands within the body. As you have previously learned, many glands are present in the body. **Exocrine glands** such as the sebaceous glands and the sudoriferous glands have ducts through which chemicals move. **Apocrine glands** are present in the groin and armpit. **Endocrine glands** secrete hormones. The endocrine glands empty hormones directly into the bloodstream. Although most people think of hormones in terms of sex hormones, sex hormones are only a few of the hormones that the endocrine system produces.

Hormones work by transmitting chemical messages to the various body cells. The hormones have special "keys" that fit the "locks" on the cell membranes that they are intended to affect. The key fitting the lock causes the cell membrane to produce enzymes that stimulate other chemical reactions within the cell. The "locks" on the cells are called **receptors** or receptor sites. Each hormone affects specific cells in different ways, and each endocrine gland produces different hormones.

THE ENDOCRINE GLANDS

There are eight major endocrine glands in the human body (Figure 5–1).

The **pituitary gland** is found in the center of the head. It serves as the "brain" of the endocrine system. It is connected to the brain by another endocrine gland called the **hypothalamus gland**.

The pituitary gland secretes many hormones called **trophic hormones**. Trophic hormones are chemicals that cause other glands to make other hormones. Trophic hormones

Hormones are special chemicals that are manufactured or secreted by glands within the body.

Secreted means synthesized or released by various cells or organs.

Exocrine glands, such as the sebaceous glands and the sudoriferous glands, have ducts through which chemicals move.

Apocrine glands are present in the groin area and armpits. They produce a thicker form of sweat and are responsible for producing the substance that, when in contact with bacteria, produces body odor.

Endocrine glands secrete hormones directly into the bloodstream.

Receptors inform T cells of what type of cell it is and that it is an "official" cell of the body and not an antigen.

Pituitary gland is found in the center of the head. It serves as the "brain" of the endocrine system.

Hypothalamus gland controls some involuntary muscles, such as the muscles of the intestines that help move food through the gastrointestinal system.

Trophic hormones are chemicals that cause other glands to make hormones.

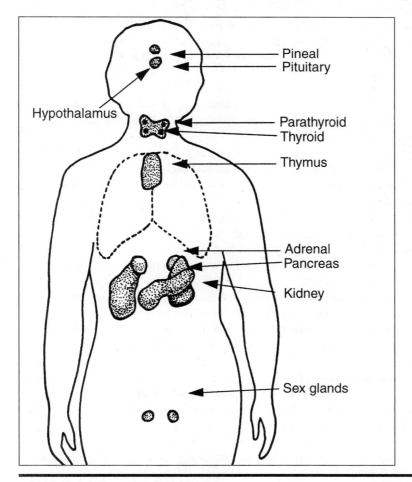

Figure 5–1 The endocrine system

are "signal hormones." Trophic hormones secreted by the pituitary gland include follicle-stimulating hormone (FSH), which is the pituitary hormone that causes production of sex hormones in the glands present in the sex organs. The pituitary gland also produces special hormones that cause regulation of the amount of fluid retained by the body, hormones that control growth, and special hormones that cause the female breast to produce milk.

Hypothalamus manufactures hormones that stimulate the pituitary gland to make other hormones. It is also able to detect needs of various parts of the body by chemically monitoring the blood.

The **hypothalamus** controls some involuntary muscles, such as the muscles in the intestines that help move food through the gastrointestinal system. The hypothalamus also manufactures a variety of hormones that cause stimulation of the pituitary gland to make other hormones. You might say that the hypothalamus is the "interpreter" between the brain and the pituitary gland. The hypothalamus is able to detect needs of various parts of the body by chemically monitoring the blood that flows through it.

Thyroid gland is located in the neck. It regulates both cellular and body metabolism and produces hormones that stimulate growth.

Thyroxine is one of the hormones secreted by the thyroid gland.

The **thyroid gland** is located in the neck. It regulates both cellular and body metabolism and produces hormones that stimulate growth. One of the hormones secreted by the thyroid gland is called **thyroxine**. Without thyroxine dwarfism occurs in children.

The thyroid gland uses a lot of iodine in its manufacture of hormones. This is why it is important to have some iodine in the diet. Iodine is present in fish, meat, and some vegetables.

Parathyroid gland is responsible for regulating calcium and phosphates in the bloodstream.

Behind the thyroid gland lies a related glandular structure called the **parathyroid gland**. The parathyroids are responsible for regulating calcium and phosphates in the bloodstream, which are necessary for proper bone growth. Vitamin D is an important element in the regulation of calcium also.

Adrenal glands are located just above the kidneys and produce hormones needed by the nervous system to transport nerve impulses.

The **adrenal glands** are located just above the kidneys. Like hair, they have an inner part called the medulla and an outer core called the cortex. The medulla makes the two main hormones called adrenaline and noradrenaline. These two hormones are needed by the nervous system to transport nerve impulses.

Adrenaline is secreted when the body is under stress.

Adrenaline is also secreted when the body is under stress. We have all experienced an "almost accident" when a car pulls out right in front of us. That feeling immediately after an "almost accident" is caused by adrenaline. You could call adrenaline the "emergency hormone." No doubt you have heard stories of people having almost superhuman strength during emergencies. This is also caused by the adrenal hormones. When a large amount of adrenaline is secreted suddenly into the bloodstream, the body responds by preparing for an emergency. The heartbeat increases, pupils of the eyes dilate, the bronchi in the lungs expand, and the body generally focuses all its attention on the impending emergency. The cortex of the adrenal glands manufactures steroids, which are very small hormone molecules that are able to penetrate cell membranes and enter cells for specific reasons. The steroid hormones produced by the adrenal cortex are called corticoids. The corticoids help regulate the metabolism and the body's use of carbohydrates, proteins, and fats. They also help to maintain water balance in the body and regulate sodium and potassium levels.

Pineal gland is located in the brain. Its function is not well understood, but it is theorized that it is related to the sex hormones.

The **pineal gland** is located in the brain, like the pituitary gland. It is very small and is funnel shaped. Its function is not well understood, but it is theorized that it is related to the sex hormones.

The **pancreas** is located in the abdomen. It has several functions. It secretes pancreatic enzymes that are delivered into the intestine. These enzymes help digest foods taken into the body.

Within the pancreas are a group of specialized cells called the islets of Langerhans. These cells manufacture a hormone called insulin, which regulates blood sugar or glucose levels. **Diabetes** is a disease that results from the pancreas not secreting enough insulin. Diabetics must take synthetically produced insulin.

The **thymus gland** has already been discussed in Chapter 2, The Immune System. As you know, it produces specialized lymphocytes to help the body fight disease. The thymus gland grows during childhood and begins shrinking in later years.

The last, but not least, of the major endocrine glands are the sex glands. These are the **ovaries** in females and the **testes** in males. The ovaries are located above the uterus and are connected to the uterus by two hollow tubes called the fallopian tubes (Figure 5–2). The ovaries contain eggs that will eventually be released into the fallopian tubes for possible fertilization by sperm. The testes are present within the scrotum. The testes are connected to another tube called the vas deferens. The vas deferens leads to a holding sac called the seminal vesicle, which holds sperm manufactured by the testes. This series of tubules continues and eventually joins the urethra, which is the tube that leads to the outside of the penis (Figure 5–3).

HORMONES PRODUCED BY THE OVARIES AND TESTES

The sex glands of both men and women produce hormones. The testes secrete testosterone. **Testosterone** is the male hormone responsible for development of typical male characteristics such as a deep voice, broad shoulders, body hair, and other male characteristics. Male hormones are called **androgens**.

The ovaries produce three hormones. **Estradiol** is one of the female hormones, better known as estrogen. **Estrogen** is the hormone that gives a woman female characteristics, such as breasts, and also helps with the development of the menstrual cycle. Another hormone secreted by the ovaries is **progesterone**, which is a steroid hormone that helps prepare the uterus for pregnancy and is an important hormone in the menstrual cycle. A third hormone manufactured by the ovaries is **relaxin**, which helps enlarge the pelvic opening during childbirth.

Both male and female sex glands receive many of their "cues" for hormone production from the pituitary and the hypothalamus. The pituitary makes a hormone called **follicle-stimulating hormone**, referred to as **FSH**. FSH from the pituitary gland causes the tests to produce sperm. Another pituitary hormone called **luteinizing hormone**, or LH, causes the testes to manufacture testosterone.

The same types of pituitary hormones cause production of female hormones in the ovaries. The FSH produced by the pituitary causes the development of the ovum, or egg. Luteinizing hormone (LH) causes the actual process of ovulation or the release of the egg (ovum) from the ovary.

Pancreas is located in the abdomen. It secretes pancreatic enzymes that are delivered into the intestine.

Diabetes is a disease that results from the pancreas not secreting enough insulin.

Thymus gland is located under the breastbone in the chest. It secretes hormones and helps to trigger synthesis of more lymph tissue.

Ovaries are located just above the uterus and are connected to the uterus by two hollow tubes called fallopian tubes.

Testes are present within the scrotum and produce sperm.

Testosterone is the male hormone responsible for development of typical male characteristics.

Adrogens are male hormones.

Estradiol is a steroid made from the hormone estrogen that gives women female characteristics.

Estrogen is the hormone that gives women female characteristics.

Progesterone helps prepare the uterus for pregnancy and is an important hormone in the menstrual cycle.

Relaxin is a hormone manufactured by the ovaries that helps enlarge the pelvic opening during childbirth.

Follicle-stimulating hormone (FSH) is a hormone secreted by the pituitary gland that causes the development of the egg, or ovum.

Luteinizing hormone causes the actual process of ovulation or the release of the egg from the ovary. It also causes the testes to manufacture testosterone.

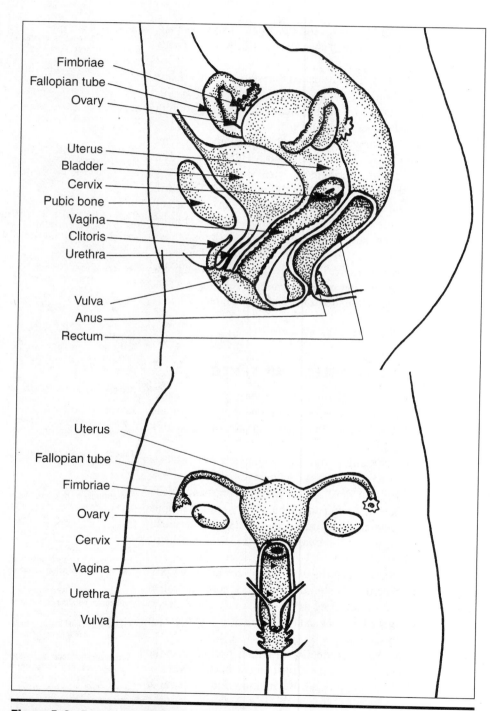

Figure 5–2 Female reproductive organs

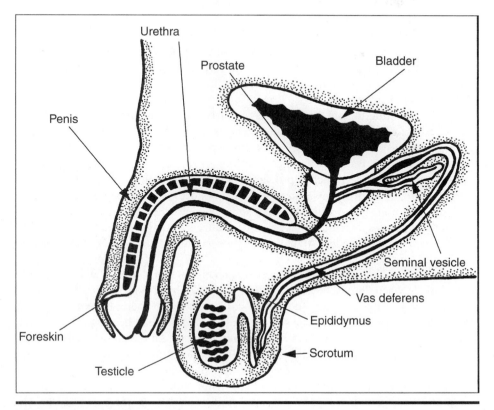

Figure 5–3   Male reproductive organs

HORMONAL PHASES OF LIFE

There are several phases of life in humans that are dramatically influenced and caused by the presence or lack of hormones. Although we produce hormones to some extent throughout life, there are several stages during which pronounced changes occur.

Puberty

Puberty is the stage of life when physical changes occur in both sexes and when sexual function of the sex glands begins to take place. Sexual reproduction is physically possible at puberty.

At the beginning of puberty, which is usually about 12 to 14 years of age (females may be earlier than males), the hypothalamus begins producing a hormone called luteinizing hormone releasing hormone, which in turn stimulates the pituitary gland to manufacture much larger amounts of FSH and LH.

The FSH and LH are trophic hormones. They cause the ovaries and testes to secrete more hormones, specifically estrogens and androgens. The sudden production of these hormones starts a number of drastic changes in physical appearance. Girls begin

Puberty is the stage of life when physical changes occur in both sexes and when sexual function of the sex glands begins to take place.

developing breasts, fat deposits form around the hips to provide feminine curvature, and the sweat glands begin producing body odor. Androgen production in females gives rise to pubic, leg, and underarm hair. In males, these changes in appearance include muscle development, development of the masculine form, broader shoulders, deeper voice, body and facial hair, and general physical growth. Puberty, of course, also triggers sexual attraction to the opposite sex.

It is interesting to note that just when sexual attraction begins, the maintenance of attractiveness gets more difficult! Many changes happen within the skin at puberty. As hormone production of the sex organs begins at puberty, many hormone changes occur that affect the skin. Probably the biggest change is related to the production of androgen, the male hormone, which is produced by both males and females. As the production of androgen begins, the sebaceous glands produce more and more sebum. Androgen is a sebaceous gland stimulant. As androgen enters the bloodstream, it carries its hormonal messages, resulting in appearance changes such as body hair growth and the development of body odor. At the same time androgen also affects the sebaceous glands.

The increase in sebaceous gland activity and production causes dilation of the follicles. This is when "pores" are first easily visible. You may notice that small children have no easily visible pore structure on the skin's surface. The pores become dilated due to increased sebum production. As the sebum fills the follicle, it begins pushing against the follicle walls, stretching them and making the pores on the surface appear larger. The nose is usually the first to develop visible pores. This development of the pore structure will continue into the bridge of the nose, then the forehead, and then the chin. You may notice that a 12-year-old client has visible follicles only in these areas. The scalp also becomes oilier due to androgen production. This is the beginning of what many refer to as the "T-zone," so named because of its pattern (Figure 5–4).

Puberty is also for many teenagers the beginning of acne and break-out tendencies. You may see a young client with large comedones in the nose, chin, and forehead areas, or occasionally only very small comedones in the nose only. The smallness of the comedones at this age is because the follicle walls have yet to stretch out much. The androgens have not yet had their full effect on the sebaceous glands.

Mothers often bring in their young teenagers with all of these problems. The young client should be advised of proper home care, but it is extremely important to keep it simple! Children of this age are often not used to daily skin care. Please be very thorough in your explanation of home care procedures. Although it is important to instruct them in proper care, they cannot be expected to perform a seven-step regime twice a day! They should be instructed to use a washable, foaming cleanser twice a day, followed by a gentle, low pH toner. A mild antiacne product should be used at night if necessary. A 2 percent salicylic or a 2.5 percent benzoyl peroxide gel is recommended.

Sunscreen should be used daily. It is important to convince young clients to start using sunblocks on a daily basis. This is the best way to prevent future sun damage. Teaching good health habits at a young age will help the client maintain good skin for a lifetime. Emphasize the dangers of excess sun and give helpful hints about using sun-

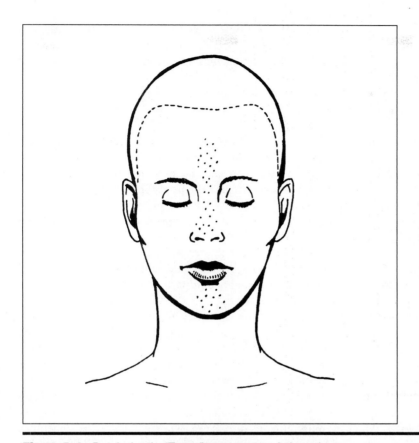

Figure 5–4   Developing the "T-zone" pore structure during puberty

screens at the beach. Moisturizers are really rarely needed by pubescent teenagers, except in very cold climates. Make sure you always recommend products that are non-comedogenic (see Chapters 12 and 13, Acne and the Esthetician and Comedogenicity, respectively).

Treatment in the salon should follow these steps:

1. Cleanse the face well with a cleansing milk for oily or combination skin. Do not use toner or astringent at this point in treatment—the follicles are usually already tight and small. Using toner on this skin at the beginning of treatment will only make extractions more difficult.
2. Presoften the clogged areas by using a desincrustant solution or pre-mask. Steam with this solution on the face for about eight minutes. It is very important that the skin is hydrated for this type of treatment.
3. Remove the pre-mask or desincrustant solution. Gently pat the skin dry.
4. Begin extraction, being careful to explain to the young client what you are doing. Explain to the client that extraction should always be performed by a professional.

You may have difficulty extracting these tightly packed comedones. Be gentle, and take your time. Remember, this is the young client's first experience with extraction! Slow, gentle pressure applied in small areas is most effective.

5. After extraction is complete, apply a toner or antiseptic astringent.
6. Apply a light hydrating fluid and use high frequency.
7. Apply a clay-based drying mask for oily skin.

The first facial treatment for a teenage client should be an educational experience, rather than a "feel-good" treatment. You should help the young client understand (in simple terms) what is happening to the skin and the need for consistent hygiene. Explain the use of noncomedogenic cosmetics and the need for professional advice in choosing the right products.

Acne development should also be explained to the teenage client so that the client is aware of possible future occurrences and their prevention.

If the young client already experiences acne flareups, you should make the proper treatment recommendations. (See Chapter 12, Acne and the Esthetician.) Treatment for most pubescent teens is only necessary bimonthly until further development of the pore structure or the beginning of acne flareups occurs.

Another problem associated with puberty is the development of a condition called **keratosis pilaris**. Keratosis pilaris appears as small pinpoint bumps, usually on the cheeks, accompanied by generalized redness. This condition is often seen in "rosy-cheeked" children. In this condition, the androgens have affected the growth of either terminal or lanugo hairs, which have started growing but are not strong enough to push through the follicle opening. The hairs remain trapped inside the follicle and as a result irritate the follicle and the surrounding skin. Although this condition is usually treated by a dermatologist who uses mild retinoids or other exfoliating agents, it is sometimes seen in the salon. You should treat this condition very gently by using mildly abrasive scrubs and light extraction. The routine use of a mild abrasive, such as granular scrubs that are not excessively drying, will help open the follicle and allow the hair to come out, cutting down on irritation. A 10 percent glycolic gel, with a pH 3.5 or above should be used in the area once or twice a day.

Keratosis pilaris is a condition in which the skin exhibits redness and irritation in patches, accompanied by a rough texture, and small pinpoint white papules that look like very small milia.

Appearance Changes in Adolescence

As the teenager gets older and further into the teenage years, the client will usually experience more problems with acne. Salon treatments should then be administered on at least a monthly basis, except in cases of more severe acne, when they should be more frequent.

The Menstrual Cycle

Menarche is a girl's first period.

Menstruation is the body getting rid of an unused ovum and accompanying endometrium.

With puberty and adolescence comes **menarche**, the beginning of the menstrual cycle in females. Menarche is the girl's first "period." **Menstruation** is the correct name for the "period." Menstruation is actually the body getting rid of an unused ovum and accompanying endometrium, which is the lining of the uterine wall, that occurs each month in females. The endometrium is formed by the uterus in response to the hormone progesterone. The menstrual cycle is a 27- to 30-day cycle in which the female's ovaries manufacture an ovum and hormonal changes take place that prepare the uterus for pregnancy in case the ovum is fertilized by sperm. When the ovum is not fertilized, the uterus sheds the lining (endometrium), which is menstruation (Figure 5–5).

There are actually six phases to the cycle:

Phase 1 occurs during the first five days of the cycle. The hypothalamus senses low levels of estrogen and progesterone and signals the pituitary gland to secrete FSH and LH. The ovaries then begin producing larger amounts of estrogen and progesterone, which prepare and release the ovum, or egg.

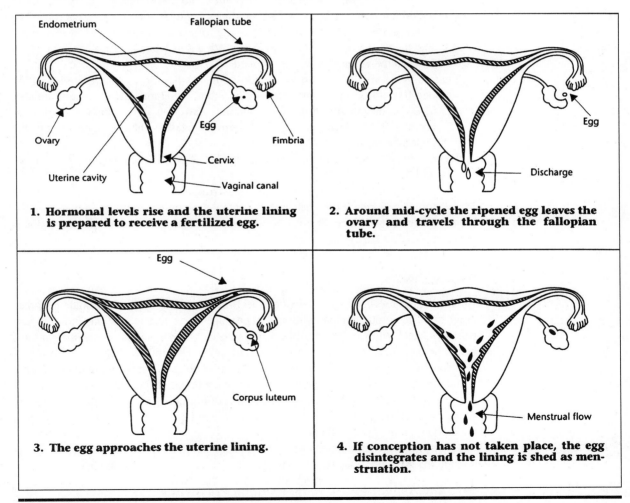

1. **Hormonal levels rise and the uterine lining is prepared to receive a fertilized egg.**

2. **Around mid-cycle the ripened egg leaves the ovary and travels through the fallopian tube.**

3. **The egg approaches the uterine lining.**

4. **If conception has not taken place, the egg disintegrates and the lining is shed as menstruation.**

Figure 5–5   The menstrual cycle

In Phase 2, the hypothalamus detects that the ovaries are secreting the right amount of estrogen necessary for ovulation, shuts down the pituitary gland's large production of FSH, and begins producing more LH. This occurs during days 6 to 12 of the cycle.

In Phase 3, the hormone levels of estrogen and progesterone are adjusted again. The estrogen level reaches a high point, which signals the pituitary gland to release a very large amount of LH, which then causes the release of the egg from the ovary. The surge in LH occurs in the 12th and 13th days of the cycle.

Phase 4 is on the 14th day, when the egg (ovum) is released from the ovaries and begins its journey down the fallopian tube to the uterus. What is left of the follicle from which the egg was released turns into a hormone-producing structure called the corpus luteum, which produces large amounts of progesterone. The progesterone produces the uterine lining, or endometrium, which is the "nest" that the uterus builds for a fetus. This 14th day is when a sperm can fertilize an egg and the woman becomes pregnant.

Phase 5 is essentially the last two weeks of the 28-day cycle. If fertilization of the egg has not occurred, the pituitary hormones FSH and LH drop substantially. The corpus luteum shrinks, substantially lowering its production of progesterone. This decrease in progesterone causes the breakdown of the endometrium.

Phase 6 begins menstruation, or the "period." The whole cycle begins again on the 28th day.

Many women experience differences in the actual days on which different phases of the menstrual cycle take place. Stress, obesity, anorexia, and other endocrine system disorders can all affect the cycle.

PREGNANCY

If the ovum is fertilized by a sperm on the 14th day of the cycle, the female becomes pregnant. The corpus luteum continues to produce progesterone, and the endometrium becomes much thicker. The fertilized egg goes through a series of transformations, begins mitotic division, and forms a mass of cells. The embryo begins to form, surrounded by a capsule-like structure called a trophoblast. The trophoblast, in simple terms, provides nutrition for the embryo. The membrane of the trophoblast eventually evolves into the placenta, which is a thick layer of hormone-producing cells that serves as the nutrient, oxygen, and waste exchange system between the growing embryo and the blood system of the mother.

The placenta manufactures many hormones, including those that affect the corpus luteum, the growth of the embryo, and the production of milk in the mother's breasts.

Skin and Appearance Changes During Pregnancy

A vast number of obvious changes takes place in the human body during pregnancy. Many of these changes affect the skin. Hyperpigmentation is often seen in pregnant women. The skin often tans much more easily than normal. Pregnancy mask is a condition in which the face develops significant hyperpigmentation, resembling a dark facial mask (Plates 5a, 5b). Light areas surround the eye areas, and the rest of the face is dark with pigment. Pregnancy masks and pregnancy-related hyperpigmentation are caused by a hormone secreted by the placenta that stimulates the melanocytes in the skin. Normally, hyperpigmentation subsides after the birth of the child, but sometimes the condition will need to be treated in the salon after childbirth. Treating hyperpigmentation during pregnancy is not advisable. Even if there is a bleaching effect achieved by the use of skin bleaches such as hydroquinone, the placenta continues production of the melanin-producing hormone, only to result in more hyperpigmentation. It is best to wait until the pregnancy is over. Observe whether the hyperpigmentation decreases significantly with the shutdown of placental hormones. If the hyperpigmentation does not fade within several months, it can then be treated. Avoiding exposure to the sun will help cut down on the amount of pigment produced during pregnancy.

Stretch marks, or striae, are marks that occur in pregnant women. These strip-like lines may be red or brown-tan in appearance and are the result of rapid weight gain during pregnancy. The skin simply stretches quickly, and the marks occur in the areas of the abdomen, breasts, buttocks, and legs. Unfortunately, little can be done for stretch marks. Many stretch marks fade after childbirth. The use of good, hydrating body creams and lubricants during the pregnancy seems to keep some women from developing stretch marks or at least lessens the severity. The creams must be applied on a daily, consistent basis for best results. In some women creams seem to have no effect. Some theories indicate that the development of stretch marks may be hereditarily or genetically connected. Research is currently being conducted using retinoids, electrical stimulation, and other methods to treat post-pregnancy stretch marks.

An increase in blood flow and blood pressure during pregnancy may lead to the development of **telangiectasias**, or small, red, enlarged capillaries on the face and other areas of the body. Avoiding sun and hot temperatures will help lessen the possibility of telangiectatic development. Telangiectasias are sometimes called **couperose** by European estheticians.

Telangiectasias usually fade rapidly after childbirth. If there are still obvious red lines after several months, they may be treated by a dermatologist or plastic surgeon using a special type of current called **diathermy**, or they can be treated by injecting saline or using a laser.

Varicose veins may also develop on the legs during pregnancy, due to weight and pressure on the legs. Resting with the legs elevated helps to prevent their occurrence. Use of support hose is also helpful in preventing varicose veins. Most varicose veins, again, fade after pregnancy, but those that do not can be treated by a dermatologist, plastic surgeon, or vascular surgeon.

Waterproof leg makeup may be used to conceal varicose veins or telangiectasias. Pregnant women may also have problems with their facial skin. Fluctuations in hormones may make problem skin worse, or significantly better. In many cases, acne-prone skin will become worse in the beginning of pregnancy, then become much better in the third or fourth month, resulting in clear skin for the rest of the pregnancy. This is the

Telangiectasias are small, red enlarged capillaries of the face and other areas of the body.

Couperose refers to diffuse redness, including telangiectasis of the face and other areas of the body.

Diathermy is a special type of current used in the treatment of telangiectasias.

result of the abundant female hormones present in the bloodstream during pregnancy. Acne will often flare up again after the baby is born, or just after the mother stops nursing. This, of course, results from a dramatic drop in female hormones in the bloodstream.

Acne in the pregnant woman should be treated as you would any case of acne (see Chapter 12, Acne and the Esthetician), except that therapy with galvanic and high-frequency current should be eliminated. Check with the client's physician if you have any doubts about treatment or products.

Precautions for Treating the Pregnant Woman

No type of electrical therapy, specifically galvanic or high-frequency therapies, should be administered to a pregnant woman, except with written permission from her physician. Physicians will often approve of electrolysis treatment, but it is important to get a written note from her doctor and keep it on file with the client's record for legal reasons.

Many topical preparations, including alphahydroxy acids, have never been extensively evaluated as to their safety when used in pregnant women. Although there is no currently available cosmetic agent known to affect the fetus, it is best to be conservative when using topical treatments and products, particularly newer functional agents. If you are in doubt about recommending a particular treatment to a pregnant client, check with her physician before administering that treatment or any questionable product for home use.

Most routine procedures may be performed on pregnant women. Special courses in body massage therapy for pregnant women are available from certified massage therapy schools. Make sure you have taken such a course before performing body massage on a pregnant woman.

Pregnant women may sometimes develop strange reactions to otherwise well-accepted treatments. Waxing, for example, may suddenly be very irritating to the skin. The only way to predict these types of reactions is to start slowly and patch-test areas for treatment. The woman's physician should supervise any internal or external drugs she takes during pregnancy. Pregnant women need lots of esthetic help during pregnancy. Pedicures may become a necessity, rather than a luxury service. Changes in the nails, skin, and hair may occur. It is also very important to be sensitive to a pregnant client's needs, because pregnancy is a wonderful, but sometimes emotional, time for some women.

PREMENSTRUAL SYNDROME

Premenstrual syndrome is a condition in which some women experience uncomfortable physical changes before menstruation.

Premenstrual syndrome is a condition in which some women experience uncomfortable physical changes before menstruation. These changes are caused by the fluctuating levels of hormone in the bloodstream. Increased estrogen levels may lead to water retention that can cause bloating, swelling of the breasts, swelling of the hands and feet, and general heaviness. The increase in hormones can also cause mood swings and may make the woman more susceptible to stress.

Controlling stress is one of the best ways to deal with premenstrual syndrome, frequently referred to as PMS. Stress-reducing techniques such as deep breathing exercises, aerobic workouts, massage, or general relaxation techniques may help reduce the symptoms. Esthetic care plays an important role in helping women with PMS feel better, both physically and psychologically. Wearing looser clothes may help constricted feelings associated with water retention.

In severe cases, hormones and other therapy administered by a physician may be warranted. Physicians may use drugs for high blood pressure or hormone-suppressing drugs to treat women with severe PMS.

PMS and Acne Flareups

Women frequently experience acne flareups seven to ten days before menstruation. The specific days in the cycle associated with acne flareups may vary in some women. The cause of premenstrual acne is not completely understood. It is theorized that large levels of progesterone, present in the bloodstream during the cycle days normally associated with premenstrual acne, somehow cause the flareups.

Premenstrual acne should be treated in the same manner as any acne flareup. Administering a good deep-cleansing facial treatment one week before the normal monthly breakout seems to help many women reduce or eliminate the flareups. Use of noncomedogenic products also can help control the breakouts, as can other therapies recommended in Chapter 12, Acne and the Esthetician. Increased stress during PMS can also cause breakouts or sudden acne flareups. Help your client choose some stress-reducing techniques or suggest that she treat herself to a body massage or other special pampering salon service to reduce stress and make herself feel better.

BIRTH CONTROL PILLS

Birth control pills work by regulating hormones normally associated with the menstrual cycle. They interfere with the normal development of the ovum by preventing or obstructing ovulation.

There are two basic types of birth control pills. One type contains both estrogen and progesterone and works by preventing the egg from maturing, therefore preventing ovulation. The other type is mainly progesterone. These are often called "mini-pills." The mini-pills work by exposing the bloodstream to extra amounts of progesterone, which causes thickening of the uterine fluids, keeping the egg from becoming fertile.

Skin Problems Associated with Birth Control Pills

The biggest problem associated with birth control pills that affects the skin is the tendency of some women to have acne flareups that are caused by hormone fluctuations due to increased levels of particular hormones present in the pills. Mini-pills, because they contain little or no estrogen, tend to be more aggravating to acne conditions. Estrogen-dominant pills tend to make acne-prone skin get better.

Starting and stopping birth control pills may have a dramatic effect on acne. Starting an androgen-dominant or progesterone-dominant pill may make acne immediately worse, whereas starting an estrogen-dominant pill may make acne-prone skin immediately better.

Stopping the pill may have like effects. Because the pill has a tendency to suppress natural hormone levels, discontinuing the pill may throw off natural hormone levels, making acne worse. It may take some time for the body to adjust to not having the hormone "supplement" present in the birth control pills. Some women take much longer to adjust.

Hyperpigmentation and the Birth Control Pill

Melasma are splotchy, pigmented complexions that may be present after use of birth control pills.

The other appearance problem related to birth control pills is that of hyperpigmentation, or **melasma**. Splotchy, pigmented complexions may be present after use of birth control pills. This hyperpigmentation usually is located in the forehead and cheeks. The upper lip is also often affected by melasma. Some women can develop a full-scale pregnancy mask associated with birth control pills.

Sunlight, especially deliberate exposure such as sunbathing, can make melasma much worse. Advise a client with melasma to stay out of the sun, and if she must go in the sun to use a strong sunblock. Sometimes the doctor can adjust the dosage or the type of the client's pill to reduce the possibility of melasma resulting from its use.

You should treat hyperpigmentation with hydroquinone and glycolic acid. See Chapter 17, The New Science of Aging Treatment, for more information on treating melasma. Paramedical camouflage cosmetics can also be used.

MENOPAUSE

Menopause is the time in a woman's life when the ovaries stop producing ova.

Perimenopause is the time before and around menopause.

Menopause is the time in a woman's life when the ovaries stop releasing ova. Menopause normally occurs when a woman is in her late forties or early fifties. The time before and around menopause is called **perimenopause**. What actually happens during menopause is that the ovaries have run out of follicles containing eggs. A female is born with 700,000 to 2 million eggs, which are contained in the follicles within the ovaries. Many die or atrophy, but at puberty about 400,000 remain. The pituitary gland secretes FSH and LH, but the ovaries stop responding. When no follicles are left to respond to follicle-stimulating hormone, no estrogen is produced in the ovary, and the preparation of the uterus does not occur.

The drop in hormone levels in the bloodstream causes a variety of physical symptoms. Hot flashes, rapid heartbeat, decreases in vaginal secretions, emotional irritability, bloating, and other signs may occur.

Osteoporosis is a weakening of the bone associated with aging that is predominant in women.

Hormone replacement therapy (HRT) uses oral or injectable female hormones to control or prevent symptoms of menopause. HRT may also help prevent skin changes or osteoporosis in women.

The same symptoms may be produced after a hysterectomy. If a woman has a hysterectomy early in life, the gynecologist will often leave the ovaries and remove only the uterus. The presence of the ovaries helps secure hormone levels in the bloodstream, at least until true menopause takes place. Medical science has discovered that women who lose their ovaries early in life are more likely to develop **osteoporosis**, a weakening of the bones associated with aging that is predominant in women. Many women have **hormone replacement therapy (HRT)** after menopause or after a hysterectomy. Use of synthetic estrogen and progesterone, taken in the sequence of the normal menstrual cycle hormone secretions, helps prevent many of the symptoms associated with menopause. It, of course, will not make women ovulate again. Estrogen is believed to have a positive effect on lessening the chances of osteoporosis development, a decreased chance of cardiac problems, and may help prevent rheumatoid arthritis.

SKIN CONDITIONS ASSOCIATED WITH MENOPAUSE

In the next two decades 40 million women will go through menopause. Esthetically, a woman may have any number of symptoms associated with perimenopause. This may include thinning hair, excess hair growth on the face or other body areas, or even increased oiliness or dryness of the skin.

Recent research indicates that the presence of estrogen has a strong influence on collagen formation. As menopause occurs, estrogen levels drop dramatically, and may have an obvious effect on the appearance of wrinkles and lack of elasticity. Use of hormone replacement therapy (HRT) may improve and reduce the loss of collagen, therefore causing skin to regain more of its previous elasticity and suppleness.

Lack of estrogen may significantly affect barrier function, increasing sensitivity of the skin, dehydration, possible hyperpigmentation, and fluctuations in blood flow. Estrogen is responsible for sending many hormonal messages to the skin, and a decrease can affect many functions of the skin, and therefore, its appearance.

Many aging problems associated with menopause may actually be the result of cumulative sun exposure earlier in life. It is coincidental that the damage of years of sun exposure happen to surface about the same time as menopause in some women. Having both sun damage and menopausal effects on the skin can cause real esthetic problems, and is even more reason why your client needs lots of care at this important time.

Hot Flashes and Flushing

Hot flashes are caused by a fluctuation in blood flow resulting from decreased estrogen, which normally helps with smooth blood flow. Without estrogen, there are sudden "spurts" in blood flow, resulting in redness and the feeling of heat in the skin. Flushing and hot flashes can be reduced or eliminated with hormone replacement therapy.

Rarely, women experience a condition called **formication**, which feel like continuous tingling and itching. Some women have described it as feeling like "bugs crawling on the skin." Again, this can be treated with HRT.

Formication is an itching and tingling feeling of the skin experienced by some women during menopause.

Use of nonfragranced creams with lipid replacement ingredients such as sphingolipids or ceramides may help with dryness and itching. The skin may be more sensitive to any stimulating product, so be careful with these, especially stimulating aromatherapy products.

Moodiness

Women may experience moodiness during menopause. Although some of this may be caused by hormonal fluctuations, it may also be stress related or may be complicated by depression. It is important that you are understanding of the needs of your menopausal client and offer stress-reducing services such as massages or aromatherapy.

Perimenopausal Acne

Clients may experience a sudden flare of acne during or just after menopause. This is again caused by a decrease of estrogen in the bloodstream, which, in turn, increases the percentage of the male hormone androgen that turns on the sebaceous glands. This results in increased oiliness, hirsutism, and acne lesions. You should treat this as you would any other acne case, but remember that the client may more readily experience dehydration and be concerned about aging skin. Be careful not to overdry the skin.

Esthetic Management of Menopausal Skin

The esthetician can play a significant role in helping the menopausal client with skin problems. The esthetician may actually notice small symptoms in the skin before the client is even fully aware that she is beginning menopause.

Keep a client's age in mind when noticing some of the symptoms we have discussed here. Adjusting a client's home care and treatment schedule may help a great deal.

For clients experiencing aging symptoms, recommend lipid-based creams, which can help improve barrier function. Soothing antioxidants can help reduce redness and discomfort. Alphahydroxy acids may also relieve various symptoms. More frequent salon treatments may help esthetic symptoms as well as help with stress management.

Menopausal Skin Symptoms

1. Dryness and itchy skin on the face and body
2. Increased sensitivity
3. Sudden flares of acne
4. Sudden hair growth on the face
5. Mood swings
6. Client complains of "suddenly aging" skin
7. Hot flashes and flushing
8. A "tired" look to the skin, with increased elastosis

ABOUT HIRSUTISM

Hirsutism refers to excessive hair growth.

Hirsutism refers to excessive hair growth. Women who have hormonal fluctuations may experience hirsutism. Excess hair growth, primarily on the face, may happen at any time in a woman's life, but especially after menopause. The dominance of the androgenic hormones after menopause is the main cause.

Hirsutism may be treated by waxing or electrolysis in the salon. Excessive facial hair growth is often best treated by electrolysis because the electrolysis is eventually permanent. Waxing may provide temporary relief in minor cases. Stiffer hairs in the chin and lip areas are best treated by electrolysis. Estheticians and electrologists should be aware of other symptoms that may require referral to a physician. Although most excessive hair is mainly a cosmetic nuisance, accompanying symptoms such as thinning of the hair, deepening of the voice, and loss of menstruation should be referred to a gynecologist.

OBESITY, ANOREXIA, AND HORMONES

Women who are extremely obese may experience a loss of hormone activity, resulting in menstrual irregularity, hirsutism, and acne. Women who are anorexic may have hormonal fluctuations and irregular menstrual cycles.

Women athletes who have a very low body fat percentage may also experience similar hormonal problems. Many estheticians have observed a correlation in avid female athletes between low body fat, hirsutism, and acne.

OTHER HORMONAL DISORDERS THAT AFFECT THE SKIN

Although it is not the esthetician's job to diagnose illness, you should be aware of some symptoms that you may connect with certain skin problems or be able to discuss a client's skin symptoms related to an endocrine illness. You should always refer suspicious skin problems to a physician. If you have a client who has multiple symptoms of any kind of illness, always refer the client to a doctor.

Hyperthyroidism is a condition in which the thyroid gland secretes too much thyroid hormone. Physical symptoms may include heart palpitations, weight loss, and fatigue. Esthetic symptoms include thinning of the skin, hair loss, and rapidly growing nails. **Hypothyroidism** is just the opposite of hyperthyroidism. The thyroid gland does not produce enough hormone. Puffy eyelids, facial swelling, and coarse skin that is very dehydrated are esthetic symptoms of hypothyroidism, if they are also associated with weight gain, poor balance, or hearing problems.

Adrenal gland disorders can also result in skin symptoms. Cushing's syndrome is a disease of the adrenal glands. Persons with Cushing's syndrome secrete too much hydrocortisone. Too much medicinal hydrocortisone can also cause the disease. Symptoms are thinning of the skin and bruises that occur easily. Addison's disease is the exact opposite of Cushing's syndrome. The adrenal glands do not produce adrenal hormones. Skin symptoms include severe hyperpigmentation on the face, dark freckles on the torso, as well as hyperpigmentation on the palms of the hands. Addison's disease is easily treated with hormone therapy.

Hyperthyroidism is a condition in which the thyroid gland secretes too much thyroid hormone.

Hypothyroidism is a condition in which the thyroid gland secretes too little thyroid hormone.

Topics for Discussion

1. What are the major endocrine glands?
2. What is puberty, and what hormonal changes take place with puberty?
3. What precautions should the esthetician take when treating a pregnant woman?
4. What are some esthetic side effects of birth control pills?
5. What are some esthetic problems associated with menopause?
6. Name several endocrine disorders and discuss their effects on the skin.

Chapter

6

Sensitive Skin, Rosacea, and Allergies

Objectives

Although allergic reactions are the domain of the dermatologist and the allergist, it is important that estheticians be very familiar with allergic reactions, sensitive skin, and cosmetic ingredient allergens. This chapter will inform you about sensitive, allergy-prone skin and rosacea. It will discuss ingredients that frequently cause allergic reactions and irritate sensitive skin. The esthetician will learn how to handle allergic reactions and how to help pinpoint ingredient allergens.

SENSITIVE SKIN

Sensitive skin is very thin, fragile-looking, pink-colored skin. People with red hair, or of Celtic or Irish, Scottish, or British descent are more likely to have sensitive skin than other ethnic groups. Because of the sensitive skin's thinness, the blood vessels and nerve endings are much closer to the surface of the skin. This is why this type of skin reddens so easily, but it is also why it becomes irritated by cosmetics more easily.

Sensitive skin is often obvious on examination. It is most often Fitzpatrick Type I, which always burns when exposed to the sun. It is often thin in appearance, bruises easily, and blanches, or turns white, easily when touched. **Blanching** is caused by pressing on the thin skin, which actually pushes the blood away from the surface tissues, thus causing a temporary white appearance. Clients with sensitive skin often report frequent irritations during their preliminary visit with the esthetician, including histories of **urticaria** (hives), allergic reactions, **pruritus** (itching), and **erythema** (redness). It is important to ask new clients if they have histories of allergies or irritant reactions to cosmetics, skin-care products and other topicals, drugs, and foods. Some clients may have already had dermatological testing to isolate allergens.

Sensitive skin will often react to internal factors such as eating spicy foods, stimulants such as caffeine or tobacco (nicotine), or niacin (vitamin B_3). These substances are called **vasodilators**. Vasodilators dilate the blood vessels, making more blood flow through the arterial systems. This dilation often shows up on the skin of a sensitive-skinned person as red, blotchy patches. They may be isolated on the face, may appear in other localized areas, or may be all over the body. Some clients may tell you that their skin gets red after drinking wine or eating Mexican food. Although this may be an allergy, it could also be a sign of sensitive skin or a symptom of rosacea.

Sensitive-skinned clients and clients with rosacea should be told to avoid spicy foods, alcohol, tobacco products, and any other stimulating foods or consumables. Hot water and any extremes in temperature should be avoided. Aerobic exercise should be done indoors in air-conditioning for these individuals. Heat, both body and infrared (sun), can cause sensitive reactions in this skin type. Long-term exposure of sensitive skin to heat, sun, stimulants mentioned previously, saunas, steam baths, or any irritating or hot environmental conditions can cause telangiectasias, or dilated capillaries, referred to by European estheticians as couperose.

Sensitive skin is becoming more and more common. Many people have "perceived sensitive skin," which means they believe their skin is sensitive. It is important to understand as much as possible about sensitive skin and know that all reactions are not fully understood by medical science.

Symptoms and Sensitive and Allergy-Prone Skin

As we discussed earlier, redness and pinkness are typical of sensitive skin. You will usually observe this, along with skin thinness, telangiectasias, and blotchiness, during routine analysis.

Skin may be **dermatographic**, which literally means "skin writing." Dermatographic skin turns red and can swell at the slightest touch or scrape. These clients can get very red just from having their makeup removed, and also get very red and some-

Blanching refers to the skin turning white when touched firmly with the fingers.

Urticaria, or hives, is due to allergies.

Pruritus is the technical term for itching.

Erythema refers to any area of redness associated with a lesion.

Vasodilators dilate the blood vessels, making more blood flow through the arterial system.

Dermatographic literally means "skin writing." Skin turns red and swells at the slightest scrape.

times swollen from extraction, waxing, hardening masks, and other physical or mechanical treatment such as microdermabrasion. Mechanical and physical treatment should be avoided on this skin type.

Subclinical symptoms are **subjective symptoms**, which means they cannot be seen through normal observation. These include chronic itching, burning, stinging, tingling, or other pains, without physical observable **objective symptoms** such as erythema, swelling, urticaria, or xerosis (dryness). Most scientists now believe that chronic subjective symptoms may be neurological in nature, which means that the nerves and nervous system are involved. Subclinical symptoms are more apparent in clients with sensitive skin or skin that has decreased barrier function, such as windburned skin or skin that has been chemically irritated.

Other symptoms may be observed during a reaction. Some of these symptoms are:

- Rash—a splotchy, red, usually flat area, sometimes associated with itching. The area is seldom raised.
- Wheal (also called a welt)—a raised red lesion associated with sensitivity or allergy.
- Hives—a group of wheals with surrounding redness. They often itch or sting. Hives are caused by the release of a hormone-like chemical called **histamine**. Hives are medically known as *urticaria.*
- **Antihistamines** are drugs that are produced to combat the formation of histamines. Nasal allergies are often treated with antihistamines, but skin reactions can also be treated with the same drugs.

Allergies can affect any area of the body, but the skin is probably the most susceptible to being affected by an allergy. An **allergy** is, clinically, the body's immune system rejection of a particular substance. The immune system, for some reason, sees a particular substance (or cosmetic ingredient) as a foreign invader. It reacts by sending out T cells to fight off the **allergen**, the offending substance. This immune response is what causes redness and irritation associated with an allergic reaction on the skin. This is the definition of a true allergy. However, a number of similar types of irritation reactions can occur that do involve the immune system, yet are not "true allergies."

When a person develops a routine allergic response to a substance, the person has become **sensitized** to that substance. The substance or product is known as a **sensitizer**. The immune system has identified this particular substance as a foreign substance. **Sensitization** to a particular product or ingredient may take place after one or many exposures or uses of that product or ingredient. This can even take place after *years* of using a product!

Generalized redness, also called **dermatitis**, which just means inflammation of the skin, may be seen in isolated or general areas.

Sensitive skin is almost always more likely to develop reactions and allergies to cosmetics. Many reactions to cosmetics on sensitive skin may not actually be true allergies. Irritations develop much more easily on sensitive skin.

Avoid any stimulating treatments such as scrubbing granules, products with large amounts of alcohol, extremely fragrant products, and stimulating masks.

Subclinical symptoms, such as stinging or tingling, have no visible appearance.

Subjective symptoms include itching or burning.

Objective symptoms, such as redness or swelling, are physically observable.

Histamine is a hormone-like chemical released during allergic reactions.

Antihistamines are drugs that are produced to combat the formation of histamines.

Allergy is the body's immune system rejection of a particular substance.

Allergen is a substance that provokes an allergic reaction.

Sensitized is having developed an allergic reaction to a substance.

Sensitizer is the substance or product a person has developed an allergic reaction to.

Sensitization refers to the process of becoming allergic to a substance and the establishment of antibodies that will always react to exposure to that substance.

Dermatitis means inflammation of the skin.

Sensitive Skin and Barrier Function

It is extremely important to protect the barrier function of the sensitive skin, which, in general, does not have a natural barrier function that is as effective as that of normal, nonsensitive skin. Decreased barrier function results in a more permeable epidermis, and irritants are more likely to cause irritations because it is easier for them to penetrate the skin surface, where they come in contact with poorly protected nerve endings. Decreased barrier function also results in **transepidermal water loss**, also known as **TEWL**, causing severe dehydration and inflammation. If skin is already irritated because of a diminished barrier function, it is much more likely to react to skin care products and cosmetics.

Transepidermal water loss (TEWL) is the evaporation of excess intercellular water.

Avoid prolonged exposure to detergents and surfactants, including desincrustation products, which should be used for shorter periods of time, and only if necessary. Surfactants and emulsifiers are used in products to keep oil-in-water solutions mixed, and as foaming cleansing agents. Unfortunately, these agents can also work on the lipids within the lipid barrier, further damaging barrier function in sensitive skin. State-of-the-art sensitive skin products are now being produced with special nonemulsifier blending agents that significantly reduce damage to the barrier function. Some of these products are emulsions that are produced using special high-pressure manufacturing techniques. The products are **physically** blended using a process called **physical emulsification**, rather than using traditional **chemical emulsifiers**, which have been known to cause irritation to sensitive skin. Inclusion of special barrier-protective ingredients, such as lipids or silicones, help protect the barrier from contact with emulsifying agents.

Physical emulsification is the process in which lotions and topical preparation are blended using physical agents to keep the preparation properly mixed.

Chemical emulsifiers are agents that cause an even blending of water and oil in a lotion or cream.

Be very careful with enzymes, "roll-off" peels, alphahydroxy acid exfoliating treatments, and microdermabrasion. All of these treatments have the potential of lessening barrier function, especially on sensitive skin.

Although a reaction may or may not be immediately detectable, a skin with lessened barrier function is more likely to react to other substances applied later. Be very careful not to overexfoliate or strip this type of skin.

The Inflammation Cascade

The **inflammation cascade** is a series of chemical reactions that occurs when the skin is irritated. When a cell is irritated, it releases special chemicals called **inflammatory mediators**, which alert the immune system to the irritation. The immune system then sends leukocytes, or white blood cells, to the site of irritation, and the leukocytes release another special chemical called a **cytokine**. The cytokine signals cells to produce "self-destruct" enzymes, which are chemicals that break down substances in the skin. These enzymes break down collagen, elastin, and hyaluronic acid, which are responsible for the smoothness, firmness, and moisture content of the skin.

Inflammation cascade is a series of chemical reactions that occurs when the skin is irritated.

Inflammatory mediators are chemicals released by irritated cells that alert the immune system to the irritation.

Cytokine is a chemical released by cells that signal other chemical immune responses.

Chronic skin irritation has a cumulative effect on skin aging and deterioration due to the irritation cascade of reactions. Therefore, it is extremely important to avoid chronically irritating the skin, whether from sun exposure or constant stripping from harsh chemicals.

Treatment Concepts of Sensitive Skin

There are three basic concepts that are widely accepted in treating sensitive skin:

1. Be very careful with the barrier function of the skin. Use products that support the barrier function, and avoid any product that might strip or impair it, including strong soaps.
2. Avoid known irritating and sensitizing material and products. This includes fragrances, certain preservatives, many "natural" ingredients (many of which have little irritancy research data), stimulating products, or products that can injure the barrier function such as strong surfactants and emulsifiers. Use products that have been shown through independent testing to have low irritancy potential. Also avoid any ingredient to which the client has had a previous allergic or irritant reaction.
3. Certain ingredients added to skin-care products for sensitive skin have been shown to decrease sensitivity. These include **chamomile extract**, **cornflower extract**, **licorice extract**, **bisabolol**, **stearyl glycyrrhetinate**, **dipotassium glycyrrhizinate**, and **azulene**, also known as **matricaria extract**. Also, the inclusion of ingredients that protect or enhance the barrier function such as lipid complexes are helpful in a sensitive skin product.

ROSACEA

In earlier editions of this book, rosacea was listed in the chapter on acne. It is now believed that rosacea is more of a problem with blood vessels and flushing of the skin than it is a true form of acne.

Rosacea is a condition of the skin in which the skin turns red very easily, known as **flushing**. This can result in eventual distended capillaries called **telangiectasias**, also known by the European term **couperose**. Originally referred to as acne rosacea or adult acne, rosacea is now the preferred name. Even though rosacea causes acne-like pimples and pustules, the actual disorder is **vascular**, or blood vessel–related (Plates 6a1, 6a2, 6a3).

Rosacea normally affects persons above 30 years of age, but can appear as early as 20 or as late as 70 or 80 years old. The sudden rushing of the blood to the face can stimulate sebaceous glands and irritate follicles, causing large red papules and pustules to form in the cheek, nose, and chin areas. When pimples and redness occur in a person who has rosacea, this is known as a **flare** of rosacea (Plate 6f). Rosacea is most prominent in light-skinned persons of Irish, Celtic, or western European origin.

Rosacea may first appear as chronically red cheeks, or a chronically red nose. A client may notice reddening of the face when drinking wine or alcohol or eating spicy foods. Clients with rosacea are more likely to redden when they are hot. Anything that causes increased blood flow to the face, or **vasodilation**, can cause a flare of rosacea (Plates 6b, 6c).

Causes of Rosacea

No one is completely sure of the exact cause of rosacea, but it appears to be hereditary and strongly related to how easily a person blushes. It is very evident that constant

---

Chamomile extract is a soothing agent.

Cornflower extract is a soothing agent.

Licorice extract is a soothing agent.

Bisabolol is an agent that is added to cosmetics designed for sensitive skin.

Stearyl glycyrrhetinate is a soothing agent derived from licorice extract.

Dipotassium glycyrrhizinate is a soothing agent derived from licorice extract.

Azulene is a hydrocarbon that is derived from the chamomile flower.

Matricaria extract is a soothing agent.

Rosacea is a condition of the skin in which the skin turns red very easily.

Flushing refers to the reddening of the skin due to stimulation.

Telangiectasias are small, red enlarged capillaries of the face and other areas of the body.

Couperose are small, red enlarged capillaries of the face and other areas of the body.

Vascular means blood vessel related.

Flare is when pimples and redness occur in a person who has rosacea.

Vasodilation is the dilation of the blood vessels resulting in flushing.

flushing of the skin makes rosacea worse and is responsible for flares. Although often treated with antibiotics, it is not clear whether bacteria or yeast are a direct cause of rosacea. Antibiotics help rosacea by controlling inflammation.

Analysis of Rosacea

When analyzing rosacea, you may notice the following symptoms:

1. Diffuse redness and distended capillaries, especially in the cheeks or nose, but sometimes also in the chin and forehead. Rosacea very rarely affects the perimeter of the face or the neck.
2. Patches of redness in the cheek area, often accompanied by enlarged pore appearance.
3. Enlarged appearance of the nose, bulbous structure, redness, with very prominent pore appearance of the nose, sometimes appearing rough and bumpy.
4. Client may report turning red very easily or redness after ingesting wine, other alcoholic beverages, or spicy foods.
5. Flares of large, red, solid-appearing, or "lumpy"-looking papules and pustules in the cheeks, nose, and chin.
6. Flares occurring after exercising, which causes heat and increased blood flow to the face.
7. Very dehydrated, sometimes flaking, red areas in the nose and cheeks. The skin may appear thick or swollen in these areas.

Rhinophyma

Severe cases of rosacea can result in a condition called **rhinophyma**, a swelling and enlarging of the nose. The comedian W. C. Fields suffered from rosacea and rhinophyma, which is why he had the famous large, red nose. Many people erroneously think that Fields' nose was caused by alcoholism. Alcohol consumption does not cause rosacea, but it certainly can cause redness and flares (Plates 6d, 6e).

Rhinophyma is an enlarging of the nose often resulting from a severe form of acne rosacea.

In severe cases of rhinophyma, plastic surgery may be necessary to reduce the tissue in the nose (Plates 7, 8).

Treatment of Rosacea

No cure is known for rosacea, but it can be managed and kept under control. Both the dermatologist and the esthetician should be involved.

Medical treatment usually involves oral antibiotics, such as tetracycline for severe flares, and routine daily application of an anti-yeast prescription medication known as **metronidazole**, commercially known as MetroGel®, MetroCream®, or Noritate®. Regular use of these topical drugs substantially reduces flares.

Metronidazole is a medication used to control rosacea and decrease inflammation.

The esthetician plays an important role as well by helping the client choose products that will not cause stimulated blood flow, will treat the skin very gently, are noncomedogenic or nonacnegenic, and that have been properly tested and documented to prevent clogged pores or follicle irritation. Teaching the client lifestyle management to avoid rosacea flares is also part of the esthetician's responsibilities (Plates 6g1, 6g2).

Many rosacea patients experience acne-like papules and pustules, and many have chronically oily areas. It is best to stick to noncomedogenic (nonclogging) products, because products containing too much emollient may contribute to breakouts. Manage oily areas with mild, yet effective, rinseable cleansers, being careful not to overstep with aggressive cleansers, which can cause irritation. Nonalcoholic, nonspicy toners are best.

Alphahydroxy acids work well on most patients with rosacea as long as they are not overused, and do not have a pH lower than 3.5. Any overly acidic product can cause irritation.

Sunscreens are a must, even though patients with rosacea should carefully avoid sun exposure because of infrared heat.

The skin of patients with rosacea often becomes dehydrated, especially if it is irritated. Stick to lightweight, nonfragranced hydrating lotions.

Management of Rosacea

1. Sun exposure is the worst culprit in causing rosacea flares. Sun must be avoided at all times. Besides ultraviolet rays, sun also radiates infrared heat, a known cause of flares.
2. Clients should wear broad-spectrum sunscreen on a daily basis. Of course, this is important for any skin, but extremely important for clients with rosacea.
3. Avoid heat as much as possible. Any sudden blood flushing of the face can cause a flare. Be careful in hot kitchens, and when opening hot ovens or dishwashers. Allow hot cars to air out before getting in.
4. Avoid saunas and steambaths.
5. Hot water should be avoided on the face. Extremely cold water can also aggravate rosacea.
6. Clients should avoid spicy foods, wine (especially red wine), and other alcoholic beverages. These all cause vasodilation, as can caffeine and hot beverages.
7. Nicotine affects blood flow and should be avoided.
8. Heat from exercise is known to cause flares. Suggest that the client try to exercise indoors in air-conditioning to avoid overheating the face. The ideal situation is to swim in a cool pool, although chlorine is also a possible aggravating factor and the skin should be rinsed thoroughly after swimming.
9. Products used on any clients with sensitive skin or rosacea should be independently tested for irritancy.
10. It is best to avoid products with fragrance because fragrances can often cause reactions.

Treatment Contraindications for Clients with Sensitive Skin and Rosacea

It is advisable to avoid the following procedures on clients with sensitive skin or rosacea:

1. Any heat exposure, including prolonged steaming. Use cool steam from the ultrasonic vaporizer or keep the steamer a minimum of 18 inches from the face.

2. Avoid paraffin or electric heat masks.
3. Prolonged or vigorous massage, such a petrissage, may be too stimulating.
4. Avoid overdrying masks or leaving clay masks on too long.
5. Many essential oils or aromatherapy products may be too stimulating for sensitive-skinned clients.
6. Extraction must be gentle and limited to a brief period to avoid redness.
7. Heavily mentholated or alcohol-based treatments should be avoided.

Treating Sensitive Skin

When treating sensitive skin, a few basic rules should be followed:

1. First and foremost, keep the treatment very simple! Do not overcomplicate by trying a large number of techniques. "The simpler, the better" is the rule of thumb when treating sensitive skin. If the client reddens during a simple treatment, it will be much easier to isolate the particular treatment technique that may have caused the irritation.
2. Use unfragranced products. Fragrances, including some essential oils, may aggravate sensitive skin.
3. Keep heat to a minimum. Prolonged steam, heat masks, and paraffin treatments should be avoided completely. Extremely cold compresses should also be avoided.
4. Massage should be very gentle. Use only effleurage, shiatsu, or gentle tapotement. Petrissage should be completely avoided, as should any rapid or deep manipulation.
5. Extraction should be very gentle, at least until you know how sensitive your client is.
6. Avoid enzyme treatments, chemical or mechanical peelings, or scrubs. For home care, follow the same recommendations for allergy-prone skin found later in this chapter.
7. Avoid SD or isopropyl alcohol–containing products on sensitive skin.
8. Be careful with essential oils because these can often overstimulate or cause reactions in sensitive skin.

Suggested Treatment for Sensitive Skin

1. Gently cleanse the skin using a cleansing milk with little or no fragrance or use a rinseable cleanser, preferably a product designed for sensitive skin. Follow with nonalcohol, low- or nonfragranced toner. The toner should be extremely gentle and nonstimulating.
2. Warm steamers should be used at a distance of 18 to 20 inches for very brief periods of time on sensitive skin. You can increase this time slowly in future treatments as you gain a better understanding of the client's sensitivities. Cool steamers that use ultrasonic vibration to create vapor without heat are now available. These machines are very helpful in treating sensitive skin, because they hydrate without exposing the skin to heat. They can be used for normal periods of time without causing irritation. Applying a lightweight hydrating fluid before steam may help cut possible irritation from steam. Hydrating fluid must also be nonstimulating and fragrance-free.

3. You may use galvanic desincrustation at a very low setting (0.2 mA) for a very short period of time. Desincrustation should be limited to clogged or acne-flared areas, and should only be performed for about two to three minutes. Again, this can be slowly increased as you progress through the weeks with the client. Dry skin should not have galvanic desincrustation treatment.

4. Brushing and vacuuming should be completely avoided on sensitive skin. Both of these procedures are very stimulating.

5. Proceed with gentle extraction, using the cotton swab technique described in Chapter 14. Avoid using a comedone extractor on sensitive skin. If the skin begins to welt, redden severely, or swell, stop extraction immediately. Extraction on sensitive clients should be limited to about three to four minutes, particularly during the first visit.

6. Spray the skin with a mild, nonalcoholic toner.

7. If the skin is very red after extraction, allow the skin to calm down before proceeding with more techniques. Allow the skin a 5- to 10-minute cool-down period after extraction. Apply a soothing gel of green tea extract, antioxidants, licorice extract, chamomile, or dipotassium glycyrrhizinate. Apply cool cotton compresses over the gel. Cool (not cold) wet cotton compresses may be helpful in reducing redness and sensitivity.

8. After the skin has sufficiently "cooled down" and is not swollen or severely red, apply a light, nonfragranced hydrating fluid and gently massage for a short period of time. Remember to use only gentle manipulations. If redness develops or increases, discontinue massage immediately. Massage should be limited to three to four minutes on the first visit.

9. Apply high frequency at its lowest setting for one to two minutes. Ionization may be used instead for one to two minutes, again at a low setting (0.2 mA). A cool compress mask or cool "globes" may be used as another alternative. Remember, any treatment should be cool, not cold!

10. Apply a non-setting gel or cream mask. Setting, drying masks should be completely avoided. If you prefer you may use more lightweight, nonstimulating fragrance-free hydrating fluid instead of a mask.

11. Allow the mask to sit for 10 to 15 minutes. Check frequently with the client to make sure it is not burning or irritating.

12. Remove the mask by spraying with a toner solution, then remove the treatment with a wet, cool, cotton pad or a cool, soft cloth.

13. Allow about three minutes before applying protectant or day cream.

It is highly advisable for sensitive clients not to wear makeup immediately after a facial treatment. A waiting period of two hours is recommended before makeup is applied.

IRRITATIONS

Irritations are inflammations of the skin that are caused by outside sources. Irritations may be caused from scrubbing the skin too hard, shaving, or certain exfoliating cosmetics or drugs.

Mechanical irritations are caused by things continually rubbing against the skin. They, too, can cause skin reactions such as urticaria. Clothing, bras, belts that are too tight, helmets, chin straps, eyeglasses, and even playing the violin can cause skin reactions and dermatitis.

Exfoliants, including scrubs and roll-off type peeling treatments, are examples of possible mechanical irritants. These should be avoided on sensitive skin.

Exfoliating or keratolytic agents such as resorcinol, salicylic acid, glycolic acid, phenol, lactic acid, retinoic acid, and benzoyl peroxide are examples of chemical exfoliants that may be irritating. The reaction they cause is an irritation due to the way the chemicals work on the skin, but it is not a true allergic reaction.

Although allergic reactions can happen while using all of the above-mentioned chemical agents, they actually exfoliate by irritating the skin. Clients may experience slight redness from these agents, particularly when they first start using them. Clients may panic because they are slightly red or peeling. The best way to keep clients from panicking is to educate them about the possible side effects of the treatment. Explain that peeling and slight redness may be a side reaction to the use of these products, but hives, rashes, and excessive itching and burning are not normal. If clients experience these more severe symptoms, they should discontinue use of the product.

ANALYSIS AND CONSULTATION WITH THE SENSITIVE AND ALLERGY-PRONE CLIENT

Very sensitive skin will begin turning red even with a mild cleansing with sponges. Redness during the very beginning of treatment is a sure-fire symptom of sensitive skin. Sensitive skin will blanch easily, or temporarily turn white when gently pressed with the esthetician's fingers. This indicates that blood vessels are close to the surface, or may indicate vasodilation. The whiting effect is caused by gently pressing the blood out of the way with the fingers.

One of the best ways to find out if your client has sensitive skin is to check her skin history and possible reactivity. Clients with sensitive skin will almost always volunteer information, because they are aware of the discomfort associated with reactions, and wish to avoid any possibility of reoccurrence. It is important to listen carefully to your clients' histories. Even if they do not know the exact cause of their sensitivities, they may be able to give you clues about what to avoid using, or what might be appropriate treatment.

Clients who have sensitive or allergy-prone skin tend to be cosmetically "gun-shy." Often the new client will have had an unpleasant reaction to a cosmetic years ago and assumes that all cosmetics are bad. The blame is placed on the cosmetic, when it is almost always the person's immune system that is the problem.

There are two ways to help calm the client's concerns. First, you must know what you're doing with allergy-prone skin, and second, you must convince the client that you know what you're doing!

It is important to be honest with the client. Promise to do your best to help the client find usable products. Try to discuss past problems. Ask the client to be specific about what products caused problems in the past. Often you will find that the client experienced an irritation reaction rather than an allergic reaction. The client may have peeled from benzoyl peroxide or retinoic acid, and assumed it was an allergic reaction, when it actually was a normal reaction.

On the other hand the client may have had an actual allergic reaction. Get a description of the symptoms. Minor redness and peeling is usually just an irritation. Hives, rash, wheals, swelling, and itching are usually symptoms of an allergy (Plate 9). Another common misconception that many clients have is confusing an allergic reaction with acne. They might say, "I tried this brand of moisturizer, but I was allergic." Upon further investigation, often you will find it was an acnegenic reaction to a product rather than an allergic reaction. It is important to tactfully explain the difference. If the client has a tendency to develop acne, the problem may have been **comedogenic** products. After reading Chapter 12, Acne and the Esthetician, and 13, Comedogenicity, you'll be able to help with that too.

Comedogenic is the tendency of a topical substance to cause a buildup of dead cells resulting in the development of comedones.

COMMON COSMETIC ALLERGIES

Allergic reactions to cosmetics are in a category of allergies known to dermatologists as **contact dermatitis**, which simply means that when an allergic person comes in contact with a particular substance, a reaction occurs. Not all contact dermatoses are cosmetic, but cosmetics often do cause allergic reactions. It is important that we be aware of the cosmetic ingredients that are most likely to cause allergic reactions (Plate 10).

Contact dermatitis is an irritation caused by either an allergic reaction or irritation to something or some substance touching the skin or coming in contact with the skin's surface.

Hypoallergenic cosmetics are cosmetics that have generally been manufactured without the use of certain ingredients that are known to frequently cause allergic reactions.

Hypoallergenic cosmetics are cosmetics that have had removed from them many well-known allergens. These ingredients have a history of causing allergic reactions in many people. Hypoallergenic does not mean nonallergenic. There is no such thing as a nonallergenic cosmetic! Somewhere in the world there is a person who is allergic to every cosmetic ingredient! More and more companies now claim that the products are designed for sensitive skin. Unfortunately, no one really governs this claim. Skin-care and cosmetic products intended for sensitive skin should be tested by an independent dermatological laboratory for potential irritancy. Obviously, fragrances, color dyes, and other known aggravating ingredients should be avoided.

TESTING FOR IRRITATION

There are several different types of irritancy testing:

1. Primary Irritation Testing, also known as a 48-hour patch test, involves the simple procedure of applying a small amount of the product (or ingredient) to be tested to the back skin of test participants, occluding it with a bandage (hence the term patch testing), and checking the area for irritation 48 hours later. This is a very simple, basic, inexpensive test, and should be administered and interpreted by a board-certified dermatologist. This test, to be truly reflective of irritation potential, should be run on at least 50 human backs. The more people tested, the more reliable the results of the test.

2. A Repeated Insult Patch Test (RIPT) is similar to the primary irritation test, but considered by physicians and scientists to be much more reliable and indicative of potential sensitivities or allergies. The human patch area is tested over and over again on the same participants. Breaks of a few days are taken between test applications. These breaks allow the body time to develop antibodies to any material being tested. repeat testing will likely reveal any delayed allergy or material that has caused sensitivity. Again, to be reliable and be considered scientifically sound, this test should be run on 50 to 200 participants.

3. Tape-Strip Irritation Testing is a relatively new test in which the skin is purposely irritated by repeatedly pulling tape off the area to be tested. Once the skin is irritated, the test product is applied and observations are made. Irritating materials should make the area more inflamed.

4. Sensitive Skin Actual-Use Testing involves using participants who are known to have sensitive skin. These individuals actually use the test product for several weeks, and the results are observed at the end of the time allotted. This is a good method of testing, but may involve many variables. This test should be run in addition to one of the more controlled procedures.

Ask your supplier to explain their testing procedures for sensitive skin products.

FRAGRANCES

Many different fragrances, derived from various sources, are used in cosmetics. Some are natural, having been extracted from plants, such as essential oils. Turpenes extracted from trees are another variety. Some musks are derived from animal by-products, and synthetic fragrances are developed.

There is no real advantage in using natural over synthetic fragrance, except perhaps in the actual odor.

Fragrance is the number one cause of cosmetic reactions. It does not matter if the fragrance is natural or synthetic. Frequent fragrance allergens include eugenol, hydroxy-citronellal, cinnamic alcohol, geraniol, and ylang-ylang. Fragrance can contain as many as 600 individual chemicals. Combining these chemicals with vehicles and delivery systems can increase the potential for skin penetration, and, therefore, increase the potential for skin reaction. There are approximately 400 essential oils, which are also fragrances or groups of fragrances. Many essential oils have had very little formal scientific testing, and may present a major problem for sensitive skin.

Another interesting fact is that so-called natural cosmetics that contain a lot of botanical ingredients actually require more preservatives to be added due to the breakdown of the plant ingredients and the presence of fungi on the plant extracts. Many people think of natural ingredients as being less irritating, but they actually can be more irritating due to the presence of so many chemicals in each extract, and the need to use larger quantities of preservative to inhibit growth of unwanted organisms in the product.

Although essential oils are widely used in esthetics, and certainly have their place in facial therapy, they are also capable of producing allergic reactions. Plant extracts of any type are made up of a variety of chemicals, from salicyclic acid to water to glucose. They may also contain very small amounts of insecticide or other contaminants. Remember that earlier in the chapter we discussed keeping sensitive and allergy-prone clients' treatments very simple. Unfortunately, when we add a large number of plant extracts, we add many new chemicals. It is best to stay with known chemicals when dealing with ultrasensitive skin. If the client experiences an allergic reaction, it will be much easier to isolate the responsible ingredient.

It is generally accepted by the medical community that fragrances cause most cosmetic reactions. If you have a client who is allergy-prone, it is always best to stick to fragrance-free products, or at least to use a cosmetic that is scented with only one plant oil.

PRESERVATIVES

The next category of cosmetic allergens is preservatives. Preservatives are necessary in cosmetic, drug, and food products. They keep harmful bacteria from contaminating these products.

Although preservatives must be used in almost all cosmetic and skin-care products, they are, unfortunately, a very frequent allergy producer. There is no strict rule of thumb to determining allergies and sensitivities to preservative ingredients.

The most frequently used preservative complex in the cosmetics industry is the parabens. Methylparaben and propylparaben are used in literally thousands of cosmetic formulations. It has been estimated that 1 percent of the United States' population is allergic to these preservatives.

Imidazolidinyl urea is the next most commonly used preservative. It is often used with methylparaben and propylparaben, because the three agents work well together against a large number of microorganisms.

Many preservatives work by emitting minute quantities of formaldehyde. Unfortunately, formaldehyde is a well-known skin irritant.

Formaldehyde-releasing preservatives include imidazolidinyl urea, diazolidinyl urea, 2-bromo-2-nitropropane-1,3-diol, DMDM hydantoin, and quaternium compounds. These important ingredients do not cause problems for most people, but may be problem ingredients for persons with very sensitive skin or poor barrier function.

The parabens (methyl, propyl, ethyl, butyl, etc.) are the most common preservatives, and are not formaldehyde releasers. Nevertheless, some clients are sensitive to them as well.

Over the last decade or two, some new preservatives have entered the market. Methylchloroisothiazolinone and methylisothiazolinone are a non-formaldehyde-releasing preservative complex, yet are primarily used in rinse-off cleansers because they have a history of some problems on certain sensitive skins when used in leave-on products such as creams or lotions. Phenoxyethanol is another non-formaldehyde-releasing preservative that has recently been coupled with the parabens as an alternative preservative for more sensitive skin formulations. However, there are some people who show sensitivity to this complex also.

Although formaldehyde-releasing preservatives are often the culprits in preservative-related reactions, there are also reactions to non-formaldehyde-releasing preservatives. If you are treating clients who have known preservative allergies, it is best to perform a patch test for all products to be used, and to have a variety of products with different preservative systems on hand. For more information on preservatives, see Chapter 8, Cosmetic Chemistry and Functional Ingredients.

COLOR AGENTS

Color agents are another source of allergies. Color agent allergies are often associated with lipstick and eyeshadow allergies. Lipstick allergy is characterized by swollen, peeling lips after using a particular lipstick. Eyeshadow allergy shows up as red, flaking upper, and sometimes lower, lids. Although it is possible to be allergic to any color agent, many people are allergic to the D & C yellow colors and D & C red colors.

SUNSCREEN ALLERGIES AND SENSITIVITY

Many clients are allergic to sunscreen ingredients. Para-amino benzoic acid, better known as PABA, has caused many allergic reactions. Although PABA is an excellent UV-B sun filter, there seem to be a lot of people allergic to PABA. PABA has "cousin" ingredients such as padimate-O, padimate-A, and amyldimethyl PABA. PABA may be present not only in sunscreens, but also in lipsticks, foundations, day creams, and moisturizers. Many cosmetic manufacturers put sunscreen ingredients in day creams routinely. Many do not make a sunscreen claim for the product, but it is nevertheless present in the product.

Salicylates

Many people are also allergic to the salicylates, a group of chemicals related to salicylic acid. Salicylic acid in its oral form is aspirin. Be careful to screen products carefully if your client tells you she is allergic to aspirin.

Salicylic acid is used frequently for treating acne and clogged pores. It is an excellent gentle exfoliant for these skin types. However, it should not be used on clients who have aspirin or other salicylate allergies. Octyl salicylate and phenyl salicylate are excellent sunscreens and may be used in conjunction with other screens in a sunscreen product or day cream.

Other Sunscreens

The two most popular sunscreens at the time of this writing are methoxycinnimate and benzophenone. These two chemicals are often used in combination to screen a wider range of ultraviolet rays. There seem to be fewer reactions to these screen agents. However, some people are allergic to these as well.

Two of the least allergy-prone screening ingredients are zinc oxide and titanium dioxide. Zinc oxide is the white cream that surfers use on their noses to prevent sunburn. These sunscreens work by reflecting the sun, rather than absorbing it.

The good thing about these two reflecting, pigment sunscreens is that very few people are allergic to them. The bad side is that they are opaque and do impart some "whiteness," and, particularly in darker skin types, can be seen on the skin. Recently, new micronization technology has made these pigment ingredients much more user friendly. These ingredients are truly excellent sunscreens, because they block large portions of both the Ultraviolet A and B rays. Zinc oxide and titanium dioxide are also often used in foundations because they provide excellent coverage. The sunscreen benefit in these foundations is just an added benefit!

Tips About Using Sunscreens and Allergies

Many clients complain that sunscreens burn their eyes. This occurs when the client gets hot and perspires while wearing the screens. Often the client has applied the sunscreen haphazardly, getting the product too close to the eyes or applying too much at once.

Advise the client to apply the screen about 30 minutes before going out. This will allow the screen to absorb better into the skin and avoid running into the eyes. Using a cream-based screen rather than a gel seems to work better for many of these clients.

Another helpful tip for clients is not to apply sunscreens on hot skin. Many clients will wait until they are already outside to apply sunscreen. Any irritating factor will be more pronounced when applied on skin that is at an elevated temperature. Again, advise the client to apply the screen before going outside.

Gel screens are lighter-weight products and are in general much better for oily, clog-prone, and acne-prone skin types. They are, however, not very waterproof. They often have a base that is an alcohol called SD alcohol, which may irritate some sensitive skins when applied.

NAIL PRODUCTS

Many nail products contain formaldehyde or a formaldehyde derivative. Many people are allergic to nail products. Nail polish, hardeners, conditioners, top and base coats, as well as other nail chemicals, often contain these allergens.

Eyelid irritations are often caused by nail products because people rub or touch thin, delicate eyelids with painted or treated nails.

ACNE PRODUCTS AND ALLERGIES

Because many acne products are also exfoliants or peeling agents, two factors must be considered to help allergy-prone or sensitive skin. Irritation caused by acne products is often necessary for the product to work. Slight redness, minor irritation, and flaking, peeling skin is a fairly normal occurrence when using peeling agents to treat acne and oily skin.

This built-in irritant can be a problem for ultrasensitive skin. You may find that your client cannot tolerate every-night use of a particular acne product. For these clients, recommend that they apply the product every other night. On the alternate night suggest that they use a noncomedogenic, fragrance-free, hydrating agent. Alternating these two products seems to work well for many sensitive oily skins. The theory is that you are peeling one night and hydrating the next. Therefore, you are reducing the amount of irritation and soothing the skin on alternate nights.

Another solution for clients sensitive to acne peeling agents is to have the client use them daily, but only for short periods of time, slowly building up to longer exposure. For example, a sensitive-skinned client may only use benzoyl peroxide for 10 to 15 minutes the first night of treatment. If this short treatment is tolerated successfully, on the next night the client can leave the product on for 30 minutes, and so on. This will slowly build the client's tolerance for the treatment. Your client will learn her tolerance level.

Benzoyl peroxide, an excellent acne treatment, is available in several strengths. The standard strengths are 2½ percent, 5 percent, and 10 percent. Sensitive clients may tolerate low strengths much better than higher ones. Unfortunately, some clients develop allergies to benzoyl peroxide and have to choose another acne treatment.

There are three alternatives for clients who are allergic to benzoyl peroxide. They are glycolic acid, sulfur combined with resorcinol, and salicylic acid.

Salicylic acid has already been discussed. It is generally a milder treatment, but cannot be used by clients with salicylate allergies. It is a good treatment, though, for sensitive clients who are not allergic to salicylates.

Sulfur, which is combined in many treatments with resorcinol, is a standard alternative to benzoyl peroxide and is one of the oldest acne treatments. Unfortunately, again, some clients are also allergic to sulfur or resorcinol, or both.

Glycolic acid is a fairly recent addition to the spectrum of acne treatment products. Glycolic acid seems to cause few allergies; however, it does sting when applied and occasionally causes irritation in sensitive clients. Many clients develop a tolerance for the burning sensation when using glycolic acid regularly.

In general, you need to be very careful when treating oily, sensitive skin. Many clients see better results with slow, nonaggressive treatments. Using gentle, rinseable cleansers, toners, and low-strength peeling agents is almost always a better solution for these clients. Try to avoid using a peeling agent in more than one product for these clients.

OTHER NONCOSMETIC ALLERGIES

Frequently, you will have clients who are allergic to products other than cosmetics, but these allergies will result in cosmetic skin symptoms. Many clients are allergic to nickel, which is frequently used in laundry detergents and jewelry. Dryer sheets or fabric softeners cause problems for some individuals.

Clients with nasal allergies will sometimes have skin reactions related to their nasal allergies. These clients should be referred to an allergist.

Hard water is water that contains a lot of minerals and lime. Hard water can contribute to dry and irritated skin, especially on the body skin, and especially in the cold winter months. If your client lives in an area with hard water, the client may want to consider installing a water softening system that removes minerals. This may be particularly advisable for clients who suffer from atopic eczema.

EYELID DERMATITIS

A frequent problem the esthetician sees is eyelid dermatitis (Plate 11). The eyelid skin is the thinnest skin on the human body and is also the most sensitive to irritants and allergens.

Red, flaky, swollen upper and/or lower lids are the signs of eyelid dermatitis. If a client comes to you complaining of eyelid dermatitis, you need to check the following:

1. Has the client started any new eye treatment, eyeshadow, liner, mascara, false eyelashes, or any other new eye products?
2. Is the client wearing nail polish? If so, is it a new color or brand?
3. Has the client had nail service recently?
4. If *yes* is the answer to question 3, did the nail technician use any new treatment?
5. Does the client have new hand cream?
6. Does the client have a history of nasal allergies?
7. Has the client had an eyebrow waxing recently?
8. Is the client taking any new prescription drugs?
9. Does the client wear contact lenses and therefore use contact lens cleaning solution?
10. Does the client use eyedrops?

All or any of these factors can cause eyelid irritation and dermatitis. If the reaction is severe, the client should be referred to a dermatologist or an allergist.

Besides cosmetic and other products used directly on the eye, nail and hand products seem to cause many of these lid reactions. Suggest that the client remove all nail products until the reaction has cleared. If the reaction clears, the nail products were probably the culprits! Clients experiencing lid irritation should be told to discontinue all treatment to the eye area until the reaction has cleared. If the client must use some product on the area, petrolatum (petroleum jelly) and mineral oil are two of the least allergenic products available. They are very unlikely to cause or worsen allergic reactions.

TREATMENT FOR COSMETIC ALLERGIES AND CONTACT DERMATITIS

Standard treatment for cosmetic allergies is topical hydrocortisone creams. These hormone-based creams relieve the symptoms. Their effect is in some cases almost immediate. Dermatologists prescribe a variety of strengths of chemical steroidal treatments for skin allergies. In more severe cases, an oral steroid or antihistamine may also be used.

Estheticians are not qualified to treat allergic reactions. Always refer the client to a dermatologist. You may, however, help the client and the doctor pinpoint the allergic substance. Help the client trace back her cosmetic rituals over the past several days to see if the client used anything that was new or out of the ordinary routine.

In severe cases of allergy, the dermatologist will test the client for individual cosmetic reactions. These tests are usually done on the client's back or forearm. The doctor paints on various cosmetic ingredients in small patches across the back and covers each with a small bandage. Either 24 or 48 hours later, the doctor removes the bandages and checks the client's "patches" for redness, swelling, urticaria, or other signs of allergy (Plate 12). The dermatologist can often pinpoint the offending allergic ingredient. Once this has been established, you can help the client by checking any present or future use cosmetics for the allergen ingredient.

This is the standard procedure for dermatological testing for cosmetic allergies. Estheticians can perform a patch test for different products on the client as well. If your client has very sensitive or allergy-prone skin, patch test new products on the client's back before trying them on the face. The procedure is simple:

1. Check the client's past allergy history. Does the client have any known ingredient, drug, or cosmetic allergies? If she does, you can eliminate using any cosmetics that have those known allergenic ingredients.
2. Type and analyze the client's skin as you normally would.
3. Select the proper home-care program for the client, taking special precaution to avoid fragranced products as much as possible and avoiding products with long ingredient lists. Also avoid essential oils and other stimulating ingredients.
4. Paint a small amount of each product on the client's back. Each application should be about the size of a nickel. Cover each patch with a bandage and write the coded number of the product being tested. Record the number and the corresponding product on the client record. For example, the test cleanser is #1, the toner is #2, and so on.
5. Instruct the client not to wash her back for the test period.
6. After 48 hours has elapsed, remove the bandages and check each patch for irritation, redness, swelling, itching, urticaria, or flaking. If you see any of these signs, avoid that product.
7. Notice what ingredients are in the offending product and compare the ingredients with the ingredient list of a product to which the client did not react. What do the two lists have in common, or more importantly, what is different about the two lists? For example, if the client reacted to her day cream, which contained a preservative like one of the parabens, but did not react to her night cream, which contained the preservative DMDM hydantoin, you may find that the client is possibly allergic to a paraben.

It takes time and experience to be good at isolating allergic ingredients. An essential knowledge of cosmetic chemistry and ingredients is also essential. If you do not feel comfortable with these procedures, refer the client to a dermatologist for patch testing.

Unfortunately, sometimes what occurs on the back does not occur on the face! The facial skin tends to be more sensitive than the body skin on most people, and, occasionally, a product that did not react on the back will react on the face! Again, it is important that both the esthetician and the client realize that allergic reactions are seldom predictable, unless it is known what specific ingredients are the allergens.

EXTERNAL FACTORS THAT INFLUENCE ALLERGIC REACTIONS

Besides general cosmetic allergies, other factors can influence allergic reactions, and possibly worsen their severity. Climate is one of these factors. Hot, humid weather or extremely cold weather can play a part in allergy. Hot, humid weather is often accompanied by a high pollen or mold count in the air, which can make persons allergic to pollen or mold more susceptible to both nasal and skin reactions. Heat alone can aggravate sensitive skin, enlarging capillaries and making the skin more reactive than normal. Extreme cold can have similar effects. Cold weather and wind tend to dehydrate the skin and make it dry and flaky. Dehydrated, thin skin is almost always more reactive to irritants and allergens. Severely dehydrated skin may burn or tingle when moisturizers are applied. Sunburned skin can also react to cosmetics or other topicals more easily.

The general rule of thumb with all these climatic effects is to stick to simple hydrating, nonfragranced products. Avoid any stimulation of the skin during these weather-induced conditions. Some drugs may make skin more sensitive. The retinoids, such as Retin-A and Accutane™ can have side effects of extreme sensitivities to cosmetics and other topical substances. See Chapter 17, The New Science of Aging Treatment, for more information on these possible reactions.

Other drugs such as tetracycline, which makes the skin more sensitive to sun, may also make the skin more reactive to cosmetics. It is very important to take a health history, including prescription medications. Advise the client to consult a doctor or pharmacist about possible skin reactions to internal medications.

LATE ONSET ALLERGIES TO COSMETICS

Late onset allergy is the development of an allergy to a cosmetic after years of use.

Occasionally, a client will develop an allergy to a cosmetic after years of use. This is called a **late onset allergy**. Constant exposure to a particular product or ingredient has caused the body to develop an allergy to that product. This may be very confusing to a client who does not understand why the product suddenly causes a reaction. Although acute reactions or immediate reactions are more likely to occur with cosmetics, delayed reactions do occur. Help the client pinpoint the allergic ingredient, and, after the reaction has cleared, try to find a good alternative. Patch test products to find the right one.

SUDDEN REACTIONS

A client will sometimes come into the salon complaining of a sudden rash or other allergic reaction or sensitivity. See if you can specify any recent changes in cosmetic habits or lifestyle. Always check for new cosmetics, nail products, and other possible topical contact allergens. If the client has not changed anything about the home care, you must try to find the allergy cause.

Have the client discontinue all home products, preferably including makeup, until the reaction has stopped and all the redness and allergy symptoms are gone. Then, one by one, have the client use products on the skin, each day adding another product. When and if the allergenic product is added, the client will know what it is.

Often a client has actually experienced some allergic reaction other than cosmetic, but because of skin symptoms it appears to be cosmetic. Sometimes these symptoms disappear, never to return. Again, as always, a dermatologist should be consulted for chronic or severe allergic reactions.

What To Do If a Client Has a Reaction in the Treatment Room

Occasionally, a client will experience a reaction in the treatment room. Most of these reactions are mild, and many are actually sensitivities rather than true allergies. A client may complain of a particular product burning or stinging. Some products, such as glycolic acid, are supposed to cause a mild burning sensation. Most of the time these minor sensations quickly dissipate.

Red, rashy, swollen skin, however, is not normal. Severe burning and stinging are not normal. If a client experiences extreme burning, redness, or swelling, remove whatever is on the face immediately. Apply cool, wet compresses or spray atomized water on the skin to soothe it. Many times simply removing the offending allergen greatly reduces the irritation. It is always best to end a treatment if a client has such a reaction. Applying further products may only aggravate the reaction. Wait until the reaction has completely subsided for a couple of days before consulting with the client about the problem. As always, severe reactions should be immediately referred to the dermatologist.

The following list of common cosmetic allergens may help you pinpoint possible allergic ingredients for allergy-prone clients or may help you pinpoint possible allergens if your client is experiencing chronic allergies or sensitivities. Remember, no ingredient is nonallergenic. These ingredients, listed by type, are simply some of the more frequent allergens.

Fragrances
Clove oil
Eucalyptus
Jasmine
Sandlewood oil
Cinnamics
Essential oils
Geraniol
Musk ambrette
Other plant extracts

Preservatives
Methyl, propyl, ethyl, or butyl paraben
Imidazolidinyl urea
Quaternium-15
Benzalkonium chloride
Triclosan
Methylchloroisothiazolinone
Methylchlorothiazolinone
2-bromo-2-nitropropane-1, 3 diol
DMDM hydantoin
Phenoxyethanol

Sunscreens
PABA
Padimate-O
Padimate-A
Methoxycinnimate
Benzophenone
Methyl salicylate
Octyl salicylate
Oxybenzone
Avobenzone

Other ingredients
Propylene glycol
Salicyclic acid
Benzoyl peroxide
Sulfur
Resorcinol
Tocopherol
Triethanolamine
Formaldehyde
Hydrolyzed animal protein
Lanolin

All of the above ingredients are extremely useful in cosmetics, and they all are needed in order to manufacture good cosmetics. Do not arbitrarily eliminate these ingredients as unacceptable.

Topics for Discussion

1. What is an allergy?
2. What is the difference between a true allergy and a sensitivity?
3. Describe sensitive skin.
4. Discuss some rules for treating sensitive or allergy-prone skin.
5. What is the difference between a reaction and an irritation?
6. Name some common cosmetic allergens and their functions in a cosmetic formula.
7. What is rosacea? How is it treated?
8. What is the irritation cascade?

Chapter
7

Essential Knowledge of Chemistry

Objectives

The esthetician is not really a chemist. The esthetician specializes in applying cosmetic chemicals and teaching clients about their uses. However, it is extremely important that the esthetician have a working knowledge of basic chemistry to better understand the biochemical functions of both the skin's cells and the cosmetics and products used in the practice of esthetics. This chapter focuses on basic principles of chemistry, providing the practicing esthetician with the basic knowledge needed to communicate better with clients about skin care and cosmetic products.

PRINCIPLES OF CHEMISTRY

Chemicals make up our whole world, from the ink on this page to the tip of your finger. Everything is made of chemicals. In the practice of esthetics, estheticians handle many chemicals on a daily basis. When you prescribe a product, or use galvanic current, or clean a steamer with vinegar you are dealing with chemistry. Because our lives, as well as our jobs, involve a series of chemical reactions and procedures, it is important that the esthetician understand the basics of chemistry.

An **element** is a chemical in its simplest form. In other words, it cannot be changed to be any purer by practical purposes and means. There are about 110 elements that make up all chemicals and all matter.

Matter is anything that takes up space and has substance. You are matter. This book is matter. Your products are matter. Essentially everything is matter! And therefore everything is chemicals!

Examples of elements are silver, gold, carbon, oxygen, nitrogen, silicon, hydrogen, sodium, chlorine, etc. Remember, these chemicals (elements) cannot be broken down by ordinary means. The chart of all the elements is called the **periodic table** (Figure 7–1).

The smallest measurable unit of an element is called an **atom**. An atom is made up of a **nucleus**, which is the center of the atom, and **electrons**, which orbit around the nucleus. An atom resembles planets orbiting the sun. The "planets" are the electrons

Element is a chemical in its simplest form.

Matter is anything that takes up space and has substance.

Periodic table is the chart of all the elements.

Atom is the smallest measurable unit of an element.

Nucleus of the cell is made up largely of protein and is also responsible for building certain proteins.

Electrons are negatively charged particles that orbit the nucleus of an atom. The exchange of these particles causes chemical reactions.

Figure 7–1   Periodic table of the elements

and the "sun" is the nucleus. The nucleus of an atom is made up of **protons** and **neutrons**. Protons are very small positively charged particles, whereas neutrons are very small particles with no real charge.

Electrons, which orbit the nucleus, are negatively charged. Remember from basic science how positive and negative charges are attracted to one another? This principle is what keeps electrons orbiting around the nucleus. The electrons which are extremely light (it takes about 1,800 electrons to equal the mass of one proton), are attracted to the nucleus because they are negative. The nucleus, of course, is positive, because it is made up of positive protons and neutrons that have no charge. Electrons orbit the nucleus in circular patterns. These patterns are called electron shells or energy levels. We refer to these orbital patterns as shells or levels. There may be one shell or many shells, depending on the size of the particular atom (Figure 7–2).

All atoms of the same element are exactly alike. They are the same size, weigh the same, and have the same number of protons. Atoms also have the same number of protons and electrons. The atomic weight of an element is the number of protons in one of that element's atoms. So if the number of protons in an atom is the same as the number of electrons in that atom, and you know the atomic weight of that element, you know exactly how many protons and electrons an atom of that element has. For example, hydrogen is a very small atom. It has a molecular weight of 1. That means that it has one proton in its nucleus and one electron orbiting the nucleus. Carbon is a bigger atom. It has an atomic weight of 6. Therefore, it contains six protons orbited by six electrons.

It takes a certain number of electrons to fill one of the shells, which are also called energy levels. The bigger the element, the more levels of electrons will be present. The first energy level holds 2 electrons; the second level holds 8 electrons; the third level holds 18 electrons. The reason this is important is because each level has a certain capacity of electrons it can hold, sort of like the capacity of a room. Atoms have a physical need to have full outer levels.

Protons are very small positively charged particles within the atom.

Neutrons are very small negatively charged particles within the atom.

Sodium atom   **Chlorine atom**

Figure 7–2 Sodium and chlorine atoms

What this means is that if an outer level of electrons is almost full, the level will "want" to fill itself up. If the outer level is almost empty, it will "want" to fill itself up. If the outer lever is almost empty, it will "want" to get rid of its few outer electrons. For example, chlorine has seven electrons in its outer level. It needs eight to complete the level. Chlorine will have a tendency to "want" to fill that level. Sodium, on the other hand, has only one electron in its outer level; it will have a tendency to "want" to get rid of that one electron, so its next level will be full. Remember, the normal configuration of atoms is to have "full" outer levels of electrons. Where can the chlorine atom find that extra electron it needs to fill its outer level? Maybe it can get one from the sodium atom that wants to get rid of its outer electron! So chlorine "steals" the electron from sodium, which sodium is glad to get rid of. Both atoms now have full outer levels of electrons. However, remember that we said earlier that each atom had the same number of positive protons in its nucleus as negative electrons orbiting the atom. Now that chlorine and sodium have exchanged electrons, doesn't that change their positive-negative electrical charges? Now that chlorine has an extra electron, it has one more electron than it has protons. That means that it has one more negative charge than it did before. Sodium has lost an electron, so it now has one more proton than it has electrons, giving it a positive charge. It has one more positive charge (protons) than it has negative charges (electrons).

Ions, or charged atoms, are the resulting atoms with new charges when atoms "steal" or "give away" electrons to each other.

When atoms "steal" or "give away" electrons to each other, the resulting atoms with new charges (and number of electrons) are called **ions**. Ions are charged atoms. The chlorine is now negative, and the sodium is now positive (Figure 7–3).

Positive and negative charges are attracted to one another. So chlorine, with its negative charge, will be closely attracted to sodium, with its positive charge. They are so closely attracted they become "locked" together because of their charges. When two or

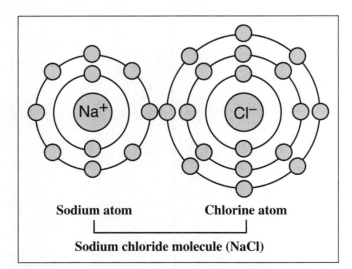

Sodium atom   Chlorine atom

Sodium chloride molecule (NaCl)

Figure 7–3   Sodium and chlorine ions

more atoms become "locked" together in this manner, they become a **molecule**. A molecule is two or more atoms joined together. Molecules have completely different properties than individual atoms. Chlorine is a gas, and sodium is a solid. Together in this molecule they are called **sodium chloride**, which is actually table salt! When two ions form a molecule by being attracted to each other's charge, the bond is said to be an **ionic bond**.

Therefore, the way atoms are joined together has a lot to do with how many electrons are present in the outer electron levels. The number of electrons in the outer level is known as that atom's or element's **valence**. Low-valence atoms are, in general, attracted to high-valence atoms.

What happens if an atom has a medium number of electrons in its outer shell? In other words, if the shell is half full, will the atom try to get more electrons or lose outer electrons? Elements with a medium-filled outer level of electrons share electrons, rather than trade electrons like ionic bonds. When atoms share electrons, the bond between the atoms is called a **covalent bond**. For example, carbon has four electrons in its outer level. It needs four more electrons to fill its outer level. So it shares electrons with other atoms. Often it shares with four other carbon atoms (Figure 7–4).

Let's go back and look again at the periodic table of the elements. The elements in vertical columns are called families of elements. The elements that are in the same horizontal column are called a period. The elements are listed from left to right in order of their atomic numbers, or the number of protons in each element's atoms. Also listed is the atomic mass, which for the purposes of this discussion is the weight of an atom of that element.

Each element has its own abbreviation, or symbol. Some symbols are the first letter or the first two letters of the element. Some abbreviations are taken from the Latin word

Molecule is two or more atoms joined together.

Sodium chloride is the compound created by combining sodium and chloride and commonly known as table salt.

Ionic bond is the bond of two ions joining to form a molecule.

Valence is the number of electrons in the outer level.

Covalent bond is the bond between atoms sharing electrons.

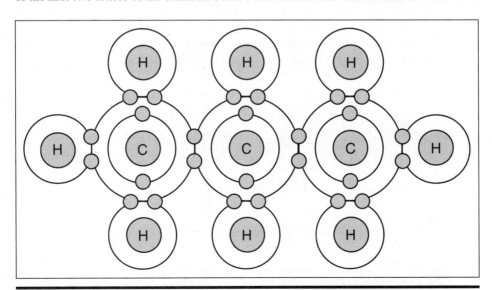

Figure 7–4 Carbon atoms "sharing" electrons with other carbon and hydrogen atoms

for that element. For example, the symbol for carbon is C, but the symbol for iron is Fe, which stands for *ferrous,* the Latin term for iron.

When atoms join together to form molecules, the number of atoms of each element in the molecule is listed beside the symbol for the element. For example, H_2O is made of one atom of oxygen and two atoms of hydrogen. Hydrogen atoms need one electron to fill the outer level. Oxygen needs two electrons to fill its outer ring. Each hydrogen atom shares an electron with the oxygen atom (Figure 7–5).

When a molecule joins two different elements together, the reaction produces what is known as a **compound**. A compound is two or more elements joined chemically to produce an entirely different substance. The new substance has completely new chemical and physical characteristics.

A **mixture** is produced when different elements or compounds are mixed together physically, but still retain separate characteristics. Most cosmetic formulas are mixtures. In other words, the ingredients do not change when mixed with other chemicals. We will discuss cosmetic formulations in more depth in Chapter 8, Cosmetic Chemistry and Functional Ingredients.

A **solution** is a mixture of other chemicals. It is an even mixture, which means the various chemicals are evenly dispersed throughout the mixture. An example of this is salt water. If you mix salt in water, the salt will distribute itself evenly throughout the water. If you keep adding more salt to the water, the salt will begin to pile up on the bottom. This means that no more salt can be dispersed evenly in that amount of water. The point at which mixtures no longer mix evenly is known as the point of saturation.

The liquid part of a solution is called a **solvent**. A **solute** is the solid part of the solution. So, in the example of salt water, salt is the solute, and water is the solvent. Salt water is a mixture, not a compound. The salt has not changed chemically, it is simply dispersed through the water. Salt (sodium chloride) is compound, and so is water (H_2O). The two compounds are mixed together but do not react chemically with one another (Figure 7–6). Many cosmetics are solutions. Makeup is a good example of pigments evenly distributed through a solvent of oil or water or both. This, too, is a solution.

Compound is produced when molecules of two different elements join.

Mixture is produced when different elements or compounds are mixed together physically.

Solution is a mixture of chemicals.

Solvent is the liquid part of a solution.

Solute is the solid part of a solution.

Figure 7–5 H_2O molecule "sharing" electrons between hydrogen and oxygen atoms

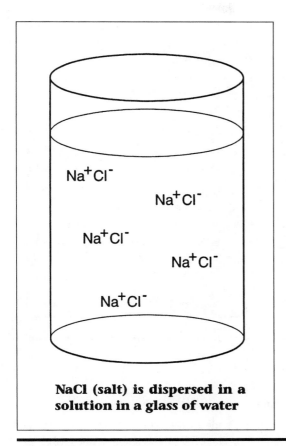

NaCl (salt) is dispersed in a solution in a glass of water

Figure 7–6 NaCl solution

pH, ACIDS, AND BASES

When water is added to certain compounds like acids, the water (H_2O) breaks up and restructures, with certain atoms joining the acid chemicals. Hydrogen chloride (HCl), for example, becomes hydrochloric acid when mixed with water. The hydrogen ions float separately in the acid. The measurement of these hydrogen ions is known as the pH of the substance. pH is an abbreviation for the negative logarithm of hydrions (positively charged hydrogen ions). Acids have a low pH, which actually means that they have a large number of hydrogen ions. Alkaline substances, or **bases**, have a low concentration of hydrogen ions. They have high pH values. Acids all have similar chemical characteristics. Bases, or alkaline substances, are also similar to each other.

Bases have a low concentration of hydrogen atoms and high pH values.

The pH scale ranges from 0 to 14. The lower the pH, the more acidic the substance. The higher the pH, the more alkaline the substance. Figure 7–7 gives examples of various substances and their pH values.

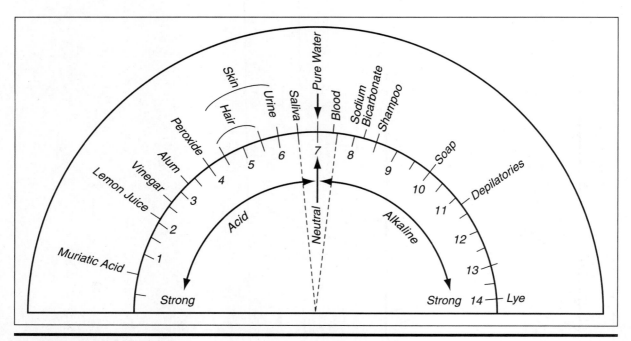

Figure 7–7   Average pH values

Why pH Is Important in Cosmetics

The skin has an acid mantle on its surface, made of a mixture of lipids, sebum, and sweat. This acid mantle has a pH of about 5.5. Therefore, it has a slightly acid pH.

Cosmetics should also have a slightly acid pH. Higher pH values tend to swell the skin and make it more permeable. This can be good or bad, depending on the circumstances. For example, desincrustant solutions and "pre-masks" used for treating clogged pores and oily areas need to have a slightly alkaline pH to slightly dilate the pores for easier extraction. They also help to conduct electricity (galvanic current) better for desincrustation.

Cleansers for oily skin may also have a slightly higher pH than that of the acid mantle. This enables these cleansers to perform a more efficient job of cutting the sebaceous secretions of oily or problem skin. Most of these high pH cleansers are followed by low pH toners. A cleanser with a pH of 6.5 or 7.0 is often followed by a toner with a pH of 4.0 or 4.5. High pH values, however, can be harmful to the skin also, particularly if they are not controlled. High pH increases the permeability of the skin, making it easier for bacteria, microorganisms, and other harmful substances to enter the body. Harsh, high pH soaps can be very irritating and can severely overdry the skin.

HOW CHEMICAL REACTIONS TAKE PLACE

Reactions between two elements or two compounds that result in chemical changes are called **chemical reactions**. During a chemical reaction, electrons of the elements or compounds involved begin either to share energy levels in a covalent bond, or form ionic bonds.

Chemical reactions are reactions between two elements or two compounds that result in chemical changes.

Some chemical reactions take place simply by mixing two chemicals together. Sodium, for example, is very reactive with water. In fact, sodium is violently reactive with water. The sodium bonds with hydrogen and oxygen to form sodium hydroxide (lye) and allows hydrogen gas to escape. In the process much energy is given off in the form of heat. The reaction is as follows:

$$2Na + 2H_2O = 2NaOH + H_2 + energy \text{ (heat)}$$

Let's talk about this equation, or symbol, for the chemical reaction taking place. Remember the chemical symbols from the periodic table. Na is the symbol for sodium; O is for oxygen; and H is for hydrogen. The number in front of each chemical stands for the number of molecules of each chemical. Numbers below a chemical symbol stand for the number of atoms of that element in a particular molecule. So, getting back to the reaction, 2Na stands for two atoms of sodium, and 2 H_2O stands for two molecules of water, which equals 2NaOH, two molecules of sodium hydroxide, plus H_2, one molecule of hydrogen.

Notice that the same number of atoms are present before and after the reaction. Before the reaction, there were two sodium atoms, four hydrogen atoms, and two oxygen atoms, 2Na + 2H_2O. After the reaction there are the same number of atoms, only with a different chemical structure. Because of the electron changeovers, we now have two totally new chemicals, lye and hydrogen. Hydrogen, of course, is a gas, and generally escapes into the air. 2NaOH, or two molecules of sodium hydroxide, have two atoms of sodium, two atoms of oxygen, and two atoms of hydrogen. The other two hydrogen atoms are given off as H_2 (hydrogen gas). So, equal numbers of the same atoms are on either side of the reaction. This is why the reaction is called an **equation**.

Equation is a chemical reaction such that equal numbers of the same atom are on either side of the reaction.

Some reactions such as the one discussed above occur very naturally, by simply combining two chemicals. Other reactions do not happen as naturally. These types of chemical reaction require what is called a catalyst. A catalyst is a substance that helps to cause the reaction, or speed up the reaction, without its atoms becoming a direct part of the reaction's products.

Another condition required for some chemical reactions is heat. Heat can trigger chemical reactions. Some reactions require exposure to ultraviolet light or pressure to take place.

CHEMICALS FOUND IN THE SKIN AND BODY

When we discuss chemicals and chemical reactions within the body, we are talking about a subject called **biochemistry**. Biochemistry is a highly complex subject that we will barely touch. So many complex chemical reactions take place in the body. Many reactions are still not fully understood.

Biochemistry is the study of chemicals and chemical reactions within the body.

As discussed in previous chapters, almost every body function involves chemical reactions. The hormones that tell our cells what to do are chemicals that react with receptor sites. The pituitary hormones that signal other glands to manufacture other hormones is another example of chemical reactions within the body.

Most of the chemical reactions within the body are called organic reactions. Organic chemistry does not mean natural chemistry. Organic chemistry is the chemistry of compounds containing carbon atoms. Carbon is an element that is a large constituent of almost all the many chemicals in the body. The chemicals that the body uses most are oxygen, carbon, hydrogen, and nitrogen. Carbon and hydrogen frequently bond together in chains. These chains of carbon-carbon and carbon-hydrogen bonds are known as **polymers**. Polymers are found in many of the body's chemicals. Proteins, DNA, sugars, and carbohydrates are just a few of the examples of polymers in the body's chemistry.

Protein is made of carbon, oxygen, nitrogen, hydrogen, and sulfur. The basic unit of a protein molecule is called an **amino acid**. Think of amino acids as modules or cars of a toy train. When many different modules are placed together, a protein molecule results. Simple proteins are groups of amino acids linked together. Sometimes the amino acids will have another chemical linked to them that is not an amino acid. These proteins with a non-amino-acid group are called conjugated proteins. Conjugated proteins make up most of the substances found in intercellular cement. Glycoproteins are amino acid chains with a carbohydrate group attached to it. Lipoproteins are amino acid chains with lipids or fats attached to the chain. Phosphoroproteins have a phosphorus or phosphate group attached to the protein chain.

The bond between amino acid groups is called a **peptide bond**. When many amino acids are in long chains, there are obviously many bonds. A chain of amino acid molecules is known as a **polypeptide**.

Simple proteins make up basic material for the body's tissues. The skin, hair, and connective tissue are made up of a protein called schleroprotein. The protein that makes up the blood and lymph are called globulins. Albumin is another type of simple protein used in the blood. Nucleic acids with protein DNA structures are another type of simple protein product. The carbohydrate groups include sugars and other compounds. Carbohydrates are formed by a chain of carbon atoms united with oxygen and hydrogen. They form units, similar to protein and amino acid units. A simple unit of a carbohydrate is called a **saccharide**. One saccharide by itself is called a monosaccharide. Two saccharides together are called a **disaccharide**. Many saccharides bonded together are called a **polysaccharide**. Examples of the various carbohydrates are illustrated (Figure 7–8).

Monosaccharides are simple sugars like glucose (blood sugar). Disaccharides include sucrose or table sugar, and maltose, the sugar used to make malted milk.

Polysaccharides are the more complex carbohydrates. They include the sugars in starch and the carbohydrates that make up vegetables and cellulose-type substances.

Lipids are basically fats. They are a third major chemical group within the body. Lipids are made up of carbon, oxygen, and hydrogen. Lipids do not form in units like proteins and carbohydrates. They are more complex. Triglycerides are the best known type of lipid. Other lipids include waxes, fats, and steroids.

Polymers are chains of carbon-carbon and carbon-hydrogen bonded together.

Protein is made of carbon, oxygen, nitrogen, hydrogen, and sulfur.

Amino acid is a protein that helps break down simple sugars, fats, and parts of proteins.

Peptide bond is the bond between two amino acid groups.

Polypeptide is a chain of amino acid molecules.

Saccharide can refer to any carbohydrate group.

Disaccharide means two saccharides are bonded together.

Polysaccharide means many saccharides are bonded together.

(a) D-Fructose (levulose)

(b) Sucrose (glucose + fructose)

(c) Amylopectin

Figure 7–8 Examples of (a) monosaccharide, (b) disaccharide, (c) polysaccharide

Again, lipids are very important chemicals in cosmetology. They can bind with proteins to form proteolipids, which are a major part of the intercellular cement. Phospholipids and glycolipids are two examples of lipid-protein compounds found in the intercellular cement.

CHEMICAL TERMS ESTHETICIANS SHOULD KNOW

There are a variety of chemical terms besides those already mentioned that estheticians should know to better interpret ingredient labels and understand more about cosmetic chemicals. Some of these words are actually suffixes or prefixes that you will see attached to different chemical names. Most of these are derived from Latin.

Proteo—(prefix) refers to protein. *Proteolytic,* as in proteolytic enzyme peelings, means protein-dissolving.

Lipo—(prefix) refers to fats, lipids, or waxes. Examples are lipoproteins, found in the intercellular cement, or liposuction, the surgical procedure used to remove fat.

Saccharides—can refer to any carbohydrate group. An example is mucopolysaccharide, a popular moisturizing ingredient.

Saturated—can either mean that a solution has absorbed as much solute as possible, or that a molecule has taken on as many hydrogen atoms as it can hold, as in saturated fat.

Aqueous—water-based, as in an aqueous solution.

Aerobic—refers to a reaction that takes place in the presence of oxygen. *Anaerobic* means without oxygen.

Hydration—water is added.

Homogenous—a mixture that is even. The solute is evenly dispersed throughout the solvent.

Suspension—the solute is suspended throughout a solvent. Suspension is usually not homogenous. A separating makeup foundation is an example of a suspension.

Alcohol—is a molecule that has a hydroxy (OH) group bonded to it. The molecule must be a hydrocarbon made of carbon and hydrogen atoms.

Amino—(prefix) refers to compounds that have an amino acid group attached; may also indicate protein derivation.

Mono—(prefix) means *one.* Example: Monosaccharide, which is a simple sugar with one saccharide group.

Di—(prefix) means *two.* Disodium means two sodium atoms that are included in a molecular structure.

Carbo—(prefix) has carbon as a base in the molecule. Example: carbohydrate.

Distilled—heated to remove one chemical from another. Water, for example, is distilled by boiling water and allowing the gas to condense back into liquid, separating the water from impurities and other contaminant chemicals.

Enzyme—a protein that is involved as a catalyst in a chemical reaction. Enzymes in cosmetics are often used to break down substances, as a proteolytic enzyme breaks down keratin protein in dead cells. The chemical names of enzymes generally end in the suffix -*ase*. Examples are *lipase* (fat-dissolving enzyme) and *maltase*, which breaks maltose, a disaccharide, into two simple glucose (sugar) molecules.

Ionized—substance has been charged by changing atoms to ions. *Deionized* means that ions have been neutralized and do not have a charge.

Poly—(prefix) means *many*. Example: *polymer, polysaccharide.*

Tri—(prefix) means *three*. Example: *tridecyl trimellitate,* an emollient.

Cyclo—(prefix) means that the molecule is in a ring structure. The carbon atoms are joined in a ring formation.

Aldehyde—a compound made of carbon and hydrogen, with a carbon, hydrogen, and oxygen group on the end of the molecule.

Topics for Discussion

1. What is an element?
2. Explain why electrons orbit the nucleus.
3. What is the difference between an element, a compound, and a mixture?
4. Describe pH. Give some pH values for various substances.
5. Explain how variations in pH affect the skin.

Chapter

8

Cosmetic Chemistry and Functional Ingredients

Objectives

It is very important that the esthetician be well informed about cosmetic ingredients. This chapter is an overview of common types of cosmetic ingredients. Discussion of their chemical functions in formulations is also included. The esthetician will learn about vehicles, including surfactants, emulsifiers, and emollients. We will also discuss preservatives, coloring agents, and other chemicals necessary to produce cosmetics.

Cosmetic chemistry is a highly complex field. Cosmetic chemists work very closely with cellular function and must be well versed in medicine, biology, chemistry, pharmacology, and cosmetology. They must be aware of the beauty needs of people, but at the same time be well trained in chemistry in order to make beauty products.

Making cosmetics is not as simple as many people think. Cosmetics vary greatly in formula. One slight variation in chemical makeup can create a whole new product texture, color, or other property. Cosmetic chemicals are divided into two basic groups. The first group is the **vehicle** group. Vehicles are spreading agents and other chemicals necessary in the formulation of a cosmetic, but they do not necessarily cause the cosmetic to alter the skin's appearance. Chemicals that cause physical changes in the skin's appearance or alter the appearance in any way are called **active agents** or performance agents. The next chapter discusses active agents. In this chapter we will primarily discuss vehicle chemicals. Vehicles include a large number of types of cosmetic ingredients.

SURFACTANTS

Surfactants are chemicals in cosmetics that cause the cosmetic to be able to slip across or onto the skin. Surfactants lower surface tension on the surface of the skin to allow cosmetic products to slip across and adhere to the skin. They are one of the biggest categories of cosmetic chemicals.

Surfactants also include detergents and soaps. **Detergents** are surfactants that are used for cleansing. They break up oils, fats, and other debris, and cause the debris to separate from the skin. When detergents are applied to the skin and are mixed with water, they begin to bubble. This bubbling is a good example of how surfactants and detergents reduce surface tension and allow water to spread more easily across the skin. Bubbling is air that has come between the surfactant and the surface of the skin. The surfactant removes surface oils from the skin, as well as makeup, dirt, pollutants, and other agents that have come in contact or adhered to the skin during the day.

Another good example of reduction of surface tension by a surfactant is in your kitchen. You cooked hamburgers for dinner and you left the pan with the hamburger grease on the stove while you ate dinner. During that time the grease, which is fats and fatty acids, has solidified in the pan. After dinner, you add hot water to the pan, which liquifies the fat. It is the temperature, not the water, that liquifies the fat. If you leave the water in the pan, the grease will remain nonsolid for the most part. But we know that hot water alone will not remove beef grease from a pan.

So you pour in some dishwashing liquid. If you look closely while you are pouring in the dishwashing liquid, you will notice that the fat has a tendency to "run" from the dishwashing liquid. This "running" is actually the surfactant or detergent improving the water's ability to remove the grease from the pan's surface. The grease will break up much faster with the detergent added to the pan.

During the process of cleaning the pan, you accidentally rubbed grease from the hamburgers on your hand. When you remove your hand from the sink, you discover that your hand is greasy. Dipping your hand into the dishwater seems to loosen the grease from your hand. This is because the surfactant (detergent) works on skin in the same way that it works on the dishes or pan.

Of course, the surfactant used in dishwashing is much too strong a detergent to use routinely on your skin. Similar detergent agents may be used in dishwashing liquids, but the concentration of detergent in the formula is far greater than that used in a facial cleanser. Detergent facial cleansers also may vary in strength and concentration. The four major types of surfactants vary with the pH of the water being used in the formulation. The four basic types of surfactants are:

1. **Anionic surfactants**, which have a negative ionic charge. Anionic surfactants are strong cleansers and are frequently used in household products.

Vehicles are spreading agents and other chemicals necessary in the formulation of a cosmetic, but they do not necessarily cause the cosmetic to alter the skin's appearance.

Active agents are chemicals that cause physical changes in the skin's appearance or alter the appearance in any way.

Surfactants are chemicals in cosmetics that cause the cosmetic to be able to slip across or onto the skin.

Detergents are surfactants that are used for cleansing.

Anionic surfactants are strong cleansers and are frequently used in household products.

2. **Cationic surfactants** have a positive ionic charge. They are frequently used in cosmetics and hair shampoos.
3. **Amphoteric surfactants** may have either a positive or negative ionic charge. They will adapt to the pH of the water used in the solution. Because they are so adaptable to both acid and alkaline water, they are frequently used in facial lotions and creams. The neutrality of the surfactant is important to the mildness of the cosmetic product.
4. **Nonionic surfactants** are used in heavier creams such as hand creams.

Some surfactant ingredients are very frequently used in cosmetic cleansers. Some of these are:

Sodium lauryl sulfate
Sodium laureth sulfate
Disodium lauryl sulfosuccinate
Ammonium lauryl sulfate
Cocoamphocarboxyglycinate
Cocamidopropyl betaine
Alpha-olefin sulfonate
Decyl polyglucoside

All of these surfactants can help remove oils, dirt, and other debris from the skin's surface. How much they remove depends on the amount of surfactant in the individual cleanser.

For sensitive and drier skin types cosmetic manufacturers often add a fatty acid, oil, or wax to cut the contact of the surfactant with the skin. The fatty substance prevents too much of the surfactant from coming in contact with the skin. Too much detergent can be irritating or dehydrating to sensitive, dry, or thin skin.

Cleansers can also vary in strength directly from the amount of surfactant that is in the formula. A cleanser for oilier skin will, in general, contain more surfactant than a cleanser for dry skin. Most cleansers are carefully prepared so that they prevent irritation on most skin types. Surfactants are also added to creams to improve the cream's slip and adhesive qualities. Some surfactants may be very irritating to the skin when used in creams.

EMULSIFIERS

Emulsifiers are chemicals that keep water and oil solutions well mixed. Let's go back to the kitchen for a moment. Remember that greasy pan? Let's pretend that the grease is in a mayonnaise jar. If you add water to the jar with grease in it, what happens to the oil? It floats to the top. This is because water and oil will not mix under normal circumstances.

If we add some dishwashing detergent to the jar, the oil will start to "break up." If we put a top on the jar and shake it, the oil will be dispersed throughout the water evenly. The water will become cloudy because the oil has saturated the water in small droplets.

The detergent is what made the oil break into small droplets and disperse throughout the water. But didn't we add a *detergent* to the water? You thought that this section was about emulsifiers? Well, it is. It just so happens that surfactants, detergents included, are also emulsifiers. They reduce the tension of the water in a cleanser and also reduce the tension of the water in a solution, or even a cosmetic lotion!

Emulsifiers work by forming a sort of "shell" around the very small oil droplets, allowing them to remain suspended in a solution of water. When a solution of water and oil is mixed, and it is mostly water, the solution is called an **oil-in-water solution**. When the solution is mostly oil, it is called a **water-in-oil** solution (Figure 8–1).

Most lotions available today are oil-in-water emulsions. They are much lighter in weight and texture, feel much less greasy, and are easier to remove. Most bottled moisturizers are oil-in-water (abbreviated o/w) emulsions. Old-fashioned cold creams are a good example of a water-in-oil emulsion. Some heavy night creams are also water-in-oil.

Have you ever found an old bottle of lotion in your cabinet? Did it look "watery"? Over time, generally a year or more, emulsifiers can stop working in an emulsion. When this happens, the lotion begins to separate back into its water and oil phases.

As a general rule, almost anything in a bottle is an oil-in-water emulsion. Almost all water-in-oil emulsions are packaged in jars. They are often too heavy and thick to be

Oil-in-water solution is a solution of water and oil that is mostly water.

Water-in-oil is a solution of oil and water that is mostly oil.

Figure 8–1 Types of emulsions

poured out of a bottle. Another way to determine a particular product's emulsion type is to check the ingredient label. The FDA requires that cosmetics list their ingredients in descending order. If oil is listed before water, it is a water-in-oil emulsion. If water is listed first, then it is oil-in-water.

Emulsifiers help to provide stability and texture to lotions and creams. They make the cream feel even and smooth. If they were not used in moisturizers the lotion would feel wet and oily when applied! Some frequently used emulsifiers are:

Amphoteric 9
Ceteth-20
Beeswax
Polyethelene glycol (PEG)
Polysorbate
Carbomer
Carbopol
Stearamide

"Water-based" generally means that the emulsion or lotion is an oil-in-water emulsion. It does not necessarily mean that the emulsion is oil-free. The main reason cosmetic companies refer to a product as being water-based is to appeal to the consumer. Consumers who have oily or problem skin and consumers who do not like greasy products look for products that are watery textured because they are lighter weight and nongreasy.

How can you tell the difference among the three basic types of surfactants? Surface active agents (which reduce surface tension of water for spreading of cosmetic products), detergents (cleansing and foaming agents), and emulsifiers (which keep water and oils in emulsion state) are all surfactants.

The difference among the three has to do with their molecular structures. The size of the molecule determines the different properties that the particular surfactant will have in a cosmetic solution. Surfactants are polymer molecules. This means that there is a chain of carbon atoms that are connected to one another. Surfactant polymer molecules have two ends. One end is attracted to water; the other end is repelled by water. The end that is repelled by water is instead attracted to fatty substances. **Lipophilic** means *fat-loving*. **Hydrophilic** means *water-loving*. The size of the lipophilic end of the polymer determines which kind of surfactant group the molecule will be. Shorter chain carbon polymers, chains with eight or ten carbon atoms, have a shorter lipophilic end and are surface active agents used in creams to improve slip (how well the product flows across the skin) and spreadability.

Medium-length chain molecules with a medium-size lipophilic end are the detergents used in cleansers that help foam and remove surface debris. Long chain polymers, which have a large lipophilic end, are the emulsifiers. This makes sense, because these molecules must have a strong attraction to fat. Remember, these molecules are the ones that "surround" or form the "shell" around the oil droplets and spread themselves throughout the water solution. The other end of the emulsifier (the hydrophilic end) is attracted to the water in the solution. So the molecule produces a "tug-of-war" between

Lipophilic means fat-loving.

Hydrophilic means water-loving.

the oil and the water. The emulsifier is attracted to the oil and is more or less wrapped around the oil, but the other end is attracted to the water in which it is floating. This constant "pulling" keeps the oil or fat evenly suspended in the water solution, or vice-versa in the case of a water-in-oil suspension. The oil droplets in an oil-in-water emulsion are referred to as **globules**. They are the dispersed part of the emulsion and are referred to as the **internal phase**. The water in an oil-in-water emulsion is called the **external phase**. A **suspension** is a liquid solution in which the internal and external phases do not stay mixed for any period of time.

> **Globules** are oil droplets in an oil-in-water emulsion.
>
> **Internal phase** is the dispersed part of the emulsion.
>
> **External phase** is the water in an oil-in-water emulsion.

We have only talked here about lotions. Many types of cosmetic emulsions are not lotions and contain other components besides water and oils. Makeup, for example, is a solid such as talc that is emulsified in a liquid. The external phase of a makeup base is usually water, possibly mixed with propylene glycol or another solvent. Aerosol hair spray is an example of a liquid that is emulsified within a gas. Mousse is an example of a gas that is emulsified within an external phase liquid.

> **Suspension** means the solute is suspended throughout a solvent. Suspension is usually not homogenous. The internal and external phases do not stay mixed for any period of time.

PHYSICAL EMULSIONS

Emulsifiers can sometimes cause problems for thin, sensitive, or dry skin types. What happens in these cases is that the emulsifiers actually start breaking down the natural intercellular lipids that form the barrier function of the skin. Although this is not a problem for all types of skin, it can cause sensitivity for already thin sensitive skin with impaired barrier function.

There is a relatively new technology that uses high-speed mixers, called **homogenizers**, to emulsify products. Most of these products are creams and lotions for sensitive skin. These products use special blends of emollients and nonsurfactant emulsifying agents that are then mixed at high speeds under pressure. This process produces a suspended effect without the use of traditional surfactant emulsifiers, eliminating further disturbance of the barrier function. These types of products are **physical emulsions** and are known as excellent moisturizers for sensitive skin.

> **Homogenizers** are high speed mixers used to emulsify lotions and creams.
>
> **Physical emulsions** are lotions or creams that use physical rather than chemical techniques to blend and suspend oil and water mixtures.

EMOLLIENTS

Emollients are ingredients that lubricate the skin and give cosmetics a soft, smooth feeling. Emollients also significantly help adhere cosmetics to the surface of the skin. Because they are so lubricating, emollients are also used as **active agents** in cosmetics. An active agent is the part of the cosmetic that actually causes a physical change, which is responsible for the change in appearance that cosmetics create. In other words, it is the active ingredient.

> **Emollients** are somewhat like occlusives in that they mostly lie on the surface of the skin and prevent water loss. They also help to "fill in the cracks" of dry, dehydrated skin.
>
> **Active agents** are chemicals that cause physical changes in the skin's appearance or alter the appearance in any way.

Emollients can sit on the surface of the skin and impede water loss (dehydration). They are generally made up of large molecules that help prevent water from leaving the surface of the skin. Therefore, they help stop water evaporation. Chemists often refer to chemicals that stop water evaporation as **protectants**. Protectants also help prevent other agents from entering the skin. For example, **silicone** is an emollient that leaves a protective film on the surface of the skin. Silicone foams are used by doctors, dentists,

> **Protectants** are chemicals that stop water evaporation.
>
> **Silicone** is an emollient that leaves a protective film on the surface of the skin.

esteticians, other health care and personal care professionals to prevent constant rubbing of the hands with latex gloves. The foam is applied before gloves are put on. Silicones are now frequently used both as protectants and as spreading agents. **Cyclomethicone**, **dimethicone**, and **phenyl trimethicone** are examples of silicone compounds now used in moisturizers, sunscreens, serums, foundations, and many other products. Silicones have been referred to as "breathable barriers." They can vary in weight or concentration, help keep the skin from becoming dehydrated, yet are noncomedogenic (not pore clogging), and nonacnegenic (will not contribute to the formation of acne lesions). Another good example of how an emollient works as a protectant is applying petroleum jelly to a baby's bottom. The petroleum jelly, also known as **petrolatum**, prevents urine and soggy diapers from irritating the baby's sensitive skin.

Petrolatum is frequently used as an emollient. Because many emollients are good at adhering to the skin, they are also frequently used as vehicles for both cosmetics and drugs. They are often excellent spreading agents. There are many different types and textures of emollients.

Petrolatum, silicone compounds, and mineral oil are **biologically inert**, which means that they will not react with normal chemical reactions within the skin, making them unlikely to produce allergic or irritant reactions. Therefore, they are excellent ingredients and are frequently used for sensitive skin, including use as drug vehicles for dermatoses such as eczema and psoriasis.

Unfortunately, all three emollients have been mistakenly accused of causing problems because they are not "natural," having been purified or derived from other sources in the laboratory. Many natural substitutes, including plant oils, are much more likely to cause irritation!

FATTY ACIDS

Fatty acids are derived from plant or animal sources. They are not corrosive acids like hydrochloric acid, and are not inflammatory to the skin. They are triglycerides that have been broken down by removing glycerin from fat. They help give a soft, firm texture to lotions and creams. They are good lubricants and smooth across the skin evenly. They also add stability to formulations. Fatty acids are a major ingredient of many soaps. When fat is mixed with sodium hydroxide, soap forms.

Fatty acids are also often used in creams, lotions, shaving creams, lipsticks, and are used as pressing agents in pressed powders and blushes. They are also used in foundations and cleansers. Each cosmetic use of fatty acids may be somewhat different.

In lipsticks, for example, the fatty acid may be used to improve creaminess or improve adherability. In shaving creams, stearic acid is frequently used because it adheres well to the skin and allows the razor to move smoothly across it. It is also a good protectant against razor burns and accidental cuts to the skin.

In makeup, it may be used for improving spreadability and texture. In pressed powders and blushes, fatty acids are used to "press" the powder into a cake, which keeps the product in a solid form until it is used.

Common fatty acids used in cosmetic formulations are:

Cyclomethicone is a type of silicone used primarily as a vehicle or emollient.

Dimethicone is a smaller, lighter version of silicone.

Phenyl trimethicone is a type of silicone emollient.

Petrolatum prevents urine and soggy diapers from irritating the baby's sensitive skin.

Biologically inert means will not react with chemicals in the human body.

Fatty acids are derived from plant or animal sources.

- **Stearic acid**—derived from animal fats and some plants.
- **Caprylic acid**—derived from coconut oil, palm oil, or animal sources.
- **Oleic acid**—from animal fats and vegetable oils.
- **Myristic acid**—occurs in coconut oil, animal fat, palm seed, and other vegetable fats.
- **Palmitic acid**—derived from plant and animal sources.
- **Lauric acid**—derived from laurel oil and coconut oil.

All of these acids are derived from fats (triglycerides) from natural sources.

Although fatty acids have many good properties for cosmetic use, many can be comedogenic. (See Chapter 13, Comedogenicity.)

FATTY ALCOHOLS

When most people think of alcohol, they think of isopropyl alcohol, poured on cuts when they were children. They may also think of alcoholic beverages. All of these forms of alcohol have negative connotations. This may explain the notorious (and undeserved) reputation that alcohol has in the cosmetic industry. Although isopropyl (rubbing) alcohol can be very drying to the skin's surface, this is only one type of alcohol. The term *alcohol* simply means that an oxygen and hydrogen atom have attached themselves to the end of a carbon chain.

There are many types of **fatty alcohols**, which are fatty acids that have been exposed to hydrogen. They have a slightly waxy feel as a raw ingredient. They are used as emollients in moisturizers. They are less sticky and heavy than many fats. Fatty alcohols are also frequently used to improve the viscosity of lotions and creams. **Viscosity** is the thickness and liquidity of a solution. There are many types of fatty alcohols:

- **Cetyl alcohol**—a widely used fatty alcohol. Cetyl alcohol is used as an emollient, an emulsifier, an **opacifying agent** (helps to turn a cream an opaque color, which helps protect the product from light exposure), and as a spreading agent. Cetyl alcohol is derived from animal tallow, but can also be made synthetically.
- **Lauryl alcohol**—derived from coconut and palm seed oils, is used as an emollient and spreading agent.
- **Stearyl alcohol**—derived from stearic acids, used as a foam-booster in detergent cleansers, as an emollient, and as a viscosity-opacity builder.
- **Cetearyl alcohol**—a mixture of cetyl and stearyl alcohols; its uses are the same as its parent alcohols.
- **Oleyl alcohol**—derived from oleic acid, is somewhat fattier and greasier than other alcohols. It is often used in superfatted soaps and dry skin emulsions.

FATTY ESTERS

An **ester** is formed when an organic (carbon chain) acid combines with an alcohol. Fatty esters are used in cosmetics as emollients and conditioning agents. One of their best qualities is that they do not feel as oily to the touch as some other types of emollient fatty ingredients. They can be used to smooth the surface of the skin or hair, to serve as a protectant, to help replace natural esters missing from older, drier skin types, and can sometimes be used as an emulsifier.

The easiest way to spot a fatty ester in an ingredient label is that they have the suffix *-ate*. An example is isopropyl palmitate. Isopropyl palmitate is a palmitic acid molecule that has been attached to the carbon chain of an alcohol, propanol.

Fatty esters vary greatly in molecular weight and size. The size can have an effect on how the ester is used in cosmetics. Again, many fatty esters are comedogenic. (See Chapter 13.)

Frequently used fatty esters in cosmetic formulations are:

Isopropyl myristate
Isopropyl palmitate
Octyl palmitate
Octyl stearate
Isopropyl isostearate
Glyceryl stearate
Propylene glycol dicaprate/dicaprylate
Cetyl palmirate
Decyl oleate

SOLVENTS

Solvents have already been discussed in Chapter 7, Essential Knowledge of Chemistry. Solvents are used in cosmetic formulations either as vehicles for the product or as vehicles for other ingredients.

Plant extracts used in cosmetics, for example, have to be extracted from the actual plant. The solvent normally used for extraction is propylene glycol. So, if you see "arnica (arnica montana) extract" on a cosmetic label, it often means that the arnica extract is present in a solution of propylene glycol or another solvent. Alcohols of various types are also often used as solvents for plant extracts.

ANTIMICROBIALS AND PRESERVATIVES

Preservatives are chemical agents that inhibit the growth of microorganisms in creams or cosmetic products.

Preservatives are chemical agents that inhibit the growth of microorganisms in creams or cosmetic products. Because of the many fats used in cosmetics, formulations are more susceptible to invasion by microorganisms than other types of chemical formulations.

The three main types of microorganisms present in cosmetic formulations are bacteria, fungi, and yeast. Cosmetics may become contaminated because of cross-contamination by the user. The user will apply the cream to the skin, re-dipping the same hand that has touched the skin into the jar of cream. When the fingers touch the cream, bacteria and other microorganisms come in contact with the product in the jar.

Preservatives must be added to cosmetics to kill these contaminating bacteria. Bacteria are also present in small amounts in the raw ingredients used to make the cosmetic.

In the making of cosmetics, preservatives are usually the first or one of the first ingredients used in the production process. This is because, if the preservative is already in the mixing tank, any bacteria introduced into the formula will be killed as ingredients are added.

Preservatives work by either directly poisoning bacteria or releasing other chemicals that poison the microorganisms. We have already discussed the allergy and irritation possibilities associated with preservatives. It is important that enough preservative be used in the cosmetic formulation to kill microorganisms without adding so much preservative that allergies will be more likely to flare.

Another trend in skin-care products is the use of botanical (plant) ingredients and other natural materials. Natural materials are more likely to break down than synthetic materials, and are more likely to be contaminated with microorganisms such as fungi. Therefore, the use of natural materials actually increases the need for more preservatives!

The most commonly used preservatives are methylparaben, propylparaben, and imidazolidinyl urea. Other paraben groups such as ethyl and butyl paraben are also used.

There are many preservative agents besides those already mentioned used in cosmetic formulations. Some of the more frequently used preservatives are:

Methylparaben
Propylparaben
Ethylparaben
Butylparaben
Imidazolidinyl urea
DMDM hydantoin
Methylchloroisothiazolinone
Methylchlorothiazolinone
Quaternium-15
Diazolidinyl urea
Phenoxyethanol

Preservatives are used in very small quantities so they do not cause unnecessary irritation. Because they are present in small quantities, they are almost always some of the very last ingredients to be listed on an ingredient label. Remember, federal law says that ingredients must be listed in descending order of their presence amount.

OTHER TYPES OF PRESERVATIVES

Besides microorganisms, chemical reactions can take place that can alter or even ruin cosmetics. **Oxidation** is one of these chemical reactions. Oxidation is the process by which oxygen is exposed to certain ingredients, which results in a breakdown of the ingredient. It is also the process by which free radicals form! Fats and fatty substances are particularly vulnerable to oxidation. Have you ever been to a picnic and noticed that the potato salad was a yellowish color on the top, but when you spooned some onto your plate, noticed that the potato salad below the surface was lighter?

Oxidation is the process by which oxygen is exposed to certain ingredients, which results in a breakdown of the ingredient.

This is oxidation. One of the main ingredients in potato salad is mayonnaise, which is mainly oil. The oil in the mayonnaise oxidizes very quickly, causing the yellow color on the top of the potato salad.

The exact same reaction takes place in the fats, fatty acids, and esters in cosmetic products. Oxygen constantly comes in contact with the cream during the manufacturing process. After the product is opened by the consumer, the product is exposed to more oxygen. Every time the consumer opens and shuts the container, the product is exposed to oxygen.

Antioxidants are chemicals that are added to cosmetic formulas to prevent oxidation. They also keep creams and other products from developing color and odor changes caused by oxidation. A bad odor may develop in creams that do not contain enough antioxidant. An oxidized cosmetic product that has discoloration and/or odor due to oxidation is said to be **rancid**. Commonly used antioxidants are:

Butylated hydroxyanisole (BHA)
Butylated hydroxytoluene (BHT)
Tocopherol (Vitamin E)
Benzoic acid

Antioxidants can also be used as skin protectants. This will be discussed in Chapter 9, Active Agents and Performance Ingredients.

CHELATING AGENTS

A **chelating agent** is a chemical that is added to cosmetics to improve the efficiency of the preservative. Chelating agents work by breaking down the cell walls of bacteria and other microorganisms so that the preservative is more easily absorbed by the microorganism.

Common chelating ingredients are disodium EDTA, trisodium EDTA, and tetrasodium EDTA. EDTA stands for the chemical name *ethylenediaminetetraacetic acid.* Again, you will see these ingredients further down on the ingredient list because they are not used in large quantities.

BUFFERING AGENTS

Buffering refers to adjusting the pH of a product to make it more acceptable to the skin. Sometimes, when products are made, the pH of the end product may be too high or too low. These pH levels may be irritating to the skin if they are not adjusted.

To remedy this problem the chemist will add a small amount of an acidic or basic chemical to bring the pH up or lower it appropriately. Citric acid is commonly used to lower the pH of a product. Tartaric acid is another acidic agent used in small quantities to bring the pH down to an acceptable acid level.

Some products have the opposite problem. The product turns out to be too acid for the skin. Ammonium carbonate, calcium carbonate, potassium, sodium, or ammonium

---

Antioxidants are topical free-radical scavengers that help neutralize free radicals before they can attach themselves to cell membranes, eventually destroying the cell. They are added to cosmetic formulas to prevent oxidation.

Rancid means discoloration and/or odor due to oxidation.

Chelating agent is a chemical that is added to cosmetics to improve the efficiency of the preservative.

Buffering refers to adjusting the pH of a product to make it more acceptable to the skin.

hydroxide is sometimes added to a product to raise the pH. These buffering agents are added in very small quantities and again will be seen lower on the ingredient label, indicating their small concentration in the product.

GELLANTS AND THICKENING AGENTS

A **gellant** is an agent that is added to a product to give it a gel-like consistency. It improves the appearance of the product and gives it more body, making it stiffer and less runny. Thickening agents make the product thicker, so that it spreads more easily, is easier to handle, and is more acceptable to the eye.

Gellant is an agent that is added to a product to give it a gel-like consistency.

Examples of thickening and gellant agents are methyl cellulose, xanthum gum, beeswax, and carbomer. Many thickening agents can also be used as emulsifiers.

COLORING AGENTS

Colors are added to products to make them more appealing to consumers. There is no other legitimate reason to use color agents in skin-care products.

In makeup, of course, color agents are extensively used. Color agents appear on the ingredient label as a variety of different names. There are two types of regulated colors, certified and noncertified.

Certified colors are pigments, also called **lakes**, that are certified and regulated by the Food and Drug Administration (FDA). They are named by listing the color name, the number assigned to that color agent by the FDA, and the metal associated with the chemical structure. An example would be *D & C* (stands for Drug and Cosmetic) *Red No. 4 Aluminum Lake.* On food packages, you may see listed on the ingredient label *F, D, & C Yellow,* for example. Some colors are approved for use in drugs, cosmetics, and foods. However, in general, you will rarely see *F, D, & C* listed on a cosmetic ingredient label.

Lakes are certified colors and are regulated by the Food and Drug Administration.

The colors certified by the FDA are blue, green, orange, red, and yellow. Noncertified colors are not metal salts. Most of these are natural plant or animal extracts, mineral pigments, and sometimes synthetic colors. Although these colors are regulated by the FDA, they do not have a specific certification number. They include a variety of common cosmetic color agents, including iron oxide, zinc oxide, carmine, beta-carotene, chlorophyllin-copper complex, annatto, ferric ferrocyanide, mica, the ultramarine colors, henna, and others.

Iron oxides are used extensively in the development of foundations. Iron oxide is frequently used to give makeup its color. There are various shades of iron oxide, and, of course, they can vary with the amount used in a particular solution. Iron oxide is actually rust, but is used in scientific formulations in makeup production.

Color agents are used extensively in the formation of foundations, mascara, eyeshadows, eye pencils, lip pencils, powders, blush, lipstick, and contour and camouflage products. Certified colors are not permitted by the FDA to be used in any cosmetics intended for the eye area. Chemists must use noncertified colors in eyeshadow, eyeliner, and other cosmetics intended for the eye area.

When the FDA first began regulating colors, there were about 116 certified colors. Over the years the FDA has determined that many of these colors are not safe for continual use, and therefore the list has dwindled to about 35 certified color agents. Some individuals are allergic to certain of the color agents. You must be careful to notice if a client tells you she is allergic to a particular color. You must check the ingredient labels of any products you wish to use on her or sell her for that particular color agent.

As discussed previously, there is no reason other than esthetics to put color agents in skin-care products. The one exception to this rule would be a moisturizing bronzer, designed to moisturize or protect and still give a slight hint of color to the skin's surface.

Many cosmetic companies now totally eliminate color from their skin-care products, because the public is becoming more aware of the lack of need for these chemicals in skin-care formulations. Also, because color agents can occasionally cause allergic reactions, eliminating the coloring agents from skin-care products cuts down on the likelihood of allergic reaction to the product.

If you use imported cosmetics, you must check to see if the import company has complied with FDA rules concerning color. Some countries do not have strong laws governing the use of color agents, and therefore may use color agents that are not permitted in cosmetics in the United States. The European Economic Community, EEC, also known as the EU, European Union, Germany, and Japan all have regulations regarding color, but even they may differ significantly from those of the United States.

ABOUT WATER

Water is the number one ingredient used in cosmetic formulations. Because most skin-care products on the market today are oil-in-water emulsions, water is extensively used, and in a lotion makes up most of the product.

Water must be prepared before it is used in cosmetics. Cosmetic factories have large tanks that prepare the water by filtering, distilling, deionizing, and sterilizing the water that is used in cosmetics.

Deionizing water before using it in a formulation neutralizes ions that can cross-react with other ingredients, or make a product unstable. **Distillation** means that the water has had minerals and other trace elements removed from it.

Deionizing is the process in which ions are removed from water before the water is used in making skin care or cosmetic products.

Distillation means that the water has had minerals and other trace elements removed from it.

You will notice that deionized water is almost always used in cosmetic and skin-care formulations. By deionizing the water before it is used, the chemist ensures a more stable formulation, particularly when using an emulsifier.

Water is both a vehicle and an active agent. It is an excellent spreading agent for creams, as well as a good rinsing product for cleaning. It also works as an active agent in moisturizers, helping to hydrate the skin. Water is, of course, the real magic ingredient in moisturizers, because it binds to the other humectants and moisturizing agents in the moisturizer. We will discuss the use of these agents more extensively in Chapter 9, Active Agents and Performance Ingredients.

HIGH-TECH VEHICLES

As we learn more about the skin's anatomy and physiology, the intercellular cement, and penetration of the skin, we learn more about formulating products that are more easily accepted by the skin and that penetrate the skin's surface better.

We know, for example, that the intercellular cement is made of various lipids. Making products and using vehicles that are compatible with the intercellular lipids can increase the product's permeability and efficacy. Lipid-based products are good examples. Of course, not every product should easily penetrate the skin. There are many examples of ingredients that would be irritating if they penetrated deeper, and many that are too large in molecular size to penetrate, regardless of what type of vehicle is used.

MICELLES

If you overemulsify an ingredient, the result is called a **micelle**. When you add emulsifier to a solution of water and oil, the emulsifier surrounds the internal phase of the solution. As the emulsifier lines up around the oil, as an example, there are small spaces between emulsifier molecules (Figure 8–2).

Micelle is an overemulsified ingredient.

In a micelle, the emulsifier completely surrounds the oil, creating a sort of bubble. The bubble encloses the oil, or whatever internal phase ingredient is being emulsified. A cosmetic that has micelles present in it is said to be micellized.

LIPOSOMES AND MICROENCAPSULATION

Microencapsulation is the process of using barrier and intercellular-compatible materials like lipids to form special microshells to protect and better penetrate certain ingredients. Many ingredients that are unstable or highly reactive can be protected from becoming unstable and can be delivered in a more effective way through microencapsulation. A good example is tocopherol, or vitamin E. Vitamin E, if unprotected, will serve as an antioxidant for the product. But if tocopherol is microencapsulated, it will serve as

Microencapsulation is the process of using barrier and intercellular-compatible materials like lipids to form special microshells to protect and better penetrate certain ingredients.

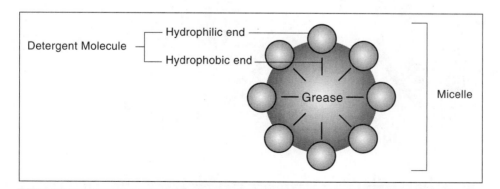

Figure 8–2 Detergent micelle

an antioxidant for the skin's protection, instead of the product's protection! A good example of microencapsulation is the liposome.

Liposomes are hollow spheres made of phospholipids. You can think of a liposome as a balloon, made out of lipids that are compatible with the lipids making up the intercellular cement.

Liposomes may be used to transport other agents, which may include moisturizers, conditioning agents, or drugs. Drugs, of course, are not used in cosmetic formulations.

The liposome may be **loaded**, which means that the liposome may be implanted with an ingredient. This ingredient, theoretically, will penetrate the skin. Eventually, the liposome will begin to dissolve, releasing the ingredient into the intercellular cement, to carry out whatever function it is meant to complete (Figure 8–3).

What you can put into a liposome depends on many factors. These include the size of the liposome, the size of the ingredient to be carried by the liposome, the shape of the liposome, the ionization of any components, and the purpose of the product. Many ingredients are simply too big to put inside a liposome.

Empty liposomes, or unloaded liposomes, are sometimes used in cosmetics to improve the penetration of a cream or moisturizer. Liposomes are not listed as such on ingredient labels—ingredients of the liposome are listed. These may include soya lecithin, lecithin, phospholipids, ceramides, or others.

Liposomes are hollow spheres made of phospholipids that are used to transport other agents.

Loaded is the term to describe a microencapsulation unit, such as a liposome, that contains a performance ingredient, such as an antioxidant.

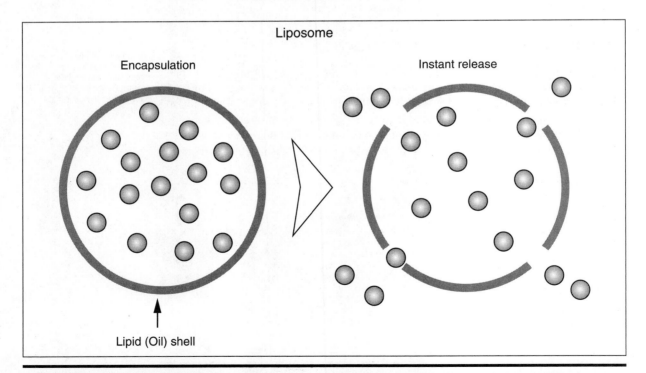

Figure 8–3 This diagram shows encapsulation methods in the liposome and the nanosphere or microsponge. (*Courtesy Thibiant International/Guinot-Paris.*)

The theories behind liposome functions are still being confirmed. Although chemists have a good idea of how liposomes work, more is being learned all the time about their value in cosmetics.

OTHER INNOVATIVE VEHICLES

Other new vehicles similar to liposomes are currently being investigated. One type involves a "microsponge" that releases an active ingredient once inside the skin. Another is the nanosphere.

Such innovations may be used for drugs before they are developed for cosmetics. As we learn more about the functions of the epidermis and the ways chemicals react with the surface of the skin, we will learn more about transport mechanisms for various cosmetic as well as pharmaceutical ingredients.

Topics for Discussion

1. What is a vehicle?
2. Discuss the difference between a surfactant, a detergent, and an emulsifier.
3. What is a suspension? List some examples.
4. How are fatty esters formed? Why are they often used in cosmetic formulas?
5. Why are preservatives necessary in cosmetics? Name some frequently used cosmetic preservatives.
6. Why are "natural" products more likely to need more effective preservatives?
7. Discuss microencapsulation. Why is it important for some ingredients?

Chapter

9

Active Agents and Performance Ingredients

Objectives

Ingredients within a skin-care product or cosmetic that actually cause changes to the appearance of the skin are known as **performance agents** or **ingredients**. They are, by far, the most important ingredients in cosmetic chemistry. Also known as **active agents**, the term performance ingredient is now preferred by some cosmetic scientists to distinguish cosmetic ingredients from drug ingredients. The chemical within a drug that causes physiological changes is known as the **active ingredient**. In this chapter, we will discuss many different performance ingredients used in cleansers, moisturizers, and treatment products as well as some of the active ingredients used in over-the-counter drugs like sunscreens and acne products.

Every cosmetic has at least one performance ingredient. Performance ingredients may also be functional ingredients, or vehicles. For example, an emollient that helps to spread the cosmetic also serves as a barrier to keep moisture from leaving the stratum corneum. This emollient is therefore both a vehicle and a performance ingredient.

In this chapter we refer to the properties of various active agents and discuss their use in various products. We need to establish here that some ingredients used in cosmetics are present because of anecdotal data. **Anecdotal** means, for purposes of this discussion, that the ingredient is supposed to provide certain benefits to the skin, but they have not yet been substantiated, or proven, by scientific means. Often, scientific studies are performed to establish what the ingredient does, but not necessarily whether it works in a particular product. The main reason you need to know this is because you do not want to make drug claims when you practice esthetics. Cosmetics are products that, by law, change the appearance of the skin, not the physiological function. We will discuss this in much more depth in Chapter 11, Claims in Cosmetics.

CLEANSING AGENTS

The active agents in cleansers may be of two types, detergents or emulsion cleansing agents.

Detergents cause cleansers to foam, as we discussed in Chapter 8. An active agent detergent is present in any foaming cleanser, most rinseable cleansers, and shampoos. They are essentially **defatting agents**, which means they remove fats and lipids, along with dirt, makeup, and debris, from the surface of the skin.

Soap also defats the skin's surface. Soaps are usually made of salts of fatty acids. There are two basic disadvantages to soap. First, most soaps have a high pH, which can irritate and dry the skin. Second, many soaps, because of their fatty acid content, leave a residue or film on the skin that is created by insoluble salts, which are formed when the soap is used. The effect of both the fatty acid salts in soap and detergents in foaming cleansers can be overdrying to dry or dehydrated skin. Therefore, fats or oils are often added to the cleansers and soaps to prevent too much of the irritating active agent from coming to contact with the skin for a prolonged period of time as well as overdrying and irritating the skin. You can think of these fats and oils as "bufferzones" set up to keep the product from stripping too much oil from the skin's surface. These products, with fat added, are often referred to as **superfatted**. Of course, the fats that are added to these products can also leave a film on the skin. This can be a problem, especially for oily skins.

Common detergent ingredients used in cleansers are:

Sodium lauryl sulfate
Ammonium lauryl sulfate
Disodium lauryl sulfosuccinate
Decyl polyglucoside
Sodium laureth sulfate
Lauramphocarboxyglycinate
Cocamidopropyl betaine

The ingredients listed above are all detergents. They may be used in any foaming or rinseable type of cleanser. Some detergents are stronger than others. Their cleansing action varies with the amount of detergent used in a particular product, as well as how long it is

Performance agents or **ingredients** are ingredients within a skin-care product or cosmetic that actually cause changes to the appearance of the skin.

Active agents is another term for performance agents.

Active ingredient is the chemical within a drug that causes physiological changes.

Anecdotal means that an ingredient is supposed to provide certain benefits to the skin, but they have not yet been substantiated, or proven, by scientific means.

Defatting agents remove fats and lipids, along with dirt, makeup, and debris, from the surface of the skin.

Soap is made of salts of fatty acids. It defats the skin's surface.

Superfatted cleansing agents have had fat added.

left on the skin. The amount of fat added to the product, of course, affects the cleansing detergent's aggressiveness.

These ingredients are frequently used soap salts, used in true bar soaps:

Sodium tallowate
Sodium oleate
Sodium cocoate
Sodium stearate

You will notice that soap ingredients almost always start with the word *sodium* and end in a fatty ester of one of the main fatty acids listed in Chapter 8: stearic, myristic, oleic, etc. Sometimes potassium is used as the reactant instead of sodium.

Emulsion cleansers are what most estheticians think of as cleansing milks. They are often used for removing makeup and are often recommended for sensitive skin because of their gentleness. Most do not have detergents, but detergents can be used in these products to help the product foam slightly, to make the product more rinseable and easier to remove, or to keep the product emulsified. Cleansing milks are made mostly of water, with an oil or fat mixed in the emulsion; therefore, they are an oil-in-water emulsion. The oil or fat is the active agent used to create a slippery surface for removal of makeup or other debris from the skin's surface. The advantage to these cleansing milks is that they are less drying and irritating to the skin and perform an efficient job of removing makeup. The disadvantage is that they generally leave a residue on the skin. This residue is usually an emollient, the same one often used as the active cleansing agent, helping to loosen the debris from the skin's surface.

The emollient film left on the skin can be good or bad. For drier skins that do not make enough oil, it can actually help condition the surface. For oily skins or acne-prone skins, it can be a problem because it leaves a residue of fat to further clog the problem skin.

Another type of emulsion cleanser is cold cream. Cold cream is often made primarily of mineral oil, making it a water-in-oil emulsion. It is certainly a more oily emulsion cleanser, although very effective for heavy makeup. It often leaves a significant amount of oil on the skin after use. Clients often complain about the greasy feeling after using a cold cream cleanser. These types of cleansers are slowly losing popularity. Emulsion cleansers should always be followed by using a toner.

Emulsion cleansers, better known as cleansing milks, are non-foaming cream-type cleansers.

PERFORMANCE AGENTS IN TONERS

The main function of toners is to lower the pH of the skin after cleansing. Secondly, toners help remove any excess cleanser or residue left on the skin after cleansing. Performance agents in toners vary greatly, depending on the skin type.

pH Adjusters

Most toners have a lower pH, usually around 4.0 to 5.5. This low pH helps to restore the normal pH of the skin's acid mantle after cleansing, which is normally around 5.5 to

6.2. Citric acid or lemon extract is sometimes added to toners to help lower the pH of the product.

Toners for Oily Skin

Astringents are functional agents, but sometimes are active ingredients if used in a drug formulation, that have a tightening effect on the skin or pore appearance. Astringent ingredients include **witch hazel** or **hamamelis extract**, **potassium alum**, **lemon extract**, and other **citrus extracts**. Astringents actually work by causing a slight swelling around the pore openings, helping to tighten the skin and minimize the appearance of the pore opening. Toner products for oily skin are sometimes referred to as astringents, although to call a product an astringent is technically a drug term.

For oilier skins, alcohol is often used as a performance agent. **Isopropyl** and **SD alcohols** are drying alcohols, unlike cetyl alcohol, which is a fatty alcohol used in creams. SD alcohol is **"specially denatured"** ethyl alcohol, also known as **ethanol**. Denaturing means the alcohol is not suitable for drinking. Bittering agents are added to the ethanol to make it taste terrible to ensure safety, so that infants who might try to ingest the product will leave it alone. SD alcohol is listed on the ingredient label followed by a number. This number indicates the technique used to denature the alcohol.

SD alcohol and isopropyl alcohol are strong cleansing agents or defatting agents that help remove excess quantities of sebum from oily skin or oily areas. In larger quantities, they are antiseptics, helping to kill surface microorganisms. This, of course, is a drug claim. Isopropyl alcohol is even a stronger drying alcohol. The drying effect of these alcohols on the skin can also have an astringent effect on the oily skin and pore appearance.

Toners for Dry Skin

Toners for dry skin often contain humectants that help restore moisture to the dehydrated skin after cleansing. A **humectant** is an ingredient that attracts water. Toner humectants may include **butylene glycol**, **propylene glycol**, and **sorbitol**. These humectant ingredients are also known for their softening effect on the skin. More on humectants will be discussed later in this chapter. Dry skin toners also have an acidic pH.

Various other performance ingredients may be added to toners. For example, **azulene**, **chamomile**, or **bisabolol** might be added for their soothing effect in a toner for dry, sensitive skin. **Salicylic acid** might be added to an oily skin toner for its keratolytic or peeling effect on the oily, hyperkeratinized skin.

A WORD ABOUT ALCOHOL

Alcohol has an undeserved terrible reputation in the cosmetics industry. Many companies tout that their products are "alcohol-free," referring to the drying effects of alcohol on the skin.

Although large amounts of SD or isopropyl alcohol can be very irritating or overdrying to dry or sensitive skin, they are very useful in helping to control oiliness in

---

Astringents have a tightening effect on the skin or pore appearance.

Witch hazel, or **hamamelis extract,** can be a soothing agent or, in higher concentrations, is an astringent.

Potassium alum is a strong astringent.

Lemon extract, or **citrus extracts,** have astringent effects.

Isopropyl alcohol is a fairly strong drying alcohol, used as a cleansing and drying agent to remove excess oil from very oily skin. Isopropyl alcohol can dehydrate and irritate if overused, or used on skin that is not excessively oily.

SD alcohol is specially denatured alcohol, also known as **ethanol.**

Humectant is an ingredient that attracts water.

Butylene glycol is a humectant often used in dry- or sensitive-skin moisturizers.

Propylene glycol is a humectant that penetrates the skin fairly easily, making it a good hydrating agent.

Sorbitol is a humectant.

Azulene is a hydrocarbon that is derived from the chamomile flower.

Chamomile is a soothing agent.

Bisabolol is an agent that is added to cosmetics designed for sensitive skin.

Salicylic acid is an antibacterial and keratolytic agent.

Natural moisturizing factors (NMFs) are hydrating agents found within the cells and within the intercellular cement.

Sodium PCA is a natural moisturizing factor ingredient.

Sphingolipids are lipid materials that are a natural part of the intercellular cement.

Glycosphingolipids are lipid materials that are a natural part of the intercellular cement.

Ceramides are lipid materials that are a natural part of the intercellular cement.

Phospholipids are naturally moisturizing humectants found within the skin.

Fatty acids are derived from plant or animal sources.

Glycerol is a humectant that is a natural part of the intercellular cement.

Squalane is a lipid material that is a natural part of the intercellular cement.

Cholesterol is a lipid material that is a natural part of the intercellular cement.

Lipid replacement involves using topical lipids to repair the barrier function.

Soy sterols are natural sources of lipid materials.

Soy lecithin is used as a moisture-binding material, also used for many liposomes.

Linoleic acid is a fatty acid that is a natural part of the intercellular cement.

Evening primrose oil is an excellent source of fatty acids, including linoleic acid.

Sunflower oil is an excellent source of fatty acids, including linoleic acid.

oily and acne-prone skin. Do not reject a product simply because it has some SD or isopropyl alcohol. Make your decision based on the skin type you are treating. For more information on alcohols, see Chapter 8.

ACTIVE AGENTS FOR DEHYDRATED SKIN

When skin is dehydrated, it is suffering from lack of water in the surface. Skin becomes dehydrated from too much sun, weather exposure, harsh cleansers, and aging. Humectants are water-binding agents that are hydrophylic, or water-loving. They have a strong attraction to water. Many chemically bind water to them, holding many water molecules.

We have already discussed the barrier function of the skin. Impaired barrier function can result not only in flaking and esthetic problems but also in increased skin sensitivity. Natural humectants, lipids, or hydrating agents found within the intercellular cement are known as **natural moisturizing factors** or **NMFs**. The NMFs in the skin help to preserve water or hydration within the epidermis, keeping the barrier function intact and keeping the skin soft and supple. Impaired barrier function can mean a lack of NMFs from missing lipids or other components, and can cause dehydration, which is sometimes severe. It can also cause a wrinkly, unfirm appearance to the skin surface.

NMFs include **sodium PCA**, **sphingolipids** and **glycosphingolipids** (also known as **ceramides**), **phospholipids**, **fatty acids**, **glycerol**, **squalane**, and **cholesterol**. These intercellular components are produced during the cell renewal process as cells migrate from the basal layer to the stratum corneum. As we age, our cell renewal slows down and, therefore, we produce fewer NMFs. This lessens the ability of the skin to hold hydration, making the skin dry, tight, flaky, and dull-looking.

In recent years, scientists have been able to isolate and prepare special ingredients that help to "repair" or "patch" the moisture barrier. These ingredients can now be used in products for dry, dehydrated, as well as aging and sun-damaged skin.

Lipid replacement is accomplished by applying a group of lipid ingredients to the skin. These include ceramides or sphingolipids, phospholipids, cholesterol, and fatty acids. These lipid ingredients can actually be derived from plant or animal sources, although most are derived from plant materials such as **soy sterols** or **soy lecithin**. **Linoleic acid** can be derived from numerous plant sources, including **evening primrose oil**, **sunflower oil**, or **borage oil**. These lipid components are naturally in the intercellular material at a ratio of 4:1:1:1. In other words, four parts ceramides to one part of each of the other components. This complex of performance lipid ingredients literally patches the impaired barrier. Its function is to hold water within the intercellular matrix.

However, lipids alone are not as effective without the use of humectants or **hydrophilic ingredients**. Hydrophilic literally means water-loving. These ingredients work like "water magnets," attracting water while the lipids hold the water within the intercellular spaces between the cells. This combination of lipid complexes with hydrators is excellent for helping restore essential moisture to dry, dehydrated, as well as sensitive skin.

Sodium PCA is an excellent hydrator. It has a strong ability to attract water and is readily accepted by the skin. Sodium PCA is used frequently in night creams, day creams, sunscreens, and other hydrating products. It can be used without lipids to hydrate oilier or combination skin. It is lightweight on the skin and does not cause clogged pores.

Glycerin is a humectant that has been used for many years. It is a very strong water binder. It is, in fact, so strong that it should not be used by itself. Glycerin can actually make the skin more dry over a period of time because it doesn't just pull water from cosmetics and the atmosphere when applied to the skin. In large amounts, it can pull water from the lower levels of the epidermis, causing transepidermal water loss (TEWL), which results in drier skin. Used in a moderate amount in a good hydrating cream, it is an excellent hydrating agent.

Propylene glycol is another widely used humectant. It penetrates the skin fairly easily, making it a good hydrating agent. Some people, however, are allergic to propylene glycol. It is used in literally thousands of cosmetics and drugs. It is frequently used in foundations. Butylene glycol is now being used more frequently in products for dehydrated as well as sensitive skin. It has less potential for sensitive skin irritation than its chemical cousin, propylene glycol. Sorbitol is another excellent hydrating agent that is frequently used in hydrating lotions.

Alphahydroxy acids, besides being surface exfoliants, are also hydrators. Lactic acid is actually used in prescription-strength moisturizers. Glycolic acid is also a hydrating agent.

OTHER HUMECTANTS

Other water binders work very differently than the standard hydrophylic agents.

Hyaluronic acid, also known as **sodium hyaluronate**, is one of these agents. Hyaluronic acid can hold up to 400 times its own weight in water. The molecule is quite large. It cannot penetrate the skin to any degree. However, because of its excellent water-binding properties, it is a frequently used hydrating performance ingredient. Hyaluronic acid is an expensive hydrator. Creams and lotions containing hyaluronic acid may be more expensive than others.

Mucopolysaccharides are carbohydrate-lipid complexes that are also good water binders. Considered a "mother-molecule" to hyaluronic acid, it is very capable of holding large amounts of water, and is an excellent hydrator. Again, it is too large to penetrate the skin.

Collagen and **elastin** are large, long-chain molecular proteins that lie on top of the skin and bind water, also helping to prevent water loss. Collagen and elastin have been used in creams for many years. They are too big to ever penetrate the skin, but they do a good job hydrating. Because they lie on top of the skin, they also help to "fill in" small lines and wrinkles, making skin look smoother.

All of the above ingredients are known as **substantives**, which are ingredients that attach themselves well to the surface of the skin, sort of spreading out across the skin, to protect and hydrate the surface.

Some of the more recent discoveries in humectants include algae and seaweed extracts. These are quite remarkable hydrators. They are substantive, forming a surface

Borage oil is an excellent source of fatty acids, including linoleic acid.

Hydrophilic ingredients, or "water-loving" ingredients, attract and bind water.

Glycerin is a humectant and is a very strong water binder.

Hyaluronic acid or **sodium hyaluronate** is a hydrophilic agent with excellent water-binding properties.

Mucopolysaccharides are carbohydrate-lipid complexes that are also good water binders.

Collagen is a large, long-chain molecular protein that lies on the top of the skin and binds water, also helps to prevent water loss.

Elastin is a large, long-chain molecular protein that lies on the top of the skin and bind water, also helps to prevent water loss.

Substantives are ingredients that attach themselves well to the surface of the skin, sort of spreading out across the skin, to protect and hydrate the surface.

gel. Some forms of algae are now being used as hydrating base materials for sensitive skin products without using traditional emulsifiers that can decrease the barrier function in sensitive skin with loss of lipid barrier.

OCCLUSIVES

Occlusives are heavy, large molecules that sit on top of the skin and prevent moisture loss.

An **occlusive** is a heavy, large molecule that sits on top of the skin and prevents moisture loss. Occlusives are exactly what they sound like, forming a barrier on top of the skin to shield the skin from transepidermal moisture loss from the inside out, much like the barrier function, except on top instead of within the skin.

Petrolatum prevents urine and soggy diapers from irritating the baby's sensitive skin.

Petroleum jelly is an excellent occlusive, preventing moisture loss from the skin.

A good example of an occlusive is **petrolatum**, or **petroleum jelly**. Petrolatum can be used by itself or incorporated into a cream or lotion. The amount of occlusion created by the petrolatum depends on the amount used in the cream formulation.

The advantages of using petrolatum in formulations are many. It is extremely hypoallergenic, rarely causing a problem with allergies or irritations. Hence, it is often used in formulas, both drug and cosmetic, for sensitive or irritated skin.

Petrolatum provides an excellent occlusive barrier both to keep water in the skin and to keep allergens, antigens, and foreign bodies out of the skin. A good example of this is the application of petroleum jelly or mineral oil to a baby's bottom to avoid skin contact with urine in the baby's diaper. Petrolatum is also very inexpensive.

There are some disadvantages to using petrolatum. First, it is extremely sticky, slippery, and greasy. Most clients do not like this greasy feeling. It is also hard to accomplish any task when your hands are too slippery to handle anything. It is extremely greasy on the face, creating esthetic problems as well. Second, it is disadvantageous to use petrolatum for oily and problem skin. Although petrolatum is not comedogenic in its pure state, it is very greasy and heavy. Besides the obvious esthetic problem for oily skin, the occlusive action of petrolatum also blocks the follicles from oil dispersement, as well as from transepidermal water loss. In other words, while it keeps the water in the skin, it does not allow sebum to leave the follicle, therefore causing a "back-up" of sebaceous secretions.

Water and sweat from sudoriferous glands also become trapped between the skin and the occlusive petrolatum, which contributes to microbial problems. This is particularly a problem when the occlusive is worn for a prolonged period of time.

Many estheticians do not like petrolatum because it is not "natural." This is simply not true. Petrolatum comes from minerals in the earth. What could be more natural? In short, petrolatum is a useful product, but it should not be used in all cases of dehydration.

EMOLLIENTS

Emollients are somewhat like occlusives in that they mostly lie on the surface of the skin and prevent water loss. They also help to "fill in the cracks" of dry, dehydrated skin.

As the skin ages, it tends not to produce as much of the essential lipids that make up the intercellular cement, or the skin produces less sebum, which helps provide a barrier on the surface of the skin to prevent dehydration. This is when emollient ingredients are used in cosmetic systems. **Emollients** are somewhat like occlusives in that they mostly lie on the surface of the skin and prevent water loss. They also help to "fill in the surface cracks" of dry, dehydrated skin.

Emollients are often used not only for dehydrated or water-dry skin but also for oil-dry or alipidic skin. Emollients have a second use as spreading agents, previously discussed in Chapter 8.

Alipidic literally means "lack of lipids." These types of skin do not produce enough lipids. This could be true of both the intercellular lipids and the sebum produced by the sebaceous gland.

Alipidic means "lack of lipids." These skin types do not produce enough lipids.

Emollients help to supplement skin that suffers from this lack of lipid production. They serve as a substitute, helping to keep the surface lubricated and protected.

These emollients are of several categories. Fatty acids have already been discussed in Chapter 8. They are emollients. Fatty alcohols and fatty esters are also emollients. We have already discussed new types of emollients that are, again, actually a synthetic version of intercellular cement lipids. These include cholesterol, ceramides, lecithin (also a humectant), squalane, and glycosphingolipids.

Lanolin is another good emollient. Lanolin has had much bad press in the past. It was thought to cause many allergies. Although this is a problem for some people, it has recently been theorized that most of the old-fashioned lanolin formula creams were also often full of perfumes and fragrances, thought to be a major source of these allergies. Purification processes for lanolin have also improved substantially over the decades, making today's lanolin a useful and relatively harmless active agent.

Mineral oil is another emollient. Like petrolatum, it is a petroleum derivative. It has many of the same advantages and disadvantages as petrolatum. It is hypoallergenic and a good emollient, helping to soothe irritated, dry, scaly skin. But it is also greasy, particularly in its pure state. However, when formulated properly into a cream, it can be an excellent active agent emollient for dry, dehydrated skin, especially when mixed with good humectant active agents.

Silicones are often used now instead of traditional fatty-type emollients. Silicones include **cyclomethicone**, **dimethicone**, and **phenyl trimethicone**, often used in combination. Often referred to as "breathable barriers," these lightweight and unique ingredients help block water to prevent it from escaping from the surface of the skin, while keeping the skin feeling light and comfortable. Another advantage is that silicones are **biologically inert**, which means they are chemicals that are unlikely to cause reactions with the skin, making them ideal for sensitive skin formulations also. The silicones are noncomedogenic and do not irritate the pores, thus are ideal for oily and acne-prone formulations. They can be used in creams, lotions, cleansing milks, foundations, and are often used in concentrated lipid serums for dry and sensitive skin with impaired barrier function.

Silicones help protect skin from epidermal water loss, and improve feel and spreadability of product.

Cyclomethicone is a type of silicone used primarily as a vehicle or emollient.

Dimethicone is a lightweight silicone emollient.

Phenyl trimethicone is a silicone emollient.

Biologically inert chemicals are chemicals that are unlikely to cause reactions with the skin, making them ideal for sensitive formulations.

INGREDIENTS FOR AGING SKIN

Although there is no way to completely avoid the aging process, there appear to be steps you can take to slow its signs. Every day more technical information is available about the aging process and measures to help appearance problems associated with aging. New ingredients are rapidly being developed.

Alphahydroxy Acids

In the history of cosmetics, no other ingredient or family of ingredients has had the impact or efficacy of alphahydroxy acids. **Alphahydroxy acids (AHAs)** are a family of naturally occurring mild acids. Most AHAs are present in fruits and vegetables, but some actually occur in human cells. Most AHAs used cosmetics have been laboratory purified or are the side product of other industrial chemical processes, such as the making of film.

AHAs have a very large number of applications in skin care and can help many conditions, including oily and acne-prone skin, sun damage, dryness, and hyperpigmentation. There are several AHAs used in skin-care treatment. These include **lactic acid**, **tartaric acid**, **malic acid**, and by far the best-known AHA, **glycolic acid**. Salicylic acid and **citric acid** are also often included when discussing hydroxy acids, but they are actually **betahydroxy acids**.

The chemical difference between alpha and beta hydroxy acids is the location of the hydroxy group on the carbon chain of the acid. *Alpha* indicates that the group is on the first carbon atom, whereas *beta* means that the group is on the second carbon atom. Glycolic acid is the smallest, molecularly, of all the alphahydroxy acids. It has been widely researched, and, because of its size, penetrates between cells more readily than the other AHAs.

AHAs are theorized to work by loosening the bond between dead corneum cells, dissolving part of the surface intercellular cement that holds dead epidermal cells together. This makes it easy to remove dead cells from the skin surface, which has a positive effect on many conditions:

1. Removal of dead cell buildup helps to smooth the surface of dry, sun-damaged, or aging skin, improving roughness, and making wrinkles appear much less deep. Results on an aging skin can become apparent in a very short period of time.
2. By removing dead surface cells, cell renewal is stimulated, bringing younger, fresher cells to the surface more quickly, and increasing the production of intercellular lipids, improving barrier function and, therefore, improving hydration of the skin. Well-hydrated skin is smoother and firmer looking and is generally healthier, helping all activities of the skin proceed more efficaciously.
3. Removing dead cell buildup from the inside of follicles helps loosen clogged pores, comedones, and other impactions on an oily skin or oily area. Continued use helps keep dead cells from accumulating on the follicle wall, which prevents impactions that can lead to inflammatory acne lesions. This property of AHAs and BHAs make them good ingredients to use for acne-prone and oily skins.
4. Removal of dead cells can mean the removal of hyperpigmented cells, which helps to lighten discolored or splotchy skin. Used in combination with a melanin suppres-

---

Alphahydroxy acids (AHAs) are a family of naturally occurring acids.

Lactic acid is an alphahydroxy acid occurring naturally in milk, both an exfoliant and a hydrophilic.

Tartaric acid is an alphahydroxy acid occurring naturally in grapes and passionfruit.

Malic acid is an alphahydroxy acid derived from apples.

Glycolic acid is the most frequently used alphahydroxy acid; exfoliant and hydrophilic.

Citric acid, or betahydroxy acid, is most often used as a pH adjuster, but can also be used as a mild exfoliant.

Salicylic acid is a betahydroxy acid with exfoliating and antiseptic properties; natural sources include sweet birch, willow bark, and wintergreen.

Betahydroxy acids are a group of organic acids used in skin care products; includes salicylic acid.

sant, such as hydroquinone, AHAs help remove stained cells, while hydroquinone helps suppress the activity of the melanocytes.

5. AHAs can also be used on body skin, removing dead, dry cells, and helping improve retention of moisture. This helps conditions such as dry, winter skin as well as aiding dermatologists in treating medical conditions such as eczema and icthyosis. Alphahydroxy acids are also helpful in removing calluses on feet, elbows, and hands.

Alphahydroxy and betahydroxy acids can be used in many products, including cleansers and toners, but are most effective when used in leave-on products such as treatment gels, serums, or moisturizing creams.

Strengths and Effectiveness of AHAs

Alphahydroxy acids can vary extensively in their strengths. Products have been formulated with as little as 2 or 3 percent to as high as 20 percent in higher strength treatment preparations, generally available only through dermatologists and plastic surgeons. There has been a great deal of controversy over the irritation potential of various higher strengths. It is generally accepted by the esthetic industry that products contain 8 to 10 percent AHA in order to show results in helping the various conditions previously discussed, although even 5 percent can show gradual improvements to the skin conditions.

The pH is also a very important factor in AHA efficacy. The lower the pH, the higher the strength of the acid, the more cells will be removed from the skin. Also, though, the lower the pH, the more potentially irritating the acid will be to the skin. AHA leave-on products of 8 percent or higher sting slightly when applied, indicating some irritancy, even though this is probably very small at this concentration.

The Cosmetic Ingredient Review (CIR) is a special panel of scientists and dermatologists who investigate cosmetic ingredient safety for the Cosmetic, Toiletries, and Fragrance Association, the largest cosmetic manufacturers association. The CIR shares its findings with the industry as well as with the Food and Drug Administration (FDA). Recently, the CIR conducted an extensive investigation of the safety of alphahydroxy acids and many derivatives of AHA. The CIR determined that home use products were generally safe, as long as they contained no more than 10 percent AHA, and had a pH no less than 3.0. Remember, the lower the pH, the stronger the acid!

Likewise, the CIR looked at salon use AHAs, and these higher strength AHAs will be discussed in Chapter 18, Chemical Peeling and Exfoliation Procedures.

Vehicles and Other Ingredients with AHAs

The cosmetic spreading agent or vehicle for AHAs can also vary greatly. AHAs can be incorporated into leave-on gels, used frequently on oily, acne-prone, and combination skin types, and lotions or creams, which are more suitable for dry skin and body skin.

Other ingredients may also be combined with AHAs in different formulations. Hydrating ingredients or emollients may be included for dry skin, hydroquinone may be included for hyperpigmented skin, and salicylic acid may be included for acne-prone skin.

Contraindications of Alphahydroxy Acids

AHAs should not be used on clients who:

- Are using or have recently used Accutane®.
- Have recently had laser resurfacing, chemical peel, dermabrasion, or other peeling procedure.
- Are using Retin-A or Renova®, or other retinoic drug or product.
- Are known to be allergic to AHA or BHA.
- Are sunburned or have visibly irritated skin.
- Have cuts, abrasions; including open acne lesions that have been scratched, or blisters.
- Are using other topical medications, unless approved by their physician.
- Are planning to deliberately expose their skin to the sun or sun beds.
- Have not had a thorough consultation and may be using products that are contra-indicated.
- Are pregnant or nursing. AHA safety has not been determined for pregnant or nursing women.

In addition, AHAs should be used carefully with other peeling agents such as salicylic acid, benzoyl peroxide, sulfur, resorcinol, or products with large amounts of alcohol.

Combining peeling agents can increase irritation. Be careful when using any stimulating product with AHAs, because this may increase irritation.

In general, it is best to supervise your client's entire home care program when using AHA products. This way you can determine exactly what they are using with the AHA product for best results and the least irritation.

Last, but certainly not least, the client *must* use a daily sunscreen with a pH of at least 15 while using AHA products!

Ingredients for aging skin:

- Alphahydroxy acids, particularly glycolic and lactic acid, help aging or sun-damaged skin by making the surface smoother, lessening lines, wrinkles, roughness, and splotchy hyperpigmentation. Long-term use improves barrier function, resulting in much better hydration, enhanced barrier function due to normal cell renewal, increased firmness, and significantly healthier looking skin.
- Lipid complexes, already discussed, are helpful for aging and sun-damaged skin in many products, including sunscreens, hydrating creams, eye creams, masks, and special concentrated serums for very dehydrated and sensitive skins.
- Hydrators have already been thoroughly discussed. They are an essential part of any program for aging skin.
- Sunscreens—because most of the damage we have discussed is caused by sun exposure, it is obviously important to shield the skin from further damage. An SPF-15 or higher broad-spectrum sunscreen should be used daily on all skins, but especially aging or already sun-damaged skin. For much more information on sun damage and protection, see Chapter 16, Sun and Sun Damage.

Liposomes

We have already discussed liposomes, which are routinely used in modern formulations to help aging skin. As we just discussed, aging skin experiences a slowdown in the manufacture of vital intercellular lipids. Liposomes, lecithin, and other similar lipid ingredients are very helpful in "filling in" these missing lipids, helping to penetrate moisturizing ingredients better, and improving the amount of time that hydrating agents retain water in the skin.

1,3 Beta-Glucan

This yeast cell membrane derivative is better known by its trade name Nayad®. It has been shown to improve wound healing. Scientists theorize that beta-glucan works by stimulating the macrophages in the skin, which, in turn, stimulate the fibroblasts, the structures within the dermis that make collagen. Beta-glucan is already in several products on the market.

Antioxidants

We have previously discussed free radicals. Free radicals may be an important factor in the aging process, including aging of the skin. Topical free radical scavengers, called **antioxidants**, help neutralize free radicals before they can attach themselves to cell membranes, eventually destroying the cell.

Antioxidants are topical free radical scavengers that help neutralize free radicals before they can attach themselves to cell membranes, eventually destroying the cell. They are added to cosmetic formulas to prevent oxidation.

One of the most popular and promising concepts in aging skin treatment is the use of antioxidant treatment. As we discussed in Chapter 2 and also in Chapter 6, free radicals cause much havoc in the skin, and are now believed by many scientists to be the primary cause of aging, both within the skin and the body. Chronic irritation to the skin by sun, pollution, smoking, chemical exposure, and other inflammations leads to cumulative damage to cells by free radicals. This results in the formation of self-destruct skin enzymes, such as **hyaluronidase**, **elastase**, and **collagenase**, which cause the breakdown of collagen and elastin fibers and the reduction in the strong supportive effects of hyaluronic acid.

Hyalurodinase is an enzyme produced during inflammation that breaks down hyaluronic acid in the skin.

Elastase is an enzyme produced during inflammation that breaks down elastin fibers in the skin.

Collagenase is an enzyme produced during inflammation that breaks down collagen in the skin.

Antioxidants work by supplying electrons to radical oxygen atoms, which need electrons to be stable. Cell membranes have an excess of electrons, therefore providing a "smorgasbord" for the "electron starving" free radical oxygen atom. Antioxidants also supply electrons, neutralizing the atoms before they have a chance to attach to the cell membranes.

Free radicals occur in normal body cellular and physiological reactions. Free oxygen atoms are given off as a result of various chemical reactions within the body. Smoking, alcohol, stress, and sun exposure also contribute to additional free radical production.

The use of topical antioxidants theoretically may be significant in helping to improve the visible signs of aging, and possibly to help prevent some of these reactions. Antioxidants are believed to be able to stop free radical cascade reactions, eventually stopping or slowing the production of these destructive enzymes. They are theorized to work by chemically "quenching" free radicals, by either neutralizing the radical by stabilizing its electron balance, or "scavenging" the reactive chemicals. At the time of this writing, there are no firm scientific studies to support this widely accepted theory as far as cosmetic skin treatment is concerned, although it is evident that antioxidants do help the appearance of the aging skin.

Antioxidants are, by nature, very unstable substances. Because they are so reactive, they must be stabilized in order to remain effective in a skin-care product. Until very recently, it was hard to stabilize these ingredients for use as performance ingredients. Antioxidants were used primarily to keep creams fresher by neutralizing free radicals within the cream or lotion. This helped prevent rancidity, but it meant that the antioxidants were a preservative, not a performance ingredient.

The invention of liposomes and other forms of microencapsulation helped provide a way to keep these reactive substances stable until they could be used. Besides acting as protective "shells" to keep the antioxidants **bioavailable**, or able to be used as a skin conditioning agent, the lipid-based microencapsulation also improved skin acceptance of the antioxidant ingredients.

Antioxidant ingredients include **superoxide dismutase**, **liposomed tocopherol** (vitamin E), **tocopheryl acetate** (another form of stabilized vitamin E), **ascorbic acid** and **magnesium ascorbyl phosphate** (vitamin C compounds), **grapeseed extract**, **green tea extract**, **retinol**, and **coenzyme Q-10**. All of these ingredients are free radical neutralizers, and are often used in combinations because some are known to work better against one type of free radical than another. Remember, a free radical reaction is always a **cascade**, or a chain of reactions, one reaction causing the next.

PRODUCTS FOR DRY SKIN

Most products designed for dry skin contain a combination of humectants and emollients and may contain some of the agents we have discussed that are designed for aging skin. They are normally water-based, or oil-in-water emulsions, although some may be water-in-oil emulsions designed for more alipidic skin.

These creams vary greatly in the amount of emollients and humectants they contain. The more oil-dry the skin is, the more emollient should be used in a treatment cream.

Treatments with large amounts of humectants are designed for oilier and combination skin types. Again, the amount of emollient will depend on the amount of oil being produced by the skin.

Hydrating fluids that are designed for younger skin types or oily adult skin may contain very little emollient. They usually contain just enough emollient to serve as a vehicle to spread the product onto the skin. Special emollients have been designed to be used in hydrating agents for oily skin. These emollients are specially designed so that they do not clog the pores or occlude the skin. Some emollient creams can cause problems for clog-prone or problem skin. More about these chemicals will be discussed in Chapter 13, Comedogenicity.

Bioavailable means able to be easily used by the skin.

Superoxide dismutase is a free radical scavenger that is an enzyme normally present in the body.

Liposomed tocopherol (vitamin E) is an encapsulated type of vitamin E that is protected from oxidation and theorized to be more beneficial to the skin than non-protected tocopherol, which tends to oxidize before applied to the skin.

Tocopheryl acetate is another protected form of vitamin E that is converted to tocopherol after it is applied to the skin.

Ascorbic acid is an acid form of vitamin C, an antioxidant; necessary for collagen production.

Magnesium ascorbyl phosphate is a stabilized ester of vitamin C, useful antioxidant and melanin suppressor.

Grapeseed extract is a powerful antioxidant with soothing properties.

Green tea extract is a powerful antioxidant and soothing agent.

Retinol is a natural form of vitamin A, appears to regulate skin function, and is theorized to be necessary for skin cell generation.

Coenzyme Q-10 is an enzyme and antioxidant that occurs naturally in the skin; presence decreases with aging. It is theorized to have revitalizing properties.

Cascade is a chain of related chemical reactions.

PLANT EXTRACTS

Hundreds of plant extracts are used as performance ingredients in cosmetics. Plant extracts are generally liquids that are pressed, boiled, or chemically extracted from different plants.

Most plant extracts are used because of their anecdotal properties.

In other words, they are reputed to cause changes in the skin. More and more of these extracts have been shown in scientific studies to be very helpful in treating different skin problems. Some have had little, if any, scientific research performed on them to determine exactly how they work.

Plant extracts are simply natural complexes of various chemicals. Many estheticians like them because they are "natural." Nevertheless, they are chemicals. Sometimes they are a large number of chemicals together in one extract. Some of these chemicals are very helpful to the skin in helping with appearance changes and conditioning.

Plant extracts are normally used in relatively small quantities in cosmetics. Usually they are listed as an extract, but if they are in a solution of water or alcohol, which most of them are, they may be listed near the top of the ingredient label. This simply means that water is the main ingredient in the extracts and that the extracts have been prepared before the formula was actually combined.

SPECIAL ADDITIVES

Special ingredients are often added to humectant and emollient products. Many of these agents are soothing agents that are added because they have the capability of reducing irritation to the skin.

Azulene is a hydrocarbon that is derived from the chamomile flower. It is an intense blue color and is frequently added to products designed for sensitive skin.

Bisabolol is another active agent that is added to cosmetics designed for sensitive skin. Aloe is also known for its soothing properties. Other agents often added for their soothing properties include:

Allantoin—derived from the comfrey root
Balm mint extract
Calendula extract
Camphor
Chamomile extract
Dipotassium glycyrrhizonate
Mallow extract
Licorice extract
Zinc oxide
Rice starch
Stearyl glycyrrhitinate
Cornstarch

These ingredients may be added not only to moisturizers and hydrating creams, but also to cleansers, masks, toners, and other cosmetic preparations.

OILY SKIN PRODUCTS

Active agents used for oily skin may be used for several purposes. They may be used as peeling agents to help prevent the buildup of cells that can cause clogged pores and acne breakouts in oily skin. Some agents serve as astringents that help to temporarily tighten enlarged pores, making the skin look smother. Other ingredients may be added for their soothing properties to help calm reddened skin associated with acne breakouts.

Lemon extract is used frequently in products for oily skin. It has good cleansing and oil removing properties. Lemon extract is less affected by the extraction process than some plant extracts. Lemon contains ascorbic acid, which is a good free radical neutralizer.

Tannic acid is an astringent ingredient found in tea and many plant extracts.

Many extracts contain **tannic acid**, which is an astringent. Some of these extracts, which are frequently used in oily skin products, are lappa extract, horse chestnut extract, birch extract, and nettle extract. Other extracts with astringent properties are cornflower extract, sage extract, saponaria, chamomile, and rosemary extract. Strong astringents may also contain isopropyl alcohol, SD alcohol, or potassium alum. These extracts may be used in toners, cleansers, or conditioning creams or lotions.

Treatment products for oily skin are usually oil-in-water emulsions, heavily water-based. They normally contain fewer emollients than those products intended for dry skin, and are often in lotion form rather than cream form, due to their large amounts of water. Other ingredients may be added as general conditioning, soothing, or healing agents. These include panthenol, allantoin, and aloe vera.

SPECIAL INGREDIENTS FOR PROBLEM AND ACNE-PRONE SKIN

Many of the same principles of product formulation are applied for problem skin as for oily skin. Problem skin more often requires the addition of chemicals that are stronger peeling agents and antiseptics. Often these ingredients are added to cosmetics designed for problem skin. However, no claim is made on these products; they are meant to be cosmetics, not drugs.

Exfoliants

Exfoliants usually come in the form of scrubs. They are water-based products with a humectant mixed with some sort of abrasive agent such as almond meal or polyethylene granules.

Keratolytic or **proteolytic** means "protein dissolving," and these agents work by dissolving keratin protein within dead surface cells, helping to remove these cells and making the skin look clearer and smoother.

An **exfoliant** is an ingredient that helps remove dead cells from the skin's surface. **Keratolytic** or **proteolytic** means "protein dissolving," and these agents work by dissolving keratin protein within dead surface cells. Alphahydroxy acids, including glycolic and lactic acids, are often grouped with keratolytic ingredients, even though they actually work by dissolving or loosening surface intercellular cement that holds cells together. Exfoliants may help the skin and its appearance by removing rough, dead surface cells, making the skin look smoother and more refined. As we have already discussed, some exfoliants help with cell renewal, improving moisture content and the barrier function of the skin. On an oily or acne-prone skin, they work by loosening pore impaction and removing dead cells within the follicles to treat and prevent hyperkeratosis that can cause acne lesions.

There are many ingredients that are exfoliants. Glycolic, lactic, tartaric, and malic acids are alphahydroxy acids. Salicylic acid is a betahydroxy acid and is used in both products for both oily skin and aging skin, and in higher concentrations as an active drug ingredient and antiseptic for acne treatment. Willow bark extract contains a large concentration of salicylic acid, as does wintergreen. Sugarcane, passionflower, apple, and grape extracts may contain natural alphahydroxy acids. Benzoyl peroxide, sulfur, and resorcinol are strong exfoliants used to help flush dead cell buildup from the follicles, helping to oxygenate the follicle and kill anaerobic acne bacteria. We will discuss more about these exfoliants in Chapter 12, Acne and the Esthetician.

OTHER SPECIAL INGREDIENTS

Clays, such as bentonite, kaolin, hectorite, and silica, are used in masks for their tightening and drawing effects and also in drying lotions for acne treatment. Another ingredient used frequently as a drawing agent is magnesium aluminum silicate.

Enzymes are used in treatments to dissolve keratin protein in dead surface cells, helping to eliminate dull, dry appearance, as well as help oily, clogged skin. These treatments are often called enzyme peels or exfoliation treatments.

Papain is a keratolytic enzyme derived from papaya. Bromelain, also an enzyme, comes from pineapple. Pancreatin is an enzyme from beef pancreas, a side product of meat processing, and is also a useful keratolytic often used in enzyme exfoliation treatment products.

CONCLUSION

Hundreds of chemicals are used as performance ingredients in cosmetics. Some active agents, as you have seen, are also vehicles and have more than one function in a cosmetic.

We have touched on only a few performance ingredients, but you will be able to use this knowledge to understand ingredient labels and their functions. With additional study, you should eventually be able to pick up a product and, simply by reading the ingredient label, know what kind of product it is and for what skin problem it is intended.

Topics for Discussion

1. What is a performance ingredient? How does it differ from an active ingredient?
2. What are the two basic types of cleansing ingredients? Discuss the products in which each is used.
3. What are natural moisturizing factors? Name some that are used in cosmetics.
4. Discuss some ingredients used to help aging skin.
5. What are free radicals?
6. Discuss some ingredients used to treat oily skin and problem acne skin.

Chapter

10

Skin-Care Products

Objectives

After the esthetician graduates from school, he or she will be amazed at the variety of skin-care products available. This chapter discusses various types of skin-care products available, products for different skin types and problems, and the chemical makeup of products for different skin types.

Although this chapter provides only an overview of the products available, it will teach the esthetician about factors involved in choosing products for various skin problems and clients' needs.

In Chapters 8 and 9 you have learned about various ingredients used in manufacturing cosmetics. Now you will learn about practical application of various formulas of cleansers, toners, creams, and other products.

There are literally hundreds and hundreds of different products available to estheticians. These are products that you will both use in the treatment room and recommend that your clients use at home. It is important to carry a variety of products to sell to your clients for home use. There are many good esthetic product manufacturers, and the most successful skin-care salons carry lines made by at least two or three of them. There is no one line that is the answer to every problem you will see.

A VISIT TO THE PRODUCT STOCKROOM

Let's take a trip to the stockroom of a successful skin-care salon. We will not talk about name brands, but we will talk about various products available in chemical terms. You will be able to use what you have learned. Remember, a primary objective is for you to be able to read ingredient labels and tell what kind of product you are examining, and for what skin type it is intended. As we look into this imaginary stockroom, we will look at various types of products. There are enough types of products in this stockroom to handle most esthetic problems (Figure 10–1).

The most important factor in prescribing the right home care for your clients is your education and knowledge of skin analysis. Make sure you receive good training in analysis. It is one of the biggest keys to success in esthetics.

Before we enter the imaginary stockroom, it must be understood that many products are available to the esthetician, and new products are developed every year. We will cover only a portion of the products available, but this will be a representative sampling of what is frequently used in skin-care salons.

CLEANSERS

As we enter the stockroom, the first thing you notice is the wide assortment of cleansers. There are both milk-type cleansers and rinseable detergent-type foaming cleansers, as well as some specialty cleansers for acne and clog-prone skin.

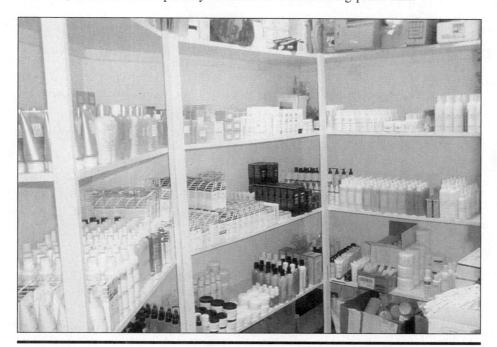

Figure 10–1   A well-organized stockroom full of supplies is important to the esthetics practice.

Let's talk about rinseable cleansers first. Rinseable cleansers usually come in a tube, sometimes in a bottle. They vary in strength and texture. Rinseable cleansers are important to carry because you will find that many clients are used to washing their faces with bar soap, like the foaming action, and do not "feel clean" unless they have "washed" their faces.

Product Profile: Rinseable Cleanser for Oily and Combination Skin

Client and Skin Type: The first rinseable cleanser we will look at is a rinseable cleanser for oily and combination skin. Clients with oily and combination skin are especially fond of rinseable cleansers because these clients need some detergent to help cut excess amounts of oil. However, we don't want our cleanser to overdry them or strip the acid mantle.

Product Characteristics: This particular cleanser is in a tube. The product consistency feels almost like soap. When the client adds water, it begins to foam moderately. It rinses completely, leaving the skin feeling fresh and clean, but not too tight. This clean but not tight feeling is a good sign that the product is pH balanced correctly for the skin type.

Chemical Action and Design: Chemically this product uses disodium lauryl sulfosuccinate as a detergent-surfactant. It also contains smaller amounts of avocado oil and cetyl alcohol, emollient ingredients added to cut the detergent action on the skin's surface so that it will not be stripping. This cleanser is also fragrance-free, a helpful characteristic when treating sensitive skin. This cleanser is a good recommendation for adult oily and combination skin or for clients who are used to heavier moisturizers but really need to switch to a lighter program for oily or combination skin (Figure 10–2a).

Product Profile: Rinseable Cleanser for Dry and Combination Skin

Client and Skin Type: This cleanser is designed for clients who have dry skin, but still want the action of a detergent cleanser. This cleanser will be good for an older client with dry skin who prefers soap over milk cleanser.

Product Characteristics: This rinseable cleanser is also packaged in a tube. It foams very slightly. It rinses well, but leaves the skin feeling very soft. This cleanser will not be aggressive enough for oily-combination skin. However, for more alipidic skin it is excellent.

Chemical Action and Design: If you look at the ingredient label of this product you will notice that its detergent agent, sodium lauryl sulfate, is listed about halfway down the list of ingredients. This means that the product is not nearly as strong a cleanser as the first cleanser. The ingredients listed after water are different types of emollients, fatty alcohols, and esters. This cleanser contains lots of emollients because it is designed for dry skin. The large amounts of emollients will keep the detergents from stripping too much lipid from the skin's surface. This product is superfatted (Figure 10–2b).

Product Profile: Rinseable Cleanser for Very Oily Skin

Client and Skin Type: This stronger rinseable cleanser is designed for clients who have very oily skin. Their skin is covered with enlarged pores, and they almost never have any dryness or dehydration. This type of client is extremely oily by 10 or 11 o'clock in the morning.

Product Characteristics: This cleanser is a liquid in a bottle. It has almost the consistency of shampoo. It foams quite strongly and rinses thoroughly, leaving the skin feeling very clean. It is much too strong for any skin type except extremely oily skin.

Chemical Action and Design: The active detergent in this rinseable cleanser is an anionic surfactant called ammonium laureth sulfate. This cleanser contains some glycolic

> **INGREDIENTS:** Deionized Water, Mineral Oil, Cetyl Alcohol,Sodium Lauryl Sulfate, Cetearyl Alcohol, Ceteth-20, Imidazolidinyl Urea, Methyl Paraben.

a

> **INGREDIENTS:** Deionized Water, Disodium Lauryl Sulfosuccinate, Cetyl Alcohol, Ceteth-20, Propylene Glycol, Avocado Oil, Methylparaben, DMDM Hydantoin.

b

Which cleanser is stronger? The first one is weaker. The surfactant (sodium lauryl sulfate) is buffered by dominating ingredients cetyl alcohol and mineral oil, which help to prevent too much contact with the surfactant. In the second formulation, the surfactant (Disodium lauryl sulfosuccinate) is diluted only by water as a larger percentage ingredient. The further the surfactant is down the list, the weaker the cleansing action. The first product is designed for dry-combination skin, and the second is for oily-combination skin.

Figure 10–2 Sample ingredient labels for cleansers

acid, which, in a cleanser, is helpful in loosening surface cells. Glycolic and other alphahydroxy acids can be used in cleansers, but, of course, are rinsed off and do not have the same long-term conditioning effects as AHAs that are used in leave-on products. This cleanser is mixed with gelling agents to form shampoo-like consistency. The surfactant concentration in a cleanser such as this is somewhat higher than other rinseable detergent cleansers that are designed for less oily skins. There are no emollients in this product, and therefore the product has no buffer against stripping oil from the skin's surface. However, this is appropriate for a cleanser that is designed for very oily skin.

Product Profile: Rinseable Medicated Cleanser for Acne

Client and Skin Type: This cleanser is made for mild to moderate acne, excessively oily, and chronic acne-prone skin. This type of skin is not sensitive and is fairly thick, due to the accumulation of corneocytes on the surface of the skin. This client may have a currently active acne condition or may tend to develop moderate acne frequently. This product may also be excellent for teenage acne.

Product Characteristics: This cleanser is very similar to the one designed for chronically oily skin, except that it contains an antimicrobial agent to kill bacteria. Medicated cleansers such as this are usually registered as over-the-counter drugs. (See Chapter 11, Claims in Cosmetics.) It is a strong foaming cleanser. It may also be made to be an exfoliant, depending on the ingredients.

Chemical Action and Design: Benzoyl peroxide may serve as the antimicrobial in a product like this, or another antimicrobial such as salicylic acid, sulfur, or hexetidine may be used. Benzoyl peroxide (see Chapter 12, Acne and the Esthetician) is also a keratolytic agent, as is salicylic acid, which serves to lightly peel away dead corneocytes from the surface of the skin as well as flush the follicular canal. Some products like this cleanser may also contain a mechanical exfoliant such as polyethylene granules. These small, bead-like granules are used in the cleanser because they are gritty and literally "bump off" dead cell buildup.

As you move across the shelf from the rinseable cleanser, you may notice a variety of milk cleansers in several different colors. As you look closer, you notice that these cleansers are designed for a variety of skin types.

Product Profile: Milk Cleanser for Oily and Combination Skin

Client and Skin Type: This cleanser is an emulsion to be used for makeup removal on oily and combination skin. Milk cleanser for acne and extremely oily skin is rarely used, at least not by itself. For acne, a milk cleanser may be used strictly as a makeup remover, followed by a rinseable detergent cleanser for extra cleansing action. This cleansing milk is a good choice for the older person with oily or combination skin who has a tendency toward oiliness and minor but persistent breakout problems. This type of client may find twice daily cleansings with detergents to be too dehydrating. Older skin tends to dehydrate much more easily than younger skin. This skin type may use a rinseable cleanser in the morning and then a gentler milk for nightly makeup removal.

Product Characteristics: This milk is a water-based fluid. It is slightly slippery to the touch and leaves the skin feeling fairly clean when removed. This product should be applied and removed with a room temperature damp sponge cloth or cleansing sponge. It is necessary with all cleansing milks to use a very soft cloth to apply and remove these cleansers, because they do not contain much detergent, if any, and do not rinse as easily as detergent cleansers. This cleanser, however, rinses well when used with a sponge or sponge cloth. Makeup is removed very easily with this product. This product should not be used on the eyes, because it is designed for oily and combination skin and is not chemically appropriate for the eye area (Figure 10–3).

Chemical Action and Design: The emollients used in this cleanser are tridecyl stearate, neopentylglycol dicaprate/dicaprylate, and tridecyl trimellitate, which are a complex of emollients designed to be a noncomedogenic oil replacement. They do not clog the skin and are easily removed from the skin. The emollients mix with the dirt,

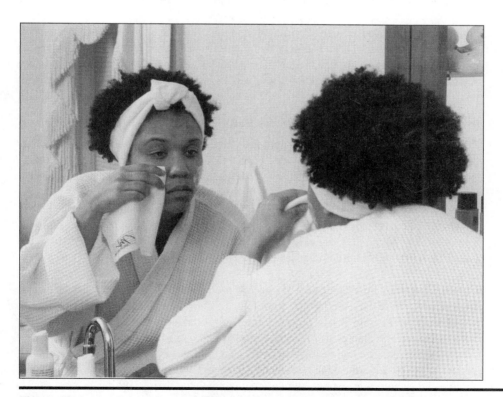

Figure 10–3   A soft chamois cloth is used for makeup removal. *Courtesy Correlations, Inc.*

makeup, and oils and work to dissolve these foreign materials so they may be removed from the skin's surface. This product has a pH of about 7.0, typical of a cleanser designed for oily and combination skin. The slightly higher pH helps the cleanser be a more aggressive solvent. The cleansing process should be followed by a lower pH toner to lower the pH and remove any film left from the emollient.

Product Profile: Cleansing Milk for Combination Skin

Client and Skin Type: This thicker cleansing emulsion is made for clients who wear heavier makeup and therefore need a more oily cleanser to dissolve the thicker, oilier makeup. This cleanser is often prescribed for older clients with combination skin. It is considerably heavier than many other cleansing milks. This cleanser may also be used frequently by actors and other performers who wear heavier stage makeup routinely.

Product Characteristics: This cleanser is a thicker liquid in a bottle. It absolutely must be used with a sponge or a soft cloth. Otherwise, it would leave a residue on the skin. Its emollients dissolve makeup very readily, making it an excellent product for heavy makeup wearers. This product should be followed by a toner designed for combination skin. The toner needs to be strong enough to remove any residue left from this cleanser.

Chemical Action and Design: Petrolatum and mineral oil are the secrets of the slipperiness of this cleanser. There is enough emulsifier in this product to make it relatively thick. The petrolatum makes the product physically heavy. Mineral oil mixed with petrolatum is an excellent makeup dissolver. Plant extracts have been added to this product for soothing.

Product Profile: Cleansing Milk for Sensitive Skin

Client and Skin Type: This lightweight milk cleanser is designed for sensitive skin. It is designed for the client with thin, fragile skin that reddens easily. It is not specifically designed for oily skin; its emollient content is meant more for dry, irritated skin. The client who has sensitive, thin skin can use this product.

Product Characteristics: This is a lightweight cleansing milk designed to be used with a soft cloth or sponge. It does not leave much residue when rinsed and has very little fragrance. It will remove liquid makeup well.

Chemical Action and Design: This water-based cleanser combines relatively large amount of water with a mixture of emollients to dissolve makeup. It does not contain a traditional emulsifier. It is a physical emulsion, blended by homogenization. As we have discussed in Chapter 8, traditional emulsifiers can impair barrier function when used on sensitive skin, increasing reactivity. Using cleansers that are physically emulsified will not further damage an already thin barrier. This cleanser contains azulene, bisabolol, and chamomile extract, which are included for their soothing properties. No fragrance is used because of allergy potentials. The only fragrance is from the plant extract used.

Product Profile: Cleansing Milk for Dry Skin

Client and Skin Type: Dry, mature skin will benefit from the use of this fairly light-weight milk for dry skin.

Product Characteristics: Again, this product should be applied and removed with a damp, soft cloth. This cleanser is slightly richer to the touch than our other milk cleansers. It does leave a residue if not carefully removed and should be used with a toner designed for dry skin.

Chemical Action and Design: The ultra-rich emollient oils in this cleanser are added to help condition the surface of the skin while cleansing, helping to avoid overstripping of the natural oils. It contains no detergents, which can strip older alipidic skin.

Some skin-care companies add expensive conditioners to cleansing product. These conditioning ingredients are normally used in creams, lotions, and fluids that are in the form of day or night treatments. In other words, they stay on the face for long periods of time. Many cosmetic scientists believe that it is useless to include expensive conditioning ingredients in cleansers, because they simply do not stay on the face long enough to do any good. Soothing agents and agents that are meant to strengthen or weaken the action of the cleanser are the only type of these agents that should be added.

TONERS

Toners, clarifying lotions, fresheners, and astringents are all basically the same type of product. Products that are titled "astringents" are considered to be OTC (over-the-counter) drugs. Toners vary in strength, drying ability, and alcohol content. They are made for three specific reasons:

1. They remove excess cleanser and residue from liquid cleansers.
2. They have a relatively low pH, helping to adjust the pH of the acid mantle after cleansing so it is not overstripped.
3. It provides a temporary tightening effect to both the skin as well as the individual follicle openings, helping to temporarily shrink "pores."

Product Profile: Toner for Oily and Combination Skin

Client and Skin Type: This toner is designed for oily and combination skin. It is good for the client who develops clogs easily but still needs a hydrating moisturizer. Adult oily-combination skin will benefit from this toner.

Product Characteristics: This toner is a clear, water-based liquid. It should be applied with a predampened cotton pad, a sponge, or a soft cloth after using a rinseable cleanser or cleansing milk, or can be atomized onto the skin with a fine-mist sprayer. Sprayers have become popular in nonalcoholic toners because they are so convenient to use. Sprayers cannot be used in toners containing alcohol because of possible accidental contact with the eyes. This toner has a lemon fragrance. After use, the skin feels clean and toned but not dry. Pores do seem to shrink after using this product. Men can also use this product as an aftershave. It is a good product for men, because it is not femininely fragranced and has enough astringent action for after shaving. This will help constrict the follicles, helping to keep the hair pointed in an outward direction so it does not become an **ingrown hair** by growing into the side of the follicle wall.

Ingrown hair is an infected follicle caused by a hair that grows into the side of the follicle wall.

Chemical Action and Design: The low pH in this toner is due to a combination of citric acid and lemon extract, which has an astringent action. It is blended into a liquid with mostly water, but also contains a glycerin derivative, which is a humectant that helps to restore water to dehydrated skin.

Product Profile: Toner for Extremely Oily Skin

Client and Skin Type: This toner is made for skin that becomes very oily after only a short period of time and has very large pores that clog very easily. This client never gets dehydrated because the skin is so oily. The client uses a strong, rinseable cleanser for very oily skin, which we discussed earlier. This toner should be applied on a predampened cotton pad or damp sponge.

Product Characteristics: This toner is a water-based liquid that is used after cleansing milk or rinseable cleanser. It has a strong astringent action. It leaves the skin feeling very clean and tight. Application to dry skin would be too drying.

Chemical Action and Design: This oily skin astringent contains plant extracts for oily skin as well as sulfur, a keratolytic peeling agent, and potassium alum, a strong astringent agent. They are in a base vehicle of water and propylene glycol, a hydrating agent.

Product Profile: Astringent for Acne-Prone Skin

Client and Skin Type: This very strong astringent is made for inflamed acne and extremely oily skin. It is a good product for teenage acne, grades II and III. (See Chapter 12, Acne and the Esthetician.)

Product Characteristics: This astringent is a light-colored liquid and has a strong medicinal (alcohol) odor. It is applied with a damp cotton ball after cleansing. It is very stripping, removes lots of sebum, and is very drying to the skin. It may burn or tingle slightly when applied, especially if applied to open acne lesions. Some extremely oily skin needs this much oil removal.

Chemical Action and Design: This product is actually an over-the-counter drug. Isopropyl alcohol is the active ingredient for its astringent properties and also for its oil-stripping action. Isopropyl alcohol and water are the main ingredients in this liquid astringent. Witch hazel distillate provides astringent properties and temporary pore "tightening." Camphor is included as a soothing agent.

Product Profile: Toner for Normal Skin

Client and Skin Type: This toner is a medium-strength tonic designed for normal and sensitive skin. It is for adult skin that basically needs moderate hydrating and has no particular problems.

Product Characteristics: This toner is a liquid and has a very mild astringent action. It does not pull on the skin. It has a moist feeling when applied. It has a slight soothing effect on the skin. It is applied with cool, wet, cotton pads after cleansing.

Chemical Action and Design: This is a very simple formula made with water, rosewater, propylene glycol (as a humectant), cucumber extract for soothing, and allantoin. It contains a smaller amount of witch hazel extract than toners for oily skin.

Product Profile: Toner for Extra-Dry Skin

Client and Skin Type: Dry, mature skin is the type of skin that this toner will help. It has moisturizing properties as well as helping gently remove traces of cleanser from dry, sensitive skin. This type of dry skin can become so dehydrated that the face becomes very tight even after a very gentle cleanser. This toner is designed for dry skin that becomes tender after cleansing. This cleanser should be used after cleansing, and applied with a cool, damp cotton pad.

Product Characteristics: This a very moist toner, almost soft to the touch. It has practically no astringent action. It is designed to moisturize the skin with humectants that provide a buffer so that the skin will not become stripped if the toner is used after cleansing.

Chemical Action and Design: A large amount of butylene glycol provides humectant effects for the skin in this water-based, fluid toner. Glycerin also has hydrating action on the surface of the dry skin. Extracts of chamomile, mallow, and cornflower are included for their softening and soothing properties. This is an unusually moisturizing toner.

DAY CREAMS AND TREATMENTS

Day creams are made for various skin types. Treatments for everything from acne to extremely dry and aging skin are available. These products vary greatly in texture and thickness, depending on the amount of fats or emollients that are added.

Sunscreen is probably the biggest health benefit that can be contained in a day cream. Besides preventing premature aging of the skin, using sunscreen is one of the best ways to help prevent skin cancer. Many day creams are also sunscreens, making them OTC drugs. Because sunscreen is such an important feature and benefit, it is becoming traditional to combine broad-spectrum UVA-UVB protection in day treatment products. Sunscreen products' ingredient labels always have the sunscreen agents listed first as active ingredients and then have other ingredients listed afterwards. It is illegal to claim sunscreen protection and not list active sunscreen ingredients on the product label.

Day creams usually contain either an occlusive agent or some sort of protectant ingredient that helps hold water in the surface layers of the skin. They may also contain various hydrating agents, emollients, or other active agents, depending on the skin type for which they are intended.

Product Profile: Day Sunscreen Protection Fluid for Oily and Combination Skin

Client and Skin Type: This product is designed for oily and combination skin. Clients who have oily skin appreciate this product because it does not feel oily or greasy and is noncomedogenic. It is a good choice for 20- to 50-year-old clients who develop clogged pores easily. This product is a good choice for people who need hydrating but become oily easily. These clients generally have trouble with their makeup not staying on well and becoming oily during the day. The lack of many emollients in this cream will benefit the client who prefers a light-textured, non-heavy day product. This will also serve well as a daytime moisturizer-protectant for oily skins during the winter months.

Product Characteristics: This lightweight day protection fluid comes in a tube. It is not a thick product and feels very light and non-greasy when touched. It absorbs quickly, helping to hydrate the skin and protect against daytime water loss, and contains SPF-15 sunscreen to shield against routine daily sun exposure during daily activities. It is applied with the fingertips in the morning before makeup, or alone. It is noncomedogenic, which means that it has been tested and found not to clog pores. This product is unusual because it hydrates, protects, conditions, contains two sunscreens, and is noncomedogenic.

Chemical Action and Design: This fluid is water-based, with small amounts of noncomedogenic emollients added. These emollients are tridecyl stearate, tridecyl trimellitate, neopentylglycol dicaprate/dicaprylate, and glyceryl stearate. The active humectants that help to bind water in this fluid are glycerin and sodium PCA. Other conditioning agents include allantoin, cornflower extract, tocopherol, and retinyl palmitate. Methoxycinnimate and titanium dioxide are the sunscreen ingredients, and dimethicone is used as a water-loss shielding agent because of its lightweight characteristics.

Product Profile: Day Cream for Dry and Dehydrated Skin

Client and Skin Type: Designed for oil-dry (alipidic), dehydrated, sensitive skin, this cream will help the client who becomes dry very easily due to lack of oil production. It is for clients who have a slight amount of oiliness through the T-zone, but the large part of the outer perimeter of the face is dry and dehydrated.

Product Characteristics: This cream is packaged in a tube. It is definitely cream, containing a substantial amount of emollient. It contains a broad-spectrum SPF-15 sunscreen and a protective agent. It is not extremely greasy or heavy, so it may be worn by clients who prefer a lighter weight day cream. It is blue due to the azulene content. It should be applied under makeup or alone during the day.

Chemical Action and Design: This cream contains propylene glycol and aloe as hydrating agents. It contains dimethicone as a shielding protective agent and benzophenone, a UVA sunscreen, as well as methoxycinnimate and octyl salicylate UVB sunscreen. These active agents are mixed into a water-based blend of emollients, including lanolin, cetyl palmitate, and beeswax. Azulene provides help for soothing sensitive dehydrated skin.

Product Profile: Day Cream for Dry Skin with Telangiectasias (Couperose—Enlarged Capillaries)

Client and Skin Type: The dry, adult, sun-damaged client will appreciate this product. This product is specifically designed to help skin with many enlarged red capillaries seen easily on the face. It helps to soothe the redness and minimizes the appearance of the capillaries.

Product Characteristics: This is a fairly heavy cream due to its emollient content. It is applied under makeup or alone. It comes in a tube. This cream is not for oily skin due to its large amount of emollients.

Chemical Action and Design: The performance ingredient in this cream that helps lessen the appearance of the redness and soothes the skin is horse chestnut extract. Oxybenzone and benzophenone are included as sunscreen agents, and titanium dioxide, a pigment, is contained for both sunscreen and coverage purposes. The main part of the cream is a water-based glycerin emulsion, with isopropyl myristate and glycerl stearate as emollients. It contains a large amount of coloring agent, designed to cut down on the appearance of redness.

NIGHT CREAMS AND TREATMENTS

Night treatment creams are normally extraintensive treatment products designed to help hydrate and condition skin during the night, a time when normal tissue repair is taking place all over the body, including the skin. Night treatments are often heavier in consistency and texture than day products. They normally contain more emollient than day cream and are not made for use under makeup. Night creams should be applied all over the skin, according to manufacturer's instructions. It is important that the skin be thoroughly cleansed before night treatment is applied.

ABOUT AMPOULES

Ampoules are designed to be extraintensive, concentrated extracts. They often contain larger amounts of performance ingredients in a water base. Occasionally they are in an oil base. They are to be applied under a night cream or fluid.

Ampoules are available for a wide variety of skin types and problems. Some are designed to be used in a series once a month or several times a year. Others are designed to be used nightly. The advantage of ampoules is they provide active ingredients in concentration in a measured amount. They generally have positive effects on the skin's appearance. They are native to Europe, where the concept was invented. Many American lines do not have ampoule treatments.

The disadvantages of ampoules are that they are more trouble to use than night cream or fluid and they are generally more expensive to use than night creams and fluids. However, clients who are extremely conscientious about their home care will often take the time to use ampoules, and not mind paying the extra expense.

Product Profile: Night Treatment Fluid for Oily, Dehydrated Skin

Client and Skin Type: This fluid is made to provide hydration to adult oily skin that is also dehydrated. It can be used on oily and combination skin. These clients are normally adults who need to use a hydrating agent, but develop clogged pores and break out easily. This fluid has been laboratory tested and found to be noncomedogenic. It is also ideal for the client who prefers a lighter weight night treatment.

Product Characteristics: Due to its low emollient content, this fluid is very light in texture and feel. It does not feel oily at all because it contains mostly humectants to attract water to the skin, rather than oils and fats that will clog this type of skin. This fluid comes in a tube and should be applied in moderate amounts to the entire skin before bedtime.

Chemical Action and Design: This fluid contains sodium PCA, a natural moisturizing factor (NMF), and glycerin as hydrating agents. It also includes allantoin, retinyl palmirate, and tocopherol in its formula for their conditioning properties. This fluid has been carefully designed without comedogenic ingredients (see Chapter 13, Comedogenicity), to avoid clogging the oily and combination skin for which it is intended. The emollients added are tridecyl stearate, tridecyl trimellitate, and neopentylglycol dicaprate/dicaprylate. This fluid adds hydration to the skin without adding excess emollients that cause buildup of cells, which cause clogs to form.

Product Profile: Night Treatment for Oily, Clogged, Adult Skin

Client and Skin Type: This product is designed for oily skin or oily, clogged areas. It is for clients who have a tendency to break out, but find that most drying agents overdry. Adult acne can benefit from this type of product because it incorporates both a peeling agent and a hydrating agent as well as a protectant. This product is also ideal for an adult oily skin client who is used to using heavy moisturizers that are clogging the skin. It feels like a moisturizer but is actually a very light peeling agent.

Product Characteristics: This lightweight product has an unusual texture somewhere between a gel and a cream. It is very light and dries quickly when applied. It has a matte dry feeling when used. It should be applied in the evening after cleansing and toning. It takes the place of moisturizer and can be used under makeup or alone.

Chemical Action and Design: Salicylic acid, a betahydroxy acid, is used in a very small quantity in this product to promote some exfoliation. This product contains glycerin and propylene glycol as humectants, and dimethicone provides protection against excess water loss.

Product Profile: Night Hydrating Cream for Combination Mature Skin

Client and Skin Type: Designed for older oily and combination skins that need hydration, but do not need extra oils, this lightweight cream is good for older clients who still have a tendency to break out. It provides hydration without oiliness. This cream could also be used as a night treatment for younger, extra-dehydrated skin types. The cream is laboratory tested to be noncomedogenic.

Product Characteristics: The cream is extremely lightweight and is absorbed by the skin easily. After use the skin feels smooth and "plumped up." It is contained in a tube and should be applied to clean skin before bedtime. It contains no color or fragrance, which is helpful for sensitive and allergy-prone skin.

Chemical Action and Design: Sorbitol is the main hydrating agent in this cream and is present in a large concentration. Sorbitol is combined with lecithin, another good hydrator readily accepted by the skin. Lecithin is the phospholipid material that liposomes are made of, but this cream is not liposomic. It uses the lecithin to retain water in the surface layers, making the cream easily penetrating. It contains the conditioners retinyl palmitate and tocopherol acetate, both reputed to help neutralize free radicals. The cream is formulated to be noncomedogenic.

Product Profile: Night Moisturizing Lotion for Dehydrated Combination Dry Skin

Client and Skin Type: This lotion is formulated to help skin that is both oil- and water-dry. This type of skin has a very narrow T-zone with little oil production or visible pore structure. Most clients will be mature women.

Product Characteristics: This treatment is a lotion and is packaged in a bottle. It is slightly oily to the touch, leaving a slight film on the surface of the skin. This characteristic is helpful for drier skin types. It is a light blue color, due to its azulene content. It should be applied before bedtime.

Chemical Action and Design: The lotion contains a mixture of oils, emollients, and humectants, providing both hydration and oils for the oil-dry skin. It contains the humectants urea, propylene glycol, and butylene glycol, and is mixed with sesame oil, peanut oil, and various emollient esters and fats. Because it contains a good amount of both hydrator and oils, it contains sodium lauryl sulfate, used as an emulsifier to keep the oils in the water-based emulsion.

Product Profile: Night Cream for Dry Skin

Client and Skin Type: Oil-dry, dehydrated, mature skin is the target for this heavier cream. This type of client is very dry for most of the year and needs a richer cream.

Product Characteristics: This cream comes in a tube. It is fairly heavy and leaves an emollient residue on the skin when applied. This film stays on skin all night. It is fragranced.

Chemical Action and Design: This cream is a mixture of humectants and emollients, containing large amounts of the latter. The active ingredient in this cream is the substantive collagen and elastin proteins, which sit on the skin's surface and help hold water. This protein is mixed with the emollients beeswax, isopropyl myristate, and cetyl alcohol. It contains petrolatum in a fairly large amount, giving it an occlusive property.

Product Profile: Night Cream for Dry, Dehydrated Skin

Client and Skin Type: This night treatment is for adult dry, dehydrated skin.

Product Characteristics: Liposomes are the feature of this cream, mixing a combination of oils, emollients, and humectants in a heavier cream that absorbs well. This fragranced cream comes in a jar. It should be applied nightly for best results. This is a sophisticated treatment complex, with many active agents, making it a more expensive cream.

Chemical Action and Design: Hydrators, emollients, conditioners, and plant extracts are present in this complex night treatment. It is designed to deliver deep hydration through its lecithin (liposome) content, helping to retain moisture for a longer period of time. It contains urea, mucopolysaccharides, and sorbitol as humectants. This is mixed into a variety of emollients including mineral oil, jojoba oil, cetyl alcohol, shea butter, and capric/caprylic triglycerides. This cream is actually available in two different formulas, one for drier skin and another for combination dry skin.

Many other types of night treatments are not covered here. Most night hydrators and creams vary in both amounts of hydrating agents and amounts of emollient. Therefore they range in design for oily, dehydrated skin to very dry skin that is both oil- and water-dry. The oilier the skin, the less emollient. The drier the skin, the more emollient. Night creams will also vary in price, mainly because of the amount and type of ingredients used. Ingredients such as lecithin, liposomes, beta glucans, and hyaluronic acid are expensive (Figure 10–4).

SPECIAL CREAMS AND TREATMENTS

Many treatment creams are available for special problems or special areas. These treatments should be used in conjunction with other day and night treatments. These include

Figure 10–4 Bottle A has more oil and emollient for dry skin. Bottle B has less oil and more hydration for dehydrated, oilier skin.

performance-oriented products like alphahydroxy acid formulations, antioxidant serums, melanin suppressant OTC formulations, and acne care treatment products.

Product Profile: Alphahydroxy Treatment for Dry, Sun-Damaged Skin

Client and Skin Type: This product is designed for dry, dehydrated mature skin that is wrinkled or sun damaged.

Product Characteristics: This is a very emollient, thicker cream that contains multiple alphahydroxy acids. It is in a jar and should be applied after cleansing and toning and before sunscreen or night hydration cream. SPF-15 sunscreen should be used daily with this product.

Chemical Action and Design: Alphahydroxy acids—glycolic and lactic—and betahydroxy—citric acid—combined with fruit-derived hydroxy acids from sugarcane, orange, and apple extracts work to exfoliate dead cells and smooth surface wrinkles and lines. Long-term use helps with barrier function and moisture retention. Emollients include hydrogenated polyisobutene, cetyl alcohol, dimethicone, and polyacrylamide, an appropriate combination for a drier skin type. Green tea extract is present in a fairly large concentration to soothe potential irritation caused by this 10 percent acid blend. Even with a large emollient base, this product has tested noncomedogenic, and has been dermatologist tested for irritancy. These results may be helpful when deciding which client is best suited for this product. The pH of this product is 3.5, in compliance with the CIR recommendations discussed in Chapter 9, Active Agents and Performance Ingredients.

Product Profile: Alphahydroxy Treatment Gel for Oily-Combination, Clogged Skin

Client and Skin Type: This product is designed for any skin with clogged pores and oily or oily-combination skin. This product is appropriate for acne patients and acne-prone skin.

Product Characteristics: A liquid gel in a bottle, this 10 percent alphahydroxy and betahydroxy blend should be used on oily to combination skin once or twice a day to help improve clogged pores and impacted areas. SPF-15 sunscreen should be used daily with this product.

Chemical Action and Design: A 10 percent mixture of alphahydroxy acids—glycolic, lactic, tartaric, and malic—with betahydroxy acids—salicylic and citric—help to exfoliate the surface as well as the follicle, removing dead cell buildup and loosening pore accumulations. The gel base contains SD alcohol 40, aloe vera gel, and hydroxycellulose, which gives the product its gel-like feel. The pH of this product is 3.5 in compliance with the CIR recommendations discussed in Chapter 9, Active Agents and Performance Ingredients.

Product Profile: Lightening Treatment Gel for Hyperpigmented Skin

Client and Skin Type: This treatment gel is intended for clients who have splotchy hyperpigmentation, melasma, or chloasma on the face or hands.

Product Characteristics: A liquid gel in an amber bottle, this product should be applied every day for best results. Clients using this product must always wear an SPF-15 or 30 sunscreen, because the symptoms being treated are caused by sun exposure. This product oxidizes very quickly, easily turning brown, indicating decreased effectiveness.

Chemical Action and Design: An OTC drug, the active ingredient in this product is 2 percent hydroquinone, which suppresses production of melanin by the melanocytes in the basal layer of the epidermis. The gel also contains 10 percent glycolic acid, which helps remove stained surface cells, as well as magnesium ascorbyl phosphate, a vitamin C derivative antioxidant known for its melanin suppressive activity. Hydroquinone is a frequent allergen, and the product should be patch-tested before using on larger areas.

Product Profile: Alphahydroxy Treatment Gel for Oily-Combination, Clogged Skin

Client and Skin Type: This product is designed for acneic skin, grades I and II. Both adults and teenagers can use this product.

Product Characteristics: A lotion in a tube-bottle, this 5 percent benzoyl peroxide lotion is used at night only on active acne papules and pustules. A light application to all areas should be followed by dabbing a small amount on any raised lesions. Do not use in the eye area.

Chemical Action and Design: This is an OTC drug. A 5 percent concentration of benzoyl peroxide is the active ingredient, which helps flush and exfoliate debris from the follicle. The oxygen released from the benzoyl peroxide kills anaerobic *Propionibacterium acnes* bacteria. The lightweight, glycerin-based lotion is a simple emulsion that serves as a spreading agent for the benzoyl peroxide. Benzoyl peroxide acts as a bleach to fabric and hair. It can be irritating if overused, and some clients are allergic to it.

Eye creams are specially designed for the skin around the eye area. This area of the skin is usually more oil-dry and more sensitive than other areas of the skin. Therefore, creams designed for these areas are generally higher in emollient and lower in humectant content. Because the skin around the eyes is very thin, if you "plump it up" by using lots of hydrating agents, you end up making the eyelid look puffy. More emollient is added to these creams to help supplement the lack of oil production associated with the eye area. Because this area is very sensitive, eye creams must be carefully designed not to irritate. Nevertheless, eye creams often do cause irritation and allergic reactions. Eye creams should be used twice daily.

Neck creams are also made with more emollients and less humectant. The neck area has thinner skin that dries easily. Neck creams should be massaged into the skin twice daily. They are available in a variety of formulations.

Masks are designed to treat a variety of skin problems, from oil-dryness to acne. They are formulated with less water than creams, lotions, and fluids and are considerably heavier than any of these products.

Masks for oily skin generally contain bentonite and kaolin; these clays are helpful in absorbing excess oil and drying the skin. These clays cause the drying of masks designed for cleansing oilier and combination skin types. These masks may contain other conditioning ingredients. For example, for acne-prone skin the mask might contain sulfur, salicylic acid, or benzoyl peroxide. For oily and combination skin it might contain camphor for soothing and antiseptic action or cornstarch for soothing action.

Dry skin masks often do not dry tightly and contain large amounts of emollients. To give substance to the mask, the chemist may use titanium dioxide or may use a gelling agent or thickener to give the mask a thicker texture. These dry skin masks may contain a variety of plant extracts, conditioning agents, emollients, and humectants. They work by adding water to surface layers as well as emollients, helping to temporarily fill in or plump up small lines and wrinkles. They can have a lasting effect on the skin, particularly if

Eye creams are designed for the skin around the eye area.

Neck creams are made with more emollients and less humectant, because the neck area has thinner skin that dries easily.

Masks are designed to treat a variety of skin problems, from oil-dryness to acne.

Exfoliants usually come in the form of scrubs. They are water-based products with a humectant mixed with some sort of abrasive agent such as almond meal or polyethylene granules.

preceded by the use of a good humectant or other active agent. The effects may last up to several days.

Mechanical **exfoliants** usually come in the form of scrubs. They are usually water-based products with a humectant, mixed with some sort of abrasive agent such as almond meal or polyethylene granules or hydrogenated jojoba oil beads. They are applied after cleansing and massaged over the skin. The granules literally "bump off" dead cells from the skin's surface. The humectant keeps the product from overdrying the skin. Exfoliants should be used several times a week for best results. They should be followed by a toner and a night or day cream. New treatments are constantly being developed. Improvements in both active agents and vehicle and delivery transport systems for active ingredients constantly help improve the quality of cosmetics and their positive effect on the appearance of the skin. For further information on other new products and developments in cosmetic chemistry, read Chapters 12, 13, 15, 16, 17, and 18.

Topics for Discussion

1. What are the differences between rinseable cleansers and emulsion cleansers?
2. What determines the difference between types of rinseable cleansers?
3. Describe some different types of toners.
4. Describe a good day cream for oily or combination skin.
5. Describe some of the various types of day creams you may find in a salon.
6. What is the difference between a day treatment and a night treatment?
7. Describe some of the different types of products that use AHAs and how they might differ for oily and dry skin types.

Chapter 11

Claims in Cosmetics

Objectives

The Food and Drug Administration is a federal agency that regulates the cosmetics industry. In this chapter you will learn about the FDA and how it functions. You will also learn about various claims made about cosmetics, and what the difference is between a drug claim and a cosmetic claim.

You will learn what kind of questions to think about when evaluating claims made by cosmetics companies about their products, which you may be using in your salon.

In 1938 the Food, Drug and Cosmetic Act was passed by the United States Congress. The act called for certain definitions of cosmetics and drugs.

The FDA, which stands for the Food and Drug Administration, is a federal government agency designed to ensure safety of consumer products, namely food, drugs, and cosmetics. They regulate the cosmetics industry. Unlike the regulation of the drug industry, where approval of drugs is necessary before they are marketed, the FDA only controls cosmetics from a disapproving perspective. The FDA does not "approve" cosmetics.

This means, essentially, that the FDA only regulates the cosmetic industry when the agency disapproves of a claim or product. This also means that cosmetic companies are not required to list their products or formulas with the FDA. They are required to register only on a voluntary basis.

When a "bad" cosmetic is found by the FDA, the agency begins investigating the cosmetic or claim. If the cosmetic is found to be unsafe, or to be making untrue claims, or to be making drug claims, the FDA will move to warn the company or remove the product from the market.

DRUG VS. COSMETIC

The Food and Drug Act of 1938 defines cosmetics and drugs as follows:

- "Drug—Articles (other than food) intended to affect the structure or any function of the body."
- "Cosmetics—Articles intended to be rubbed, poured, sprinkled, or otherwise applied to the human body or any part thereof for cleansing, beautifying, promoting attractiveness or altering the appearance."

Now, we have discussed how functional or performance agents work on the skin in the last few chapters. But even if these performance agents do affect the function of the skin, we cannot make this claim if the product is a cosmetic. We can, however, say that the product "improves the skin's appearance."

Does this sound silly? Many cosmetic scientists agree, but this is the law as it exists. Cosmetics affect the appearance. If it is claimed that they affect the body or the skin's physiological function, they are considered drugs.

The key words here are *claims* and *intention*. If your product does affect the skin's function, and you do not mention it while selling the product as a cosmetic, you have not broken the law. You are selling the product and claiming that it only improves the appearance.

In other words, what you *intend* for the product to do makes it a cosmetic or a drug. Let's look at a few examples. A toner for oily skin contains an antiseptic ingredient. Killing bacteria is a drug claim because it affects the skin's function and rids the body of possible disease-causing microorganisms. But if the toner contains the antiseptic ingredient and no claim about the antiseptic action is made, then it is not a drug claim. You can say that the toner "helps reduce the appearance of enlarged pores" or "helps remove excess oil" or "improves the appearance of oily areas." These are all claims about the appearance. The fact that the toner also probably kills bacteria is just not mentioned.

Now, if you register the same product as a drug, you can say "This product helps kill bacteria," or "Kills germs that can cause infection." You are permitted to make these physiological claims if the products registered with the FDA as a drug. OTC means over-the-counter drugs. These are drug products for which a physician's prescription is not needed. Prescription drugs require a written prescription from a licensed physician. Dentists and veterinarians are also permitted to write prescriptions. Estheticians only use OTC drugs unless they are working directly under the supervision of a licensed physician. OTC drugs that are used by or sold by estheticians may include sunscreens, melanin suppressants for hyperpigmentation, acne medications, and hydrocortisone creams.

Let's explore another possibility. A cream is made with good vehicle ingredients that are very acceptable to the intercellular cement, making the probability of deeper penetration of the product higher. The cream includes the free radical scavengers tocopherol and grapeseed extract that help reduce irritation and redness. It also contains alphahydroxy acids, shown to stimulate new collagen production when used routinely.

Now these theories may be true, but if the claim is made that "this cream makes cells healthier by reducing free radicals with vitamins A and E, and stimulates the production of new collagen," a drug claim has been made! You are saying that the product (1) contains vitamins, which are known to affect body functions; (2) "makes cells healthier," which is a physiological claim; and (3) "stimulates the production of new collagen," another physiological claim.

So you have three drug claims in just one descriptive phrase. In order to make these claims, the product would have to be registered as a drug. If you claim that the cream makes skin look healthier and helps to smooth the appearance of rough textures, you have made a cosmetic claim. You have simply made the claim that the product improves appearance and have not said anything regarding physiological function.

Registering a product as a drug means that the product must have had substantial testing to support its ingredient claims, efficacy, and safety. It takes years to have new ingredients approved.

Drug ingredients that have been used for long periods of time safely and effectively are permitted for the uses for which they are approved. Salicylic acid, for example, has long been approved for use in OTC acne products. It is recognized as safe and effective for treating minor acne. Because of its long history of safety, manufacturers may use it in acne products, and must register the product if they are making a drug claim. They do not need to file for "new ingredient" testing, though.

VERBAL CLAIMS

As a licensed esthetician or cosmetologist, you must be careful of what you say to clients regarding claims for products. If you say that a product affects the physiology of the skin, then you intend for that product to have drug effects, and you are therefore making drug claims!

You must be careful never to make a claim about a cosmetic that is a drug claim. Always describe products as "improving the appearance," "reducing the visible signs of wrinkles" (intention: you are reducing the appearance of the wrinkle, not the wrinkle itself), "lessening the appearance of puffy eyes" (you are treating the appearance of puffiness, not the physiological factors that caused the puffiness). Good key words include

- "help to . . ."
- "reduces the appearance of . . ."
- "diminishes the visual signs of . . ."
- "improves the appearance of the skin . . ."

Any words that imply that the skin looks better are usually appropriate. Remember, a cosmetic cleanses, beautifies, promotes attractiveness, and alters the appearance.

But what about how cosmetics really affect the skin? It is the opinion of this author and many other cosmetic and health scientists that we need a new product classification with the FDA. It has been proposed that a "cosmeceutical" category be established. A **cosmeceutical** would be defined as a product that is designed for appearance improvement, but may have positive physiological effects on the skin, on a cellular level. Because cosmetic scientists, as well as scientists from the medical community, do have evidence that many cosmetic ingredients affect the behavior and function of the skin, it is felt by many that this new category is needed. Cosmetologists and estheticians cannot legally explain the actual chemical reactions that occur in products.

Cosmeceutical is a product that is designed for appearance improvement, but may have positive physiological effects on the skin, on a cellular level.

THE LABELING LAW

In 1977 the Federal Packaging and Labeling Act was instated by the FDA. This package of regulations required all cosmetic manufacturers to list ingredients used in their products. The initial reasoning for this package of regulations was to protect consumers who suffered from allergic reactions to particular ingredients.

In theory, the consumer could check the ingredient label for allergen ingredients and thus, theoretically, avoid a potential allergic reaction.

The ingredients are required to be listed on the outermost part of the packaging. If the product is in a box, the ingredients must be listed on the box. Products that are marketed in jars or containers without using a box or other outer packaging must list ingredients on the container itself. The reason for the requirement for the ingredients to be on the outermost surface of the packaging is so the consumer can easily find the list.

Again, in this author's opinion, this is both helpful and hurtful. It is true that a consumer can check for ingredients to which he or she is allergic. But the consumer often reads other chemical names that he or she does not understand or knows nothing about. As an example, a consumer once said that she did not want to use a particular moisturizer because it contained methylparaben, and she did not like to use products with oils in them! The consumer had mistaken the preservative *paraben* for the oil *paraffin*. An easy mistake, perhaps, but nevertheless this illustrates the fact that consumers do not, in general, know enough about chemistry to read an ingredient label, much less know what it means.

The names of the chemical listed must be registered in the CTFA compendium, which is essentially a directory of generic chemical names agreed upon by the CTFA, the Cosmetics, Toiletries, and Fragrance Association (which is the largest association of cosmetic manufacturers), the FDA, and other interested consumer and manufacturing groups. These names are used so that any two companies who use a particular ingredient will list it in the same way on their ingredient labels. These names are the industry standard. It is not acceptable by the FDA to list chemicals by their trade names or functions.

The ingredients listed on the label must be in the order of concentration that they are present in the product. In other words, a cream that is a mixture of 70 percent water,

10 percent mineral oil, and 5 percent sodium lauryl sulfate must list the ingredients in descending order of concentration such as, "water, mineral oil, sodium lauryl sulfate. . . ."

The exception to the concentration listing rule is that any ingredient that is less than 1 percent concentration in the product can be listed in any order. In other words, toward the end of the list, after ingredients with 1 percent concentration are listed, any ingredient (at less than 1 percent concentration presence in the product) may be listed in any order.

The sources of the ingredients are also illegal to use on the ingredient label. Some "natural" cosmetics manufacturers will list cetyl alcohol, for example, and then afterwards list in parentheses *(coconut oil),* indicating that cetyl alcohol is derived from a "natural" source. This is an illegal listing, because it may be confusing to the consumer. Secondly, just because a chemical is naturally derived does not necessarily mean that the quality is better.

Extracts from plants are usually listed by the plant name and the word *extract.* Plant extracts or derivatives must include the Latin genus and species of the particular extract. For example, aloe extract must be listed as "aloe *(Aloe barbadensis)* extract." This rule is intended to designate exactly what specific type of plant was extracted. For example, there are numerous types of seaweed. Different types may have very different functions. The extract may or may not contain a solvent such as oil, propylene glycol, water, or alcohol. The term *extract* implies, according to the industry rules, that there may be solvent ingredients in this plant extract constituent. It is generally accepted that this is an acceptable labeling practice. Sometimes extracts will be listed as "essence of . . ." or "infusion of. . . ." This means that the extract is in a suspension of water or that extracts have been added to water used in the formulation.

DRUG LABELING

On OTC products, the manufacturer must list first the active ingredient(s) and then list the other ingredients used in the vehicle for the cream or topical product. A sunscreen product, for example, may read:

- Active ingredients: Methoxycinnimate, Benzophenone.
- Other ingredients: Water, Proplyene Glycol, Carbomer 940, Cetyl Alcohol, Methylparaben, Propylparaben, Fragrance.

The actual active ingredients are listed separately, and vehicle ingredients are listed second. Products registered as drugs must list the active ingredients first on the ingredient label.

There are other rules regarding claims for OTC drugs. Often, there are standard phrases that must be used for usage instructions or to describe functions of the drug, along with warnings. These are mandated by the FDA.

Once again, the FDA is a disapproving agency, meaning that they only investigate a cosmetic if it is believed that a fraudulent or medical claim is being made, or if the product is unsafe or contaminated. The FDA does not approve cosmetics. Claims that a particular cosmetic is "FDA approved" are false, misleading, and illegal.

OTHER COSMETIC CLAIMS

Hypoallergenic

Hypoallergenic cosmetics are cosmetics that have generally been manufactured without the use of certain ingredients that are known to frequently cause allergic reactions.

A cosmetic that is claimed to be **hypoallergenic** has generally been manufactured without the use of certain ingredients that are known to frequently cause allergic reactions. Fragrance is generally left out of the hypoallergenic cosmetics, because fragrance is one of the main causes of allergic skin reactions.

The term *hypoallergenic* does not mean nonallergenic. There is no such thing as a nonallergenic cosmetic. Somewhere in the world there is a person allergic to every single ingredient used by the cosmetic industry. Although there is no way to guarantee a product as nonallergenic, hypoallergenic cosmetics statistically cause fewer allergic reactions.

Some companies run sophisticated allergy tests on their products to demonstrate their hypoallergenic status. This unfortunately still does not guarantee nonallergenicity; it simply shows that the company cares and believes in their product enough to have it tested.

The truth is that most cosmetics today are hypoallergenic and are designed that way. Most companies take great care to make sure their products can be used by most people. It is in their financial interest to do so as well.

Fragrance-Free Cosmetics

As discussed earlier, many cosmetic manufacturers purposely do not use fragrances in their products to reduce the chances of allergic reaction. Such products may still actually have an odor or smell. This is the odor of the actual ingredients used in the product formulation. However, not adding fragrance to a cosmetic is a generally good idea, when possible.

Preservative-Free Cosmetics

Anhydrous products are treatment products that do not contain water.

Recently, thanks largely to the advancement in silicone technology, some preservative-free cosmetics have been developed. These treatment products are **anhydrous**, which means they do not contain water. Water is an essential element to sustain life of pathological bacteria. Most of these products are serums, based with silicone mixtures or petrolatum. Most cosmetics and skin-care products do contain preservatives, which are necessary to inhibit growth of harmful bacteria.

Noncomedogenic

This means that certain ingredients that are known to cause comedone development and acne flareups have not been used in these cosmetic formulations. Fats and emollients are the principal agents that cause these reactions.

Unfortunately, there is no standard industry definition of the word *noncomedogenic,* and the FDA does not require that testing be performed to make such a claim. Unfortunately, certain companies take advantage of lack of rules and make claims that their products are noncomedogenic without performing the proper testing. For much more information on noncomedogenic testing, see Chapter 13, Comedogenicity.

Nonacnegenic

Often this term is used interchangeably with noncomedogenic, but *nonacnegenic* means that the product has been designed not to cause comedones to develop or follicle irritancy that can cause immediate acne flareups. It takes sometimes as much as six months for comedones to form, whereas follicle irritancy potentially can cause an acne flareup much more quickly.

Again, a variety of tests for follicle irritancy can be run, but some companies make the claim without proper testing.

Dermatologist Tested

Once again, this can be a very confusing term. Generally, ethical companies mean that the product has been tested for irritancy under the supervision of a dermatologist. One writer asks the question, "Dermatologist tested—for what?"—a good question. This can be a misleading term.

Natural Cosmetics

One of the latest rages in cosmetic development is the so-called "natural" cosmetics. Naturally derived ingredients in cosmetics have been used for decades. Although nature has some wonderful chemicals to contribute to the cosmetics industry, they are not sufficient by themselves, nor are they always superior to synthetic chemicals.

The fact is that in one form or another everything comes from the earth! Think about it. Even the ingredients used to make plastic come from Mother Nature!

Natural products can also cause allergic reactions. For more on this, see Chapter 6. Do not choose a cosmetic solely on the basis of its "naturalness."

Organic Cosmetics

This is probably also supposed to mean that the cosmetic ingredients used are derived from "natural" sources. The term *organic* actually means that the chemistry of a substance involves the element carbon.

Puffing

Puffing is a term used to describe the way some companies make their products sound better. This is actually an insulting term, because it usually used to mean that the cosmetic company is making the product sound better than it actually is.

Most companies want their products to sound good. Companies that use outrageous claims to promote their products, like "face-lift in-a-jar," make the entire industry suffer. Companies that promote their cosmetics for their real benefits are fortunately in the majority. However, there is always one unscrupulous company that will make outrageous claims in order to make money. Fortunately, consumers soon find that their claims aren't true.

Animal Testing

Some companies claim that they do not perform testing on animals. Although many companies do not believe in excessive animal testing, certain tests must be performed to ensure a safe product.

Formulas often are not tested on animals, but almost all ingredients used in cosmetics have, at one time or another, been tested on animals. This is the only way to make sure that the individual ingredients are safe for human use.

In general, cosmetics companies have made a legitimate effort to reduce animal testing, eliminating excessive and unnecessary testing. However, some important tests cannot be performed without using animals.

Some estheticians are single-mindedly against animal testing. Many of these estheticians do not understand that it is vital to ensure ingredient safety. Some of these safety tests cannot be run without the use of animals.

Rapidly developing technology may eventually eliminate animal testing. Laboratory-produced skin, and other **in vitro** tests, not performed on live organisms, are being discovered. Progress is being made, but as of this writing there are still a few very important safety tests that cannot be run without the use of animals. We all hope that, eventually this will no longer be an issue, but we also must be scientific enough to understand the need for nontoxic products that are safe for human use.

In vitro refers to scientific testing that occurs outside of a living organism. It has not been tested on a live specimen.

International Companies

Some products are imported from other countries where laws regarding cosmetics may be different than those of the United States. Because of this, some companies make claims that are legitimate by their country's standards, but are illegal or misleading by U.S. standards. Importers of these products should be aware of these differences and change claims that are not permitted in the United States. Although many companies are extremely conscientious about this, a few companies, out of ignorance, do not make the proper changes.

Today's consumer is generally better informed than consumers of years past and knows better than to believe unrealistic claims. Unfortunately, enough "bad guy" companies have "cried wolf" often enough that the consumer is often wary when buying cosmetics.

Discussing Claims with Clients

Always try to be honest with clients about a product's true benefits. Hard selling only offends clients. Estheticians should educate their clients about proper products for their skin. The client is only interested in making the skin look the best it can look. Do not make promises you can't keep. Each client has unique problems and conditions, and clients will not always react to products in the same way. There is no way an esthetician can absolutely be sure any product will work. All an esthetician can do is give the best advice possible.

BUYING PRODUCTS FOR YOUR SALON

You will, no doubt, attend many trade shows throughout your career where cosmetics companies display their products for you to purchase. You should do your homework before you purchase products from any company.

You should ask many questions before buying a product line. Some of these questions are:

1. Are the theories used by the company's products rational?
2. Do they make legitimate claims? If the product sounds too good to be true, it probably is too good to be true!
3. How much care do they take in developing cosmetics?
4. Are their products formulated with allergies and comedogenicity in mind?
5. If they make claims about hypoallergenic or noncomedogenic products, do they test their products?
6. Are these tests run by the company or by an independent testing company? (It is better if they are performed by an outside company—they are less likely to be biased.)
7. Are they willing to let you see the test results?
8. Are their prices competitive with similar products?
9. Do they use ingredients that you have never heard of? If you are current on your skin-care journal reading, you should be aware of new and innovative ingredients that are legitimate.
10. What is the company's history? Who is its founder, and what are the founder's credentials?

The more education you have, the better you will be at selecting the best reputable companies. Be careful not to be pressured. Good solid companies don't mind if you think about a purchase before making it.

Many more questions should be asked of companies before you choose a line. You should investigate their reputation with colleagues you respect. You should look into their marketing programs and find out if they are accessible if you have questions, and how fast their service is.

The bottom line is are they honest, and do they have a quality, legitimate product?

Topics for Discussion

1. What does the FDA regulate?
2. Why is the FDA called a "disapproving" agency?
3. Discuss the Food and Drug Act's definitions of cosmetics and drugs. How do these definitions differ?
4. What is the reason for listing ingredients on a cosmetic label?
5. What are the labeling laws for drug products?
6. Discuss the terms *noncomedogenic* and *nonacnegenic*. What tests should be run to legitimately make these claims?

Chapter

12

Acne and the Esthetician

Objectives

In this chapter you will learn about factors that influence the development of different types of acne. You will learn to identify the different types of acne lesions and will learn about several acne-like medical conditions. You will learn how dermatologists treat acne and when you should refer a client to a dermatologist. A variety of treatments, ingredients, drugs, and products will also be studied.

Acne is a skin condition that results in inflammatory and noninflammatory lesions. Commonly associated with teenage and adolescent skin, it actually affects many age groups at different stages of life. There are many forms of acne and acne-related conditions that the esthetician sees every day. Although many forms of acne require the care of a dermatologist, many clients can benefit from esthetic treatments for problem skin.

COMMON ACNE

The most common form of acne is called **acne vulgaris**. This is the type of acne so often associated with teenagers. It usually begins at the inset of puberty, at which time teenagers begin producing larger amounts of sex hormones. (See Chapter 5.) These hormones cause stimulation of the sebaceous gland, which produces an overabundance of sebum.

This extra oil adds to a condition called **retention hyperkeratosis**. As we learned earlier, the epidermal cells, particularly the corneum, is constantly shedding and being replaced by younger cells. Retention hyperkeratosis is a hereditary condition in which these cells are retained, stick to the surface of the skin, and begin lining the inside walls of the follicles. We will, for simplicity, refer to retention hyperkeratosis as "cell buildup." The cells build up inside the follicles much like wax has a tendency to build up on the surface of furniture.

This process of buildup is complicated by the fact that the cells continue to push to the surface of the epidermis at a faster rate. *Hyper* means more than normal, so hyperkeratosis means the process of keratinization (turnover of cells) occurs at a rate much faster than normal.

Retention hyperkeratosis is a hereditary condition. If a child's parents both had acne, there is a very good chance that the child, also, will have a strong tendency to develop acne.

Some researchers believe that retention hyperkeratosis is caused by an inability of the body to produce intercellular structures called lamellar granules. These granules are theorized to release an enzyme that causes dead cells to break away from the corneum in the normal manner. It has been determined that chronic acne patients do not have as many of these active structures present in their follicular cells.

As cells build up on the inside of the follicle wall they form a small impaction called a **microcomedo**. Microcomedones (plural) are actually a mixture of dead cells, bacteria, fatty acids from sebum, and other cellular debris. Microcomedones are not visible to the naked eye. They cannot be seen without a microscope. They continue to retain more and more of the mixture of dead cells, sebum, and bacteria, until they become a visible lesion on the surface of the skin (Figure 12–1).

Noninflammatory and Inflammatory Acne Lesions

There is a point in the development of the impaction where the microcomedo either becomes an inflammatory or noninflammatory lesion. **Noninflammatory** means that the impaction is not red or inflamed. Examples of noninflammatory acne lesions are **open comedones** (blackheads) and **closed comedones** (whiteheads) (Plate 13).

Open comedones occur when the follicle is large enough to hold all of the debris retained by the follicle. The **ostium**, or opening, in these follicles is dilated by the mass of the impaction, allowing the comedo to push toward the surface opening.

Proprionbacterium acnes (P. acnes) is the scientific name of the bacteria that causes acne vulgaris. These bacteria are **anaerobic**, which means that they do not need oxygen to grow and survive. These bacteria are constantly present in all follicles in small numbers. They are kept from reproducing to large numbers by the oxygen that is constantly aerating the open follicle. However, when the follicle gets blocked from oxygen

Acne is a skin condition that results in inflammatory and noninflammatory lesions.

Acne vulgaris is the most common form of acne that is often associated with teenagers.

Retention hyperkeratosis is an overabundance of sebum that often begins at the time teenagers begin producing larger amounts of sex hormones.

Microcomedo is a small impaction formed by cells that have built up on the inside of the follicle wall.

Noninflammatory means that the impaction is not red or inflamed.

Open comedones are noninflammatory acne lesions usually called blackheads.

Closed comedones are noninflammatory acne lesions called whiteheads.

Ostium is the opening in follicles.

Propionibacterium acnes (P. acnes) is the scientific name of the bacteria that cause acne vulgaris.

Anaerobic bacteria are bacteria that do not need oxygen to grow and survive.

circulation, these bacteria multiply in great numbers, feeding off the sebum produced by overactive sebaceous glands (Plate 14). Open comedones do not encourage development of this bacterial growth because the follicle opening is large enough to expose the follicle to oxygen. The oxygen is also what causes the "blackhead" to form at the exposed part of the impaction. This darkening is caused by the exposure of the top of the comedo to the oxygen in the air outside the follicle. The sebum turns a brown color, similar to the way mayonnaise will turn yellow if left out on a picnic table for a period of time. The darkness is also caused by clumps of **melanin** (skin pigment) present in the dead cells in the comedo. This theory is easily demonstrated by observing an extracted open comedo. It is a solid cylindrical plug, topped by a dark area that gets lighter as the deeper parts of the impaction are extracted.

Melanin is the pigment of the skin.

Open comedones, therefore, rarely develop into inflammatory lesions. Unfortunately, the same cannot be said for closed comedones. Closed comedones have very small pore openings, which prevents oxygen from readily penetrating the follicle. The walls of the follicle stretch to hold the contents of the impaction, but the follicle opening does not. Because of this lack of oxygen, the lesions can easily become inflamed due to the increasing number of bacteria multiplying in the anaerobic environment.

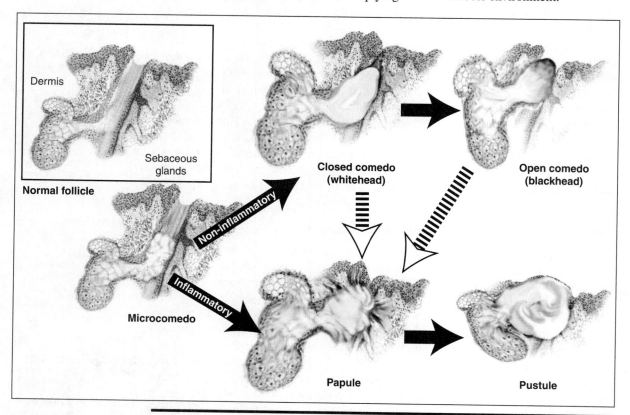

Figure 12–1   The progression of acne

Closed comedones are easily recognizable. They are frequently seen in adult women, often in the blush line of makeup users. They are small "underground" bumps and are not easily extracted. They are frequently associated with the use of comedogenic cosmetics (see Chapter 13, Comedogenicity), as indicated in the blush line of some women.

When enough bacteria form inside the closed comedo and the impaction becomes large enough, a small tear occurs in the follicle wall, which stimulates the immune system to investigate (see Chapter 2), releasing white blood cells into the area. This begins the inflammatory process.

A **papule** is a red, sore bump without a "whitehead" (no pus) (Figure 12–2). This is the beginning of the "rescue" by the white blood cells. When enough white blood cells arrive, they may form a "clump" and rise to the surface, creating what is known as a **pustule** (Plate 15). *Pus* is the common name for this "clump" of white blood cells. For practical purposes, a papule is often described by the client as a large, red, sore bump that never "comes to a head." Papules seem sometimes to "magically disappear." This is because the immune system has "won the battle" and disposed of the impaction through enzymes and absorption, and the body has disposed of the remains through normal blood excretion. Papules affect the nerve endings more than pustules because they are deeper in the skin. This explains the soreness. Pustules have "migrated" the impaction toward the skin surface, dilating the follicle opening and relieving the pressure on the nerve endings, resulting in less pain.

A **nodule** is similar to a papule, but is deeper in the skin and feels very solid and sore. **Cysts** are deep infections caused by a deep, massive invasion of white blood cells. They are very pustular and very large (Plate 16).

Papule is a raised area on the skin that is generally smaller than 1 centimeter.

Pustule is a clump of white blood cells that have formed and risen to the surface of the skin.

Nodule is a raised lesion that is larger and deeper in the skin. A nodule looks like a lump, but the skin can be moved over the lesion.

Cysts are deep infections caused by the deep, massive invasion of white blood cells.

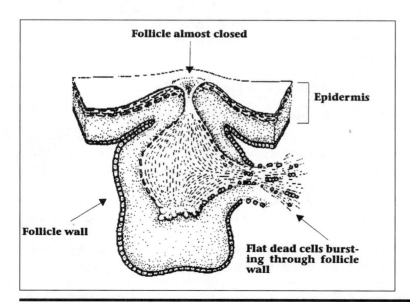

Figure 12–2   The papule

The Grades of Acne

Acne is "graded" by dermatologists on a four-point scale. (See Plates 17a–d.)

- **Grade 1 acne**—mostly open and closed comedones with an occasional pimple. Grade 1 acne is typical of a teenager just beginning puberty.
- **Grade 2 acne**—very large number of closed comedones, with occasional pustules or papules.
- **Grade 3 acne** is thought of by most people as "typical teenage acne." It involves large number of open and closed comedones and many papules and pustules as well. It is very inflamed and red.
- **Grade 4 acne** is commonly referred to as cystic acne, with many deep cysts and scar formation.

Why Scars Form

Scars form when the skin, in a desperate attempt to heal itself, produces lots of collagen to try to compensate for the lack of normal skin functioning. This type of scar is usually raised. Acne "pit" scarring occurs from actual destruction of the tissue during the inflammatory process. Cystic acne is almost always associated with scarring (Plate 18).

Hormones

Androgens are male hormones largely responsible for oily skin and acne.

Testosterone is the male hormone responsible for the development of typical male characteristics.

Dihydrotestosterone (DHT) is a form of male hormone that stimulates the sebaceous glands to produce sebum.

Hormones, specifically male hormones, or **androgens**, are the mechanism that cause stimulation of the sebaceous glands, which, in turn, produce more sebum. This sebum causes inflammation in the follicles, coating the cell buildup and providing a source of fatty acids, which is the food of *P. acnes* bacteria.

Testosterone, an androgen, converts to **dihydrotestosterone (DHT)**, another form of male hormone that "switches on" the oil gland. The oil gland is stimulated via receptor sites on the cells of the sebaceous glands, which are little "switches" that are "turned on" by hormonal stimulation.

As we discussed in Chapter 5, males and females produce both male and female hormones, which are transported around the body via the blood system.

Premenstrual, Hormonal, and Adult Acne

Premenstrual acne flares are often referred to as adult acne. Often, women who have never had problems with acne as a teenager suddenly develop a problem in their 20s or 30s. Although this can be related to comedogenic cosmetics, stress, and hereditary acne factors, hormones play a significant role in adult female acne.

Again, the male hormone, or androgen, flares in the bloodstream cause this type of flareup. Premenstrual flares are caused by a sudden predominance of androgen, which corresponds with the eventual loss of the egg during menses.

The elevation of testosterone in the bloodstream begins eight to ten days before a woman's period. This elevation is actually not an increase in androgen as much as a decrease in the female hormone estrogen. Nevertheless, there is suddenly a larger percentage of androgen in the bloodstream, and therefore a sudden likely increase in stimulation of the sebaceous glands.

A sudden flow of sebum in the follicle causes **perifollicular inflammation**, inflammation around the inside of the follicle. This irritation causes swelling inside the follicle, decreasing the flow of oxygen to the lower part of the follicle and creating an "anaerobic pocket," an ideal environment for the *P. acnes* bacteria. The bacteria multiply, feeding off the sebum and causing a sudden flare of acne papules and pustules.

Perifollicular inflammation means inflammation around the inside of the follicle.

Chin Acne

Many women suffer from premenstrual acne flares predominantly in the lower part of the face, the chin, and the jawline. Many researchers believe that this is the area most responsive to male hormone sebaceous stimulation. It is also believed that many women have very large sebaceous glands in these areas and relatively small follicles. When a sudden sebaceous stimulation occurs, these follicles fill very quickly, causing inflammation due to the large amount of sebum.

Stress

Stress is what causes "pimples on prom night." Many acne sufferers, as well as dermatologists and estheticians, have noticed acne flareups when a patient is under stress. A final exam at school, dating problems, financial problems, or difficulties at work seem to frequently accompany breakouts.

There is a fairly simple explanation for this relationship. Stress causes the brain to manufacture a hormone that, in turn, causes the adrenal gland to make more hormones, which causes an abundance of oil to be produced. The reaction is very similar to the premenstrual reaction.

Birth Control Pills

Birth control pills can cause an androgenic flareup that can contribute to acne. When starting birth control pills the skin may get better or worse. The same may be true when discontinuing birth control pills. Women using birth control pills may find that their monthly premenstrual breakouts occur at a different time in the cycle.

The reasoning here is simple. Birth control pills affect hormone levels and may affect different women in different ways. (See Chapter 5 for more information).

Pregnancy

Pregnancy may also produce unpredictable flareups or clearing of acne. The usual course is that acne gets worse during the first three months of pregnancy, then gets dramatically better. The acne may flare up again after childbirth or after breastfeeding is discontinued. Theoretically, this is due to obvious hormone changes, but stress levels may be partially responsible.

Menopause

During menopause, similar hormonal changes are very prominent and may cause flares. Because menopause is a time of more permanent hormonal change, some women will experience even more acne flares and other androgen-induced symptoms, such as facial hair growth.

Treatment of Hormonal Acne

In many cases, hormonal acne flares can be handled using topical treatments to manage these flares. Regular deep cleansing facial treatments, as described later in this chapter, are helpful in decreasing the instances in many cases.

Many of these women also have very oily or oily combination skin. Proper use of a good rinseable foaming-type cleanser, gel-based 10 percent alphahydroxy acid used daily, and the elimination of comedogenic (clog-pore causing) products (see Chapter 13, Comedogenicity) help to prevent comedones from forming and cut down on acne flares.

In chronic cases of hormonal acne, hormonal therapy using special kinds of birth control pills may be prescribed by a dermatologist, gynecologist, or family physician. Tricyclen® is a birth control pill approved by the FDA as a management drug for hormonal acne. In extreme cases, chronic hormonal acne may also be a symptoms of more serious illnesses such as ovarian polycystic disease and adrenal growths. If you notice chronic hormonal breakouts that are not responsive to topical treatment, do not hesitate to suggest that the client consult her physician.

Inflammatory vs. Comedonal Acne

Many women also notice that premenstrual flares result in sore, inflamed papules. Hormonal acne is more inflammatory and less comedonal. In other words, it is the sudden irritation, rather than the traditional and slower buildup of cells in a comedo, that causes these papular lesions. The soreness is due to the swelling and relatively deep inflammation inside the follicle. This deep swelling is more likely to cause pressure on nerve endings, creating a painful lesion.

Inflammatory acne is not just caused by hormones. Acnegenic skin-care products that cause overnight flares of pimples are a good example of inflammatory acne. Overtreated skin that has had too many peeling agents, or peeling agents applied too often, will show signs of dry irritation and often flares of inflammatory acne. Be very observant of your clients' habits in these cases. Often they are overtreating their skin or may be using a new product that causes a flare.

Unfortunately, professional products are not immune from being acnegenic. "Natural" products also do not mean nonacnegenic. Check to make sure that the products you use and sell have been properly tested for irritancy to make sure they do not cause acnegenic or follicle irritancy reactions.

The Beginning of Teenage Acne

The beginning of teenage acne is characterized by minor breakouts in the nose area. Small blackheads and clogged follicles, small papules, and small milia are found. The esthetician will only notice the beginning of visible pores in the nose and chin and sometimes the forehead. This is the beginning of adolescent pore structure, and usually, puberty and adolescence. Usually within six months more pimples will develop. Boys may notice small pimples in the lower cheeks. This may be caused by the beginning of beard hair growth. The hair is beginning to grow, but the follicle is not large enough to accommodate the hair.

This condition is known as **keratosis pilaris**, which essentially means there is a very small hair trying to force its way out of the follicle, resulting in irritation. This condition, which may affect girls or boys, is usually red or pink and has a "sandpaper" texture. It is often seen in the lower cheeks. If you look carefully at the area, you may notice very small whiteheads, responsible for the bumpy feel. Keratosis pilaris also frequently occurs on the upper arm, and is more likely to affect adults in this area. Keratosis pilaris is best treated with alphahydroxy home care lotions and gels, and use of mild mechanical exfoliating cleansers helps bump off dead cells to allow the hair to come out. Salon treatment using softening and extraction techniques is also helpful.

Young teenagers should be treated every two to three months until breakouts become persistent. At that time regular treatments are recommended. Recommend a gentle, nonmedicated, foaming cleanser, a toner for oily/combination skin, and a mild gel of alphahydroxy or salicylic acid or 2½ percent benzoyl peroxide. Used regularly, these products will help prepubescent teens through this period. Teenagers usually do not need a moisturizer except in cold weather. Regular use of noncomedogenic, daily-use broad-spectrum sunscreen is also advised.

Lack of Care

Young teenagers may not be disciplined when it comes to a regular facial care routine. Sit them down and gently explain the need for consistent care. They usually will take advice from you before they will from Mom at this age.

Teenagers are not the only age group that suffers from lack of skin hygiene. Even though acne is not caused by dirt, many adults neglect their skin. Sleeping in makeup is not only unhygienic, it also means that the night treatment is not applied. Explain to the client that she may come to have a treatment at the salon twice a month, but she is responsible for the other 60 times a month that the skin is cleansed and conditioned! Help her find simple routines that she enjoys doing. Teach her to clean her face as soon as she gets home for the evening. This is also a good time to floss her teeth, right after dinner. When she gets sleepy later in the evening, she can walk past the bathroom guilt-free!

ENVIRONMENTAL FACTORS THAT INFLUENCE ACNE

Heat and Humidity

There is no question that acne is more likely to flare up in the summer months when heat and humidity are high. Heat causes the skin to swell slightly, and humidity causes tremendous swelling of the outer epidermis. It is reasonable to assume that this could possibly exert enough pressure on the follicles to further complicate an already existing condition.

It has been observed over the years that people who live in tropical, warm climates with high humidity experience a fairly predictable seasonal pattern of flareups. Estheticians should bring this to the attention of their clients and encourage them to come to the salon more often for treatments during this type of weather if the client notices a consistent relationship.

Keratosis pilaris is a condition in which the skin exhibits redness and irritation in patches, accompanied by a rough texture, and small pinpoint white papules that look like very small milia.

Sun Exposure

Although sun exposure may have an immediate drying effect on acne lesions, sun damages skin and is documented to cause more "cell buildup," which can add to or increase the chances of acne flareup.

Many acne patients claim their acne improves with sun exposure. Tanning masks the redness, and as the buildup of tan cells occurs on the surface of the skin, acne may appear better. As soon as beach season is over, however, these same patients notice reoccurrence of their acne. What actually happens is that the tan fades and the cell buildup subsides, suddenly exposing a tremendous number of clogged follicles and closed comedones. The most unfortunate part of this situation is that these clients have a strong tendency to neglect treating their acne during beach season, making it more complicated when the tan fades. It is up to the esthetician to educate the client before sun season to avoid this problem.

Greasy Workplaces

Acne patients who work in environments where their skin is constantly exposed to large amounts of occlusive grease or airborne grease, such as that present in fast-food restaurants, may notice a strong flareup in their conditions. Occupations such as car mechanics and short-order cooks are good examples of such situations. It is best for these individuals to avoid working for prolonged periods of time under these conditions. Advise clients who must work in these types of jobs to cleanse their skin at regular intervals (about twice during an eight-hour period) with a mild cleanser that will remove the environmental oil without drying the skin too much.

OVERCLEANING

Clients are constantly under the impression that acne is directly caused by lack of cleansing. Although keeping skin as clean as possible is certainly important, acne is not caused by dirt. In fact, acne can be aggravated by too much cleaning. Repeated exposure to detergents in facial cleansers, for example, can aggravate acne if the client is using the cleansers too often. Estheticians often find that their clients are cleaning the face numerous times daily (eight to ten times). This causes enough irritation to precipitate not only an acne aggravation, but other sensitivities as well. Instruct these clients to cleanse two or three times a day only.

SELF-TRAUMA EXCORIATIONS

Acne excoriée is a condition in which a person picks at their acne lesions, causing scrapes and possible scars and hyperpigmentation.

This essentially means that the client is scratching or picking at the skin until the raised portion of the acne lesion is literally scraped off the face (usually with the fingernails). This condition is known as **acne excoriée**. Most clients pick at their lesions subconsciously. These lesions appear red, flat, and raw on the surface of the skin, similar to a freshly scraped knee or brush burn (Plate 19).

▲ PLATE 1

Herpes Type II in an HIV-positive patient.
(Courtesy Rube J. Pardo, M.D., Ph.D.)

PLATE 2 ▶

Shingles on the neck and face of an
HIV-positive patient. *(Courtesy
Rube J. Pardo, M.D., Ph.D.)*

▲ PLATE 3

Seborrheic dermatitis in an HIV-
positive patient.*(Courtesy Rube J.
Pardo, M.D., Ph.D.)*

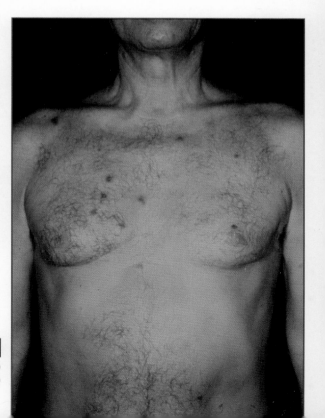

PLATE 4 ▶

Kaposi's sarcoma in an AIDS (HIV-positive)
patient. *(Courtesy Rube J. Pardo, M.D., Ph.D.)*

◄ **PLATE 5a**

Mask of pregnancy with hyperpigmentation.
(Courtesy Timothy G. Berger, M.D.)

PLATE 5b ►

Melasma in a male patient is very unusual.
(Courtesy George Fisher, M.D.)

a1

a2

a3

PLATES 6a1-3

The beginning stages of rosacea. The first symptoms of rosacea may be just a redness pattern across the nose and cheeks, or a red, slightly swollen nose.

▲ PLATE 6b

Nose telangectasias. Dilated capillaries called telangectasias, and a coarse textured appearance of nose ostia are typical of the rosacea client.

▲ PLATE 6c

A rosacea flare in an adult. Note the redness and papules. This patient also has ocular rosacea, affecting the eyelids.

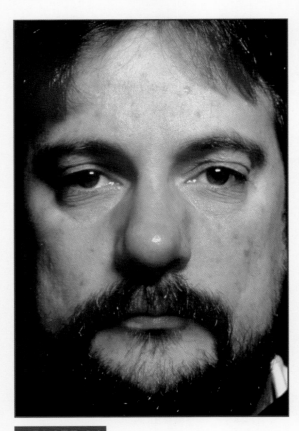

▲ PLATE 6d

Red, swollen noses can be the beginning of rhinophyma.

▲ PLATE 6e

Dark and red distended capillaries, enlarged pores, and enlargement of the nose are shown in this photo of rhinophyma. This nose will also have large amounts of sebaceous filaments and secretions.

▲ PLATE 6f

An example of a severe flare of rosacea, which can affect the whole face.

g1

g2

PLATES 6g1, 2

Before and after rosacea treatment. Rosacea can be kept under control by using prescribed topical and/or oral medication, controlling flushing, avoiding heat, spicy foods, and other triggers, and using non-irritating skin care products. *(Rosacea photos courtesy of National Rosacea Society and Mark Lees Skin Care, Inc.)*

▲ PLATE 8
Rhinophyma.
(Courtesy Rube J.
Pardo, M.D., Ph.D.)

▲ PLATE 7
Rhinophyma in rosacea. *(Courtesy Rube J.
Pardo, M.D., Ph.D.)*

▲ PLATE 10
Severe contact dermatitis as a reaction to cosmetics.
(Courtesy Rube J. Pardo, M.D., Ph.D.)

▲ PLATE 9
Urticaria (hives). *(Courtesy Rube J.
Pardo, M.D., Ph.D.)*

PLATE 11 ▸

Eyelid contact dermatitis from cosmetics.
(Courtesy Rube J. Pardo, M.D., Ph.D.)

◂ **PLATE 12**

(a) Dermatologist-administered patch tests for various contact allergies.
(b) Positive patch test indicating allergy to nickel. *(Courtesy Rube J. Pardo, M.D., Ph.D.)*

12a

12b

PLATE 13 ▸

Open and closed comedones.
(Courtesy Michael J. Bond, M.D.)

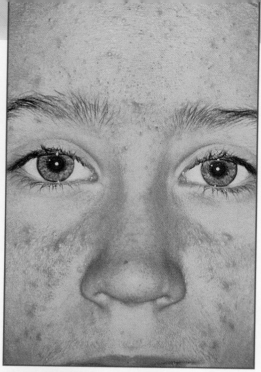

The development of acne in a young girl

The pustule

The cyst

Grade 1 acne. *(Courtesy Mark Lees Skin Care, Inc.)*

▲ **PLATE 17b**

Grade 2 acne. *(Courtesy Mark Lees Skin Care, Inc.)*

▲ **PLATE 17c**

Grade 3 acne. *(Courtesy Melvin L. Elson, M.D.)*

PLATE 17d ▸

Grade 4 acne.
(Courtesy Melvin L. Elson, M.D.)

PLATE 18 ▸

Facial scarring

▲ **PLATE 19**

Self-trauma excoriation. (*T. Fitzgerald,* Color Atlas and Synopsis of Clinical Dermatology, 3e *(1996) reprinted by permission of The McGraw-Hill Companies.*)

▲ **PLATE 20**

Seborrheic dermatitis. (*T. Fitzgerald,* Color Atlas and Synopsis of Clinical Dermatology, 3e *(1996) reprinted by permission of The McGraw-Hill Companies.*)

◄ **PLATE 21**

Typical pattern of perioral dermatitis on the chin. Perioral dermatitis can also appear on the cheeks or anywhere around the mouth area. (*Courtesy Mark Lees Skin Care, Inc.*)

a

b

▲ **PLATES 22a,b**

This case of grade I acne was improved significantly in only six weeks of home care by eliminating comedogenic products, using daily follicular exfoliants to loosen and prevent hyperkeratosis, and using an effective foaming cleanser to control sebum. (*Courtesy Mark Lees Skin Care, Inc.*)

PLATES 23a–d

This client had problem skin for 15 years and was using comedogenic product before starting treatment. All comedogenic products, including makeup, were eliminated and replaced with non-comedogenic products. Home care included sunscreen, hydrator, a 10 percent alpha/betahydroxy gel, a drying lotion for blemishes, a sulfur-based mask, and effective surfactant cleansers. No salon treatment was performed. Results photographed after six weeks of home care. Note improvements in redness, comedones, texture, and coloration. *(Courtesy Mark Lees Skin Care, Inc.)*

a

b

▲ **PLATES 24a, b**

Treatment for clogged, dehydrated skin includes non-comedogenic hydration fluid and sunscreen with low levels of emollient, along with an alphahydroxy acid gel. This home care was used for six weeks in this case study. Note the differences in texture, tone, clarity, and even coloration. (*Courtesy Mark Lees Skin Care, Inc.*)

◀ **PLATE 25**

Sebaceous filaments, often called clogged pores, are follicles filled with solidified sebum. The black tip is oxidized sebum in the top of the follicle. (*Courtesy Mark Lees Skin Care, Inc.*)

PLATE 26 ▶

Cotton swabs are used to gently extract comedones and sebaceous filaments by gently lifting and slightly twisting the skin. Careful preparation of the skin with desincrustation is essential for ease in extraction.

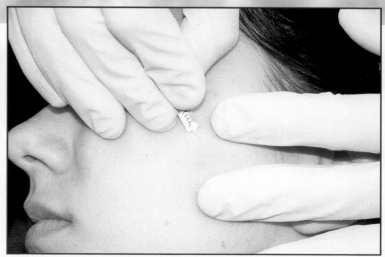

PLATE 27 ▶
Dilation using a lancet.
*(Courtesy Mark Lees Skin
Care, Inc.)*

PLATE 28 ▶
Milia are often seen around the eye area,
as seen on this client's upper lid.
(Courtesy Mark Lees Skin Care, Inc.)

▲ **PLATE 29**
Xanthalasma. *(Courtesy Timothy G. Berger, M.D.)*

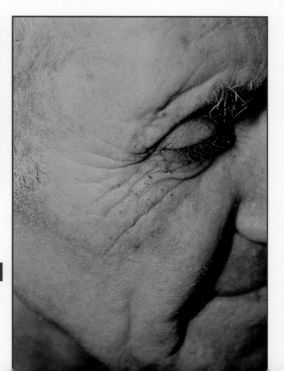

PLATE 30 ▶
Favre Racouchot (senile solar comedones) in a
typical pattern on a sun-damaged individual.
(Courtesy Rube J. Pardo, M.D., Ph.D.)

PLATE 31a–h

Samples of skin tissues from the buttocks and faces of people in different age groups. a) and b) are photographs of a 2-year old girl; c) and d) are of a 49-year old woman; e) and f) are of a 77-year old woman; and g) and h) are of an 80-year old woman. *(Photographs reprinted courtesy of J. Bedford Shelmire, Jr., M.D., author of* The Art of Looking Younger*, St. Martin's Press, New York.)*

Hyperpigmentation, often caused by cumulative sun exposure, can be improved with the use of alpha and beta hydroxy acids, and lightening or brightening agents such as hydroquinone or magnesium ascorbyl phosphate. In this case study, a series of 30 percent alphahydroxy acid exfoliation treatments showed this improvement in three weeks. *(Courtesy Mark Lees Skin Care, Inc.)*

a

b

Tinea versicolor. *(Courtesy Rube J. Pardo, M.D., Ph.D.)*

◄ PLATE 34

Basal cell carcinoma.
(Courtesy Rube J. Pardo, M.D., Ph.D.)

◄ PLATE 35

Squamous cell carcinoma.
(Courtesy Michael J. Bond, M.D.)

a

b

▲ PLATES 36a, b

Actinic keratosis is frequently seen in sun-damaged clients. *(Courtesy Michael J. Bond, M.D.)*

PLATE 37 ▸

Multiple sebaceous hyperplasia in an adult male with oily skin and sun damage. Sebaceous hyperplasias are typically found on the forehead, temple, and upper cheeks, but can appear anywhere on the face. *(Courtesy George Fisher, M.D.)*

PLATE 38 ▸

Proper application of a well-formulated DHA self-tanning product produces beautiful results in a short period of time and is the only safe way to "tan." *(Courtesy of St. Tropez Tanning Essentials.)*

Before Application **Following Application** **12 hrs After Application**

a

b

▴ PLATES 39a, b

Glycolic treatment is popular for lessening the appearance of facial wrinkles. Shown here are before and after photos of the eye area. *(Courtesy Murad Skin Research Laboratories, Inc.)*

a

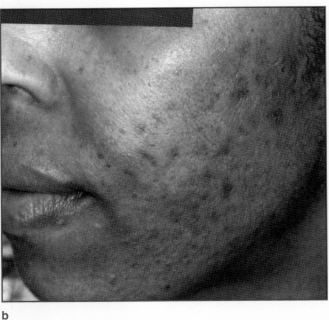
b

Glycolic treatment can significantly improve the appearance of problem and acne-prone skin (before and after). *(Courtesy Murad Skin Research Laboratories, Inc.)*

a

b

Glycolic treatment can help the appearance of hyperpigmented skin conditions. *(Courtesy Murad Skin Research Laboratories, Inc.)*

PLATE 42 ▶

Glycolic acid is applied to the skin of a client who has been using a lower strength glycolic treatment product for at least two weeks at home. This treatment is applied with cotton swabs and carefully monitored according to manufacturer's directions. *(Courtesy Mark Lees Skin Care, Inc.)*

▲ PLATE 43a

Phenol solution is used on the wrinkled lip of this patient. Shown here is the "frosting" effect after application of the phenol solution.

▲ PLATE 43b

Several months after the peel, the lip is much smoother. *(Courtesy Kirk Smith, M.D.)*

a

PLATES 44a, b

In-depth phenol peel (before and after). *(Courtesy Melvin L. Elson, M.D.)*

b

Application of salicylic acid using
a large swab.

a

b

This series of photos illustrates exfoliation treatment using 20 percent
salicylic acid. Notice the frosting on the skin where the treatment has
been applied. Before any treatment, cumulative sun damage results in
uneven pigmentation and hydration.

c

d

Note improvement after two treatments, six weeks apart.
(Courtesy Mark Lees Skin Care, Inc.)

e

PLATES 46e, f

Temporary hyperpigmentation and discoloration can occur during the first one or two weeks following salicylic treatment. In this more extreme case, dark splotches exfoliate to reveal a smoother texture and tone. *(Courtesy Sotheys, USA.)*

f

Rhytidectomy, or face lifting, can dramatically improve the appearance of sagging facial skin and elastosis. A forehead lift has also been performed on this patient. *(Courtesy Samuel J. LaMonte, M.D.)*

PLATES 48a–d

Blepharoplasty, or eyelid surgery, along with a facelift, can help to significantly restructure the eye contours, achieving a more alert, youthful look. *(Courtesy Samuel J. LaMonte, M.D.)*

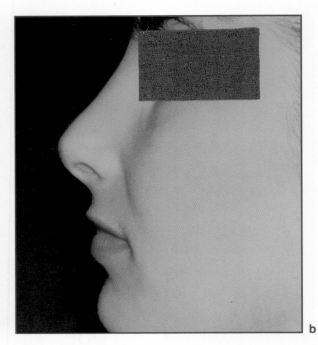

These views feature the patient before and after a rhinoplasty. Note the reduction of the nasal bone protrusion, the straightening of the nostrils, and the softer look of the face in general after surgery. *(Courtesy Samuel J. LaMonte, M.D.)*

a

b

a) Acne scarring in the cheek of this former acne patient. b) After dermabrasion, the cheek area is much smoother. c) This patient needed both dermabrasion and revision of this large surgical scar. d) Notice how much smoother the appearance.

c

d

Case Studies in Post-Laser Care:

◀ PLATE 51a

The patient arrived 11 days post-CO_2 laser resurfacing, concerned with extreme redness and dry, tight skin.

▲ PLATE 51b

The patient complained of extreme tightness around the mouth, and dryness was evident from crusty flaking above the upper lip. The patient was instructed in the use of proper camouflage makeup and how to achieve as natural a look as possible. The patient was instructed to use a fragrance-free moisturizer along with a lipid-based serum to increase hydration. The patient was also instructed in proper cleansing of the skin, using a non-foaming gentle cleanser.

A facial treatment using a lipid-based hydrator with hyaluronic acid and sodium PCA and a gentle steam treatment to increase hydration were administered. Cool steam was applied over which high-frequency current was applied to provide a gentle massage. After this, cold cryogenic globes were applied over gauze. These are special glass or Pyrex® balls filled with cold refrigerant chemicals, like those used in chemical ice packs. Another layer of hydrator was applied over the entire face and allowed to sit for 20 minutes. After the treatment a lipid serum was applied.

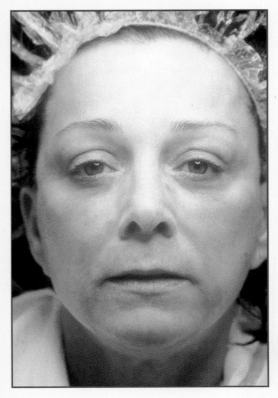

◀ PLATE 51c

The patient experienced significantly lessened redness in five days.

▲ **PLATE 51d**

Flakiness and dryness was lessened and smoothness was achieved in five days. The patient reported ease of dryness and discomfort almost immediately.

▲ **PLATE 51e**

This patient had an extreme amount of redness after full-face CO_2 laser resurfacing and full facelift. She had an important engagement in only a few weeks and was very concerned about having a natural appearance for this event.

Again, this patient was given the same hydrating cream, lipid serum, and gentle cleanser, and was instructed in the use of camouflage makeup to cover the redness.

◄ **PLATE 51f**

The patient had tremendous improvement in only five days. Within a short period of time, she was able to discontinue the heavier camouflage makeup and return to the use of a lighter weight liquid makeup.

◄ **PLATE 52a**

Note the deep nasolabial folds on this patient.

PLATE 52b ►

By injecting collagen, the surgeon achieves a remarkable reduction in wrinkles.
(Courtesy Kirk Smith, M.D.)

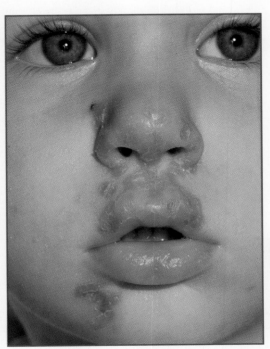

◄ **PLATE 53**

Impetigo is commonly seen on the face. *(T. Fitzpatrick,* Color Atlas and Synopsis of Clinical Dermatology, 3e *(1996), reproduced with permission of The McGraw-Hill Companies.)*

PLATE 54 ▶

Folliculitis on the back.
(Courtesy Rube J. Pardo, M.D., Ph.D.)

◀ PLATE 55

Facial cellulitis. Note the severe
swelling and inflammation.
(Courtesy Rube J. Pardo, M.D., Ph.D.)

PLATE 56 ▶

Tinea corporis infection on the leg.
(Courtesy Rube J. Pardo, M.D., Ph.D.)

▲ **PLATE 57**

Herpes simplex causes common cold sores.
(Courtesy Timothy G. Berger, M.D.)

▲ **PLATE 58**

Typical case of herpes zoster (shingles). Note the lesions follow a typical nerve-route pattern. *(Courtesy Rube J. Pardo, M.D., Ph.D.)*

▲ **PLATE 59**

Molloscum contagiosum. *(Courtesy Melvin L. Elson, M.D.)*

PLATE 60 ▶

Warts. *(Courtesy Rube J. Pardo, M.D., Ph.D.)*

Pityriasis rosea. *(Courtesy Mark Lees Skin Care, Inc.)*

Contact dermatitis in a hairstylist due to parapheneline-diamine.

Contact dermatitis due to nickel allergy. *(Courtesy Rube J. Pardo, M.D., PhD.)*

PLATE 63

Discoid lesion in systemic lupus.
(Courtesy Rube J. Pardo, M.D., Ph.D.)

PLATE 64

Psoriasis.
*(Courtesy Rube J.
Pardo, M.D., Ph.D.)*

PLATE 65 ▸

Skin tags are often seen on the
neck and in the chest area.
(Courtesy Michael J. Bond, M.D.)

These clients usually pick at the skin as a habit. It must be pointed out to these clients that the lesions will never heal properly as long as they continue to pull off the scabs, and that the fingernails carry many germs that can cause other types of infections besides acne. Encourage these clients to use a mask treatment at home routinely (but not too often). Suggest that they wear loosely fitting gloves while reading or watching television. The touch of the glove material will signal them and make them aware when they are scraping at their skin.

It should be pointed out here that although a number of clients pick absentmindedly, many "self traumatizers" are troubled mentally or are under a tremendous amount of stress. Handle these clients gently. They need lots of understanding as well as good skin care.

NUTRITION AND DIET

There are numerous falsehoods regarding the effects of food on acne. Chocolate, nuts, seafood, greasy "teenage" foods such as burgers and french fries, milk, and milk products have all been falsely accused at one time of causing or worsening acne. Although some of these foods are not healthy in large quantities because they may be high in sugar, cholesterol, or triglycerides, they do not directly or indirectly cause acne. Many acne patients and, unfortunately, estheticians are still under the mistaken impression that these foods cause acne.

It is important to have a properly balanced diet to have good skin and good health. The only food group that has consistently been implicated in aggravating acne conditions is iodides. Foods that are high in iodides include some types of shellfish, kelp, squid, asparagus, and iodized salt in salty foods. Iodine causes a follicular irritancy when ingested in large quantities. Consumed in reasonable quantities occasionally, these foods probably do not cause serious problems. It stands to reason, though, that excessive consumption of foods high in iodides can cause acne to flare up.

Zinc supplements are furnished to some acne patients by dermatologists. Prescribed in inflamed acne to reduce redness and inflammation, the usual dosage is 100 mg per day. It is best to check with a dermatologist before suggesting zinc supplements to your clients, because estheticians are not registered dieticians and therefore are not authorities on nutritional science. It is best to leave advice to the specialists in this area.

ACNE AND COSMETICS

Probably the best service an esthetician can render to an acne patient is helping the patient choose cosmetics and skin-care products that are noncomedogenic (see Chapter 13, Comedogenicity).

So many factors cause or contribute to acne, but the esthetician has control over only a few. Heredity and hormones are not part of the practice of esthetics. Even though we may know a lot about these subjects, there is little the esthetician can do to control or affect these factors. Estheticians can temporarily reduce stress by administering soothing treatments, but the stress-reducing effects of these therapies are not long lasting when the client gets in an argument with the boss or forgets when a term paper is due.

The point here is that the only real factors over which estheticians have control are how the client cleanses the skin and what cosmetics and skin-care products the client uses routinely.

It is imperative that the esthetician fully understand comedogenicity for acne and problem-skin clients. It is the best service we can offer them. The client may come in for treatment only once a month but she exposes herself to cosmetics and skin care up to 60 times a month.

The esthetician must eliminate all possible comedogenic factors from the home care and cosmetic regime of the acne patient. Cosmetics, skin care, and topical drugs are the only things that are in constant, direct contact with the skin.

ACNE-RELATED CONDITIONS

Seborrhea (Seborrheic Dermatitis)

Seborrhea is an irritation associated with oily skin and oily areas. Dandruff is a type of seborrhea. Seborrhea is characterized by dry-looking, flaky, crusty patches. Redness is often apparent under these crusty patches. Seborrhea is normally seen in the scalp, around the hairline, along the sides of the nose, and in the ears (Plate 20).

Seborrhea is often misdiagnosed by the client or an inexperienced esthetician as "dry skin," when it is actually associated with oily skin. Seborrhea is best treated by a dermatologist, but the esthetician should be involved in choosing the correct skin-care program. Again, it is important to avoid comedogenic products. Suggest a gentle but thorough cleanser, toner, and very light, noncomedogenic moisturizer. Overmoisturizing can be a contributing factor to seborrhea.

Low humidity and poor, or lack of, cleansing both contribute to this irritating condition. This is one situation when small amounts of sun exposure actually seem to help. If the client does not improve immediately, the client should be referred to a dermatologist, because this condition can be chronic and volatile. Typical dermatological treatment includes the use of hydrocortisone, coal tar shampoos, salicylic acid, selenium sulfide, and zinc pyrithione medications. In the salon, avoid excessive massage and stimulating treatments. Use soothing, nonirritating treatments. Mild extraction of the areas often helps reduce follicle inflammation by removing impactions.

Perioral Dermatitis

Perioral dermatitis is dermatitis around the mouth.

Perioral dermatitis, which is dermatitis around the mouth, is also considered an acne-related disorder. Red papules and pustules in the mouth, nose, and chin area, usually small in size and in clusters of several lesions, are apparent. Almost always found in women, perioral dermatitis often occurs during the childbearing years, 20 to 35 years (Plate 21).

The condition is sometimes accompanied by scaliness and stinging dehydration. Moisturizers may complicate the condition. If a moisturizer is used, it should be water-based, noncomedogenic, and used sparingly. Perioral dermatitis is, again, in the domain of the dermatologist. Mild cortisone creams, antibiotics, and acne medications are often prescribed.

Avoid massage and instruct the client not to touch or rub the area, because this can worsen the condition. Mild sulfur acne preparations may be helpful.

In the salon, avoid massage or overstimulation of the area. Esthetic treatments can help the client's other problems, but you must refer the client to a dermatologist for treatment of the perioral dermatitis. Mild foaming cleansers and toners for oily and combination skin are recommended. Concealing color toner, such as green underbase, is recommended.

TREATMENT PRODUCTS AND INGREDIENTS FOR ACNE

Benzoyl Peroxide

Benzoyl peroxide works well on most forms of acne vulgaris and occasional pimples. Benzoyl peroxide works by peeling off excess cell buildup, temporarily dilating the follicles, and breaking up follicle impactions and debris. Benzoyl peroxide also releases oxygen in the follicle, helping to kill bacteria. Benzoyl peroxide is available in a variety of bases, from drying clay bases to masks, creams, gels, and lotions. The lotions and gels are most frequently used by estheticians.

Benzoyl peroxide is a frequently used acne medication; both an exfoliant and antiseptic.

Benzoyl peroxide normally is made in three strengths:

- 2½ percent for mild acne and thin, sensitive skin
- 5 percent for moderate acne
- 10 percent for more severe acne

Additional strengths are available by physician's prescription. Scrubs and foaming washes containing benzoyl peroxide are also widely used. Unfortunately, many people are or become allergic to benzoyl peroxide (see Chapter 6). Benzoyl peroxide is also a bleach and may bleach fabric and hair if contact is made. Benzoyl peroxide may also be used in the treatment room as a treatment after extraction.

Recommended Usage of Benzoyl Peroxide

1. First and most important, check to see if the client has ever experienced an allergy to benzoyl peroxide. Many clients will overuse a benzoyl peroxide product, resulting in peeling and irritation, which the client may assume is an allergy. But, when in doubt, don't.
2. Benzoyl peroxide may be used as a keratolytic (see Chapter 8) to loosen impactions (open and closed comedones), or as a treatment for papules and pustules. Therefore, benzoyl peroxide can be used on present pimples or used as a preventative for development of future lesions.
3. Benzoyl peroxide can be a very aggressive drying agent. Visible peeling of skin will often occur. Some clients, especially older women, will confuse this peeling with "aging." Tightness of the peeling skin may accentuate lines and wrinkles for a short

period of time. As the dead skin buildup is removed, the visible peeling lessens or subsides with continual use of benzoyl peroxide. Unfortunately, these clients will often stop using the benzoyl peroxide just as it is beginning to work. It is best to explain this peeling procedure to the client at the first consultation before it actually begins. Explain that the peeling will be temporary and is not the same type of drying that occurs with aging. Many older clients find that, with continued use of a peeling agent, their aging skin looks better, and their acne is controlled. With many clients, especially older ones, it is good to recommend a light, noncomedogenic moisturizer that they can use to combat the visible flaking and peeling from drying agents, which will make the skin more comfortable as well as make the drying areas look smoother.

4. Occasionally, a client will call complaining of severe itching, burning, urticaria (hives), and rash. This is most likely an allergic reaction. Tell the client to discontinue treatment immediately. Severe allergic reactions should be seen by a dermatologist. Overuse of benzoyl peroxide products, as previously discussed, can cause an irritation reaction similar in appearance. The client should wait until the irritation completely subsides before retrying benzoyl peroxide. The client should then try applying the benzoyl peroxide to a small area for the first day or two of application. If the irritation returns to the small test area, she should completely discontinue use.

5. Benzoyl peroxide should be used with extreme caution on black skin. It is recommended not to exceed 5 percent benzoyl peroxide in these clients. The area around the mouth should be treated very lightly, because occasionally black clients will experience darkening (hyperpigmentation) of this area.

Sulfur and Resorcinol

Sulfur and resorcinol are often combined in an acne-drying product. These products are usually available in gels, creams, masks, and clay-based "spot" treatment products. They are ideal for use when a client is allergic to benzoyl peroxide products. These products are also irritants and can cause irritations or allergic reactions. They can be used in the same way as benzoyl peroxide products. They help peel away excessive cell accumulations and loosen follicle impactions. They do not, however, release oxygen as benzoyl peroxide does. As a general rule, they are not quite as aggressive as benzoyl peroxide, but are also less irritating. Although benzoyl peroxide is usually the more effective treatment, sulfur-resorcinol products are very helpful in drying acne lesions. If an allergy occurs, follow the same procedures as recommended for benzoyl peroxide.

Salicylic Acid

Probably the mildest of the drying agents, this chemical is ideal for use on older, drier skin types. It usually comes in lotion form and can be incorporated in a moisturizing base. It is available in various strengths. Many companies automatically include salicylic acid in their moisturizers for problem skin. In thin or sensitive skin, it is often used as a day treatment, whereas benzoyl peroxide or sulfur-resorcinol is used as a night treatment.

Some people are very allergic to salicylates, the family of salicylic acid-type products. Salicylic acid, in its oral form, is aspirin. If your client is allergic to aspirin, avoid using salicylic acid.

Glycolic and Alphahydroxy Acids

Alphahydroxy acid at 8 to 10 percent in a gel base is very effective at helping remove impactions. Alphahydroxy acids help acne by removing dead cell buildup and loosening impactions in the skin. Coupled with salicylic acid, and in more serious acne, benzoyl peroxide or sulfur and resorcinol, this treatment can really help clogged skin and problem acne. After the acne has cleared, regular use can help keep follicles clearer of hyperkeratosis, helping to prevent comedones and other acne lesions.

PRODUCTS FOR HOME CARE FOR ACNE CLIENTS

Scrubs and washes are very popular treatment cleansers for the acne patient. There are several types of these rinseable cleansers available.

The base of most of these washes is water and a mild-to-aggressive detergent. These detergents (see Chapter 8) are surfactants that help remove excess oil from the skin's surface, which helps keep the oil from further clogging follicles. Examples of detergents are ammonium lauryl sulfate and disodium lauryl sulfosuccinate (a milder detergent used for more sensitive skin and less drying).

Acne medications such as benzoyl peroxide, sulfur-resorcinol glycolic acid, and salicylic acid are sometimes added to these detergent bases. These are referred to as **medicated cleansers**. They can be considerably more active than regular cosmetic detergent cleansers. For extremely oily, problem skin, these medicated cleansers sometimes contain small, bead-like granules made of polyethylene or ground nuts, seeds, or hulls. These **exfoliating cleansers** help to mechanically remove surface cell buildup, helping the detergents or medication penetrate the surface better. However, they can be very abrasive on red, sensitive, thin skin, and are not recommended for Retin-A or Accutane patients or patients using any other prescription peeling agent. They should only be used on the thickest, oiliest skin types.

Cleansing milks for acne are generally only recommended for makeup removal. Their use should be followed by a mild-to-moderate detergent cleanser to remove any traces of the cleansing milk. These cleansing milks are generally used at night only and should be made of noncomedogenic ingredients.

Medicated cleansers are acne cleansers, in which medications such as benzoyl peroxide, sulfur-resorcinol, and salicylic acid have been added.

Exfoliating cleansers are acne cleansers in which small, bead-like granules made of polyethylene or ground nuts, seeds, or hulls have been added.

Cleansing milk is an emollient, non-foaming cleanser, generally used for makeup removal.

Astringents and Toners

Astringents and toners are usually recommended for acne clients to use after cleansing. These toners are helpful in controlling surface oils and in lowering the pH after cleansing. They are always water-based, with astringent chemicals such as witch hazel, isopropyl or SD alcohol, lemon extract, or citric acid. Some toners are made with antiseptics such as salicylic acid, which also exfoliates the skin.

Toners containing more aggressive drying agents such as alcohol and salicylic acid should be avoided on sensitive skin or the skin of someone using Retin-A or other prescription peeling agents.

Day Treatment for Acne-Prone Skin

Acne and oily skin are not immune from sun damage. In fact, sun protection is often neglected in the acne patient. The use of peeling agents increases this need for suncreen protection.

Advise your client to use a lightweight broad-spectrum screen that has been tested for comedogenicity and follicle irritancy. This should be applied every morning after an application of 8 to 10 percent alphahydroxy gel.

Night Treatments

Medicated gels have already been briefly discussed. These gels or creams contain peeling agents to help remove cell buildup and are extremely beneficial to acne clients. They contain benzoyl peroxide, salicylic acid, sulfur, resorcinol, or glycolic acid.

Hydrating fluids are sometimes needed by acne clients to combat flaking caused by the medicated gels. Adult acne patients frequently require the use of these hydrating fluids. A good hydrating fluid for problem skin is extremely light in texture, made without comedogenic ingredients. They are often alternated with peeling treatments, used on skin with acne tendencies and during colder seasons.

Masks for Acne

Bentonite is an oil-absorbing clay frequently used in clay cleansing masks.

Masks for acne clients are almost always in a clay-type drying base. The clay most frequently used is **bentonite**, which has excellent oil-absorbing qualities. Masks for acne are frequently also medicated, containing benzoyl peroxide, sulfur, or sulfurated lime. They are available in a variety of strengths. Camphor is a popular ingredient for more sensitive and adult skins, because it is less drying than the keratolytic agents. Some clay masks also contain a mechanical granule such as pumice or polyethylene to help exfoliate during application and rinsing.

Masks should be applied for 15 to 20 minutes after night cleansing. After drying, they should be removed by wetting the mask, then gently wiping off with a very soft cloth or sponge. Toner and night treatment should then be applied.

Masks are used two or three times a week, depending on the client's condition and oiliness. Weather and climate may also influence use frequency.

Home Care Treatment for Beginning Teenage Acne

1. Wash the face thoroughly with rinseable foaming cleanser. Use a sponge or soft cloth to help exfoliate surface cells. Rinse thoroughly.
2. Apply mild antiseptic toner with a damp cotton ball or gauze to the entire face.
3. Apply an 8 to 10 percent alphahydroxy gel to the entire face, avoiding the eye area. Please explain to the teenager that it is normal for this to sting slightly when first applied.
4. After the alphahydroxy has absorbed, apply a noncomedogenic, lightweight broad-spectrum SPF-15 sunscreen. Most sun damage occurs before age 18; therefore sunscreen must be used daily!

Night Treatment

1. Remove any makeup thoroughly with noncomedogenic cleansing milk.
2. Wash face thoroughly with rinseable cleanser as shown above. Apply toner.
3. Apply alphahydroxy gel as in the morning treatment.
4. Apply a small amount of 2½ or 5 percent benzoyl peroxide gel to clogged areas. Gently massage until the gel penetrates. Apply additional dabs of gel to individual raised lesions (papules and pustules). The only medication seen should be on the lesions. Excessive peeling may result, particularly in young, sensitive skin if too much medication gel is used.

Salon Treatment

Salon treatment should be administered whenever clogs and comedones are present. Sometimes treatment is necessary only every month or two during the very beginning stages of the teenage years. Treatment should be more frequent when apparent blemishes are more frequent. Parents should be consulted and advised when treating very young skin, so that they may advise children at home. It is often best to consult with the young client without the parent present, and then discreetly talk to the parent afterwards. Teenagers will often perform home care better if they do not feel "supervised." It is important to advise parents to bring the young client in as soon as pimples start to develop. Unfortunately, many parents neglect a child's acne, thinking they will "outgrow it," until the teenager has a more serious condition. "An ounce of prevention is worth a pound of cure!"

Home Care Treatment for Grade 1 Acne

Morning

1. Wash the face with granular (nongranular if sensitive or thin skin) medicated cleanser, with wet fingertips, then with a wet sponge or very soft cloth. Rinse thoroughly with room temperature water.
2. Apply moderate strength toner to the entire face (except eyes). Allow to dry briefly.
3. Apply an 8 to 10 percent alphahydroxy gel to the entire face, avoiding the eye area.
4. After the alphahydroxy has absorbed, apply a noncomedogenic, lightweight broad-spectrum SPF-15 sunscreen.

Afternoon

It is sometimes advisable in very oily skins to repeat the morning procedure in the mid-afternoon, or after school for teenagers. Cleansing should be repeated in the afternoon if working in a greasy environment or after exercising.

Evening

1. Remove makeup thoroughly with noncomedogenic cleansing milk.
2. Wash the face again with medicated cleanser. Nonmedicated foaming cleanser can be substituted if the skin is irritated, sensitive, or peeling.
3. Apply toner as in the morning.

4. Apply alphahydroxy gel as in the morning.

5. Apply 5 percent benzoyl peroxide, sulfur-resorcinol, or salicylic gel or lotion to all clogged and oily areas lightly. This treatment should penetrate almost immediately. Apply additional dabs to pimples and raised lesions. It is important that the client understand that they are not only to treat raised lesions. Treating unaffected but oily areas routinely with light applications will help break up "cell buildup" and help prevent future lesions (Plates 22a, 22b).

Frequency of Salon Treatments

Weekly or biweekly treatments are advised until the acne clears substantially. This normally takes between three and six months. After clearing, the client should be treated every three to four weeks in the salon and should use masks two to three times a week at home. The client should be reminded that acne is a controllable, not curable, condition, and that upkeep is very important.

Home Care for Grade 2 Acne

The home care routine is the same as for grade 1 acne; however, avoid very strong toners. Remember, there are usually many closed comedones in grade 2 acne. These lesions have smaller pore openings, and astringents may prevent these follicle openings from loosening with home care therapy.

Grade 2 acne is one of the hardest types to clear. It requires diligent attention from both client and esthetician. Treatments in the salon should be weekly or biweekly. Extensive extraction is necessary. After the first consultation, allow the client to use products two weeks before the second salon treatment. The closed comedones usually will be much easier to extract after two weeks of proper home care. It is especially important that these clients avoid comedogenic products. The esthetician should check every product carefully for comedogenic ingredients (Plates 23a–d).

Home Care for Grade 3 Acne

Most grade 3 acne cases should be seen by both the dermatologist and the esthetician. The esthetician must pay careful attention to the dermatologist's instructions and prescriptions. Benzoyl peroxide granular washes, stronger astringents, and 10 percent benzoyl peroxide gel may be used, if not contraindicated by the dermatologist. Oral medication is often required for these clients. They will also need help choosing noncomedogenic products and makeup.

Treatment is advised weekly, unless otherwise directed by the dermatologist. Once clear, the client should be seen for salon treatment every three to four weeks.

Home Care for Grade 4 (Cystic) Acne

Grade 4 acne always requires a dermatologist. This is the oiliest and worst acne condition. Home care should be the same as for grade 3 acne, again following any specific instructions from the dermatologist. Salon treatment should be frequent to help prevent lesions by removing clogs and open and closed comedones. Be very careful if cysts or nodules are present during treatment. Refer the client to the dermatologist immediately for treatment of any cysts, nodules, or deep papules. Again, avoidance of comedogenic ingredients is a must for these clients.

DRUGS OFTEN PRESCRIBED BY THE DERMATOLOGIST FOR ACNE TREATMENT

Retin-A

Tretinoin, better known as Retin-A, is a vitamin A acid that was developed in the late 1960s at the University of Pennsylvania by a team of researchers headed by Dr. Albert Kligman. Retin-A works by helping "flush out" follicular debris, helping to clear the follicles of comedones. It also is an excellent drying agent for oily skin and pimples. It is used extensively as a prescription in all grades of acne and is often used for other skin problems. (See Chapter 17, The New Science of Aging Skin Treatment.) Retin-A requires a physician's prescription, because it is a potent topical acid. It is available in cream, gel, and liquid forms.

> **Tretinoin** is a form of vitamin A acid, also known as Retin-A, a prescription drug for treating acne.

Because it is a powerful keratolytic, it is usually not used with other keratolytics such as benzoyl peroxide, sulfur-resorcinol, alphahydroxy, or salicylic acid, except by dermatologist recommendation. Occasional cases do well with benzoyl peroxide and Retin-A. This is a dermatological decision. Do not add keratolytics to a Retin-A user's regime without consulting the dermatologist.

Tretinoin, also known as retinoic acid, does not have a substantial direct effect on bacteria within the follicle, however. It is often used with a topical antibiotic called **clindamycin** (trade name Cleocin-T™), which is a powerful antibiotic. It is in an alcohol base, and by itself can be quite drying. The theory here is to use a powerful "follicle flusher" along with an antibiotic to kill bacteria and remove comedones and impactions. Because Retin-A is such a powerful keratolytic, it is also an irritant. It is not unusual for clients beginning Retin-A to experience flaking, dry skin, redness, irritation, and slight discomfort. The prescribed dosage varies with the client and the dermatologist, but many dermatologists start patients on Retin-A every third night, slowly increasing the frequency to nightly applications.

> **Clindamycin** is a topical prescription antibiotic used for acne treatment.

Because of the irritating side effects of this drug, clients often find that their present skin-care program and cosmetics may be irritating or overdrying. It is up to the esthetician to work with the client or dermatologist to find products that work with retinoic acid therapy.

Adapalene, commercially known as Differin®, is a chemical cousin of retinoic acid. Adapalene produces similar effects and side effects as tretinoin, but it is reputed to be less irritating in some patients.

> **Adapalene** is a form of vitamin A, also known as Differin®, that is a topical prescription drug used for acne treatment.

Azelaic acid, commercially known as Azelex®, is a different type of acidic agent that helps flush follicular debris. Azelaic acid also has a melanin suppressive effect on hyperpigmented skin, but is not, at the time of this writing, officially approved as a melanin suppressor for prescription drug use. It is approved for acne treatment.

> **Azelaic acid** is a form of acid, also known as Azelex®, a topical prescription drug used for acne treatment.

Products for Users of Retinoic Acid and Other Prescription Exfoliators

1. First, eliminate any other keratolytics from the client's home-care program. As discussed previously, avoid benzoyl peroxide, sulfur, resorcinol, salicylic, and glycolic acid. Use these products with Retin-A clients only with the approval of the dermatologist.
2. Eliminate high alcohol products, particularly those containing isopropyl alcohol.
3. Avoid fragranced products.
4. Avoid spicy, stimulating products.
5. Avoid large amounts of citric acid.
6. Eliminate essential oils from the regime. Large amounts of many plant extracts may cause further irritation.
7. Sometimes it is necessary to totally eliminate the use of astringents or fresheners, particularly during the first six to eight weeks of Retin-A therapy.
8. Encourage the use of sunscreens, because Retin-A also makes the skin photosensitive.
9. Eliminate the use of granular scrub cleansers or tight drying masks, particularly during the first part of the Retin-A therapy. Later in the therapy (six to eight weeks), a gentle granular exfoliant, diluted with cleansing milk, may be beneficial in helping to remove dry, dead cells.
10. Highly stripping cleansers, soaps, and abrasives must be discontinued.

Basic Home Care for Acne Clients Using Tretinoin and Other Prescription Peeling Agents

Morning
1. Cleanse the face with a gentle foaming cleanser for oily or combination skin.
2. Apply a gentle, nonalcoholic toner if not too irritated from beginning treatment.
3. Apply a noncomedogenic SPF-15 sunscreen. If using clindamycin, apply sunscreen after clindamycin application, or follow the dermatologist's specific instructions.

Evening
1. Remove makeup with a gentle cleansing milk. Extremely oily skin may need to be washed gently with a foaming cleanser. Apply toner if not too sensitive.
2. Wait 20 minutes.
3. Apply the topical drug as directed by a physician.

If the skin is very dehydrated, a light, nonfragranced, noncomedogenic, hydrating fluid may be applied 20 minutes later. Check to make sure that this is approved by the physician. If Retin-A is used on alternate nights, the client may choose to use the same noncomedogenic hydrating fluid on alternate nights to combat dehydration.

Salon Treatment Changes for Clients Using Prescription Peeling Agents

1. Do not use wax on these patients. Waxing is extremely irritating to retinized skin. Electrolysis is usually acceptable to continue.

2. Avoid enzyme treatment, particularly when starting the prescription. After eight weeks or so, these may be acceptable.
3. No mechanical abrasion, brushing, or "rub off" type masks.
4. Avoid all keratolytics previously discussed during treatment.
5. Camphor masks can usually be tolerated if the skin is not red and irritated.
6. Avoid excessive massage.
7. Electrical therapy should be shortened in duration and performed at a lower intensity.
8. Avoid heavy, thick creams, as with all acne clients.

Tetracycline is an oral antibiotic often prescribed for patients with chronic and persistent acne. Minocycline (Minocin™) is another oral antibiotic often used for chronic acne sufferers. Erythromycin is prescribed in both oral and topical medications. It is also an antibiotic.

Accutane

Accutane is a cousin of retinoic acid. It is an oral medication prescribed for patients with severe, chronic, grades 3 and 4 acne with multiple cysts. It is very useful when treating this type of patient.

Accutane has numerous side effects, including severe drying of the skin and mucous membranes, nosebleeds, and severely dry, cracked lips. More severe side effects include birth defects in children of women who take Accutane during their childbearing years. Many doctors insist on a pregnancy test for women planning to undergo Accutane therapy. Other side effects include muscle aches. Periodic blood, kidney, and liver function tests are administered during Accutane therapy. These side effects may sound frightening, but Accutane can be the most effective acne drug for hard-to-treat cases. Every precaution is taken by dermatologists. Under these circumstances it can be a safe, effective treatment.

Skin Care for the Accutane Patient

Follow the same precautions as recommended for Retin-A patients. No waxing *on any part of the body* should be done during or for several months after Accutane is discontinued. You may need to administer soothing hydrating treatments to the Accutane patient, using light, noncomedogenic, hydrating fluids and gentle gel or cream masks.

Again, avoid all keratolytics, excessive massage, and any stimulating treatments. Extractions on Accutane patients should be extremely gentle, because the skin becomes extremely thin and fragile and reddens and bruises easily.

Help the Accutane patient with light hydrating fluids and gentle cleanser. This may be the first time this type of client has ever used a moisturizer. Take some time to re-instruct the client in the uses of the new products.

After Accutane therapy, the skin usually returns to being somewhat oily—rarely is it as oily as it was before treatment. Within two or three months after Accutane is discontinued, reevaluate the skin and recommend the correct home-care regime.

DERMATOLOGICAL TREATMENT OF CYSTS

The dermatologist treats cysts by a number of different methods. Extraction is used, using a small incision to drain the cyst. This technique is known as acne surgery.

Sometimes the dermatologist injects the cyst with a steroid. The steroid usually clears the lesion in between one and three days of injection. It is an extremely effective treatment for cysts. The doctor usually also prescribes an oral antibiotic for these patients. Avoid pressure or extraction around a freshly treated cyst. Sometimes the dermatologist will suggest avoiding facial treatment until the cyst is completely healed.

ANALYSIS TECHNIQUE FOR ACNE OR PROBLEM SKIN

Before treating problem skin, the esthetician should take a thorough health history of the client. This is best accomplished by having the client fill out a health form. On your form you should include:

1. Client name, address, and phone numbers.
2. The client's occupation. This tells you if the client is in a high-stress job, or if the client is employed in a situation where there is constant exposure to "greasy air," such as a fast-food restaurant.
3. Is the client already seeing a dermatologist? If so, was medication prescribed? Is the client using the medication as instructed by the dermatologist? (Often a client is not using the medication correctly, or has discontinued it because of excessive drying or irritation. Do not interfere with a doctor's prescription or attempt to instruct about medication! Refer your client back to the dermatologist for further instruction. Never instruct a client to discontinue prescribed medication!) If questions arise, call and consult with the dermatologist.
4. How long has the client experienced problem skin? (This may tell you if it is a long-term hereditary problem or if it is caused by short-term factors such as comedogenic cosmetics, hormones, drugs, stress, etc.)
5. When does the client have flareups? Shortly before her period? During stressful times?
6. Is the client under a lot of stress?
7. What cosmetics and skin-care products does the client use presently? Request that the client bring in products presently used during the first visit. This will allow you to check for comedogenic products and to see what steps the client is taking to help.
8. Is the client using birth control pills, and what type?
9. Has the client had any history of hormone problems? Is she experiencing menopause? Is she taking prescribed hormones?
10. Is she pregnant?
11. Does the client have allergies to any cosmetics, foods, or drugs?
12. Does the client have any other health problems or use any other form of medication?
13. Does the client eat a balanced diet?

14. Does the client take vitamin supplements?
15. Does the client have a history of acne in the family?
16. How often does the client clean the skin and with what product?
17. Does the client pick at acne lesions?
18. The client's age. Sometimes this will indicate the nature of the problem.

These standard questions should also be asked on the preliminary form completed on the first visit. It is generally recommended that any client who has not visited in six months fill out a new health evaluation form. Make sure you check for any other health problems or contraindications for home-care or salon treatments (such as electrical therapy, heart problems, etc.) just as you would on any client.

Hands-On Analysis

Remove the client's makeup and cleanse the skin's surface thoroughly. Analyze the client's skin through a magnifying lamp. It is a good idea at some point in the beginning of analysis to look at the skin with the client in a magnifying mirror. The best way to accomplish this is to use one of the two-way mirror devices available through equipment manufacturers. This interaction will allow the client to see what you are describing. Explain each type of problem to the client as thoroughly and simply as possible. Remember, the client is a consumer, not a professional. The bottom line of interest for the client is how you can help with beauty problems and problem skin.

Ask the client lots of questions about any skin problems:

• How often are you having breakouts?
• Where do they occur?
• Do they seem to come at certain times of the month?
• What do the blemishes look like when they occur?
• Do you normally have more or less breakout than this?
• Explain what you are doing now at home.

Even though the client may have written some of these answers down on the health form, it's a good idea to discuss them. Clients sometimes forget to write something down, or the esthetician may discover that the client is doing something incorrectly. This is also a good opportunity to review any experiences that the client has had with previous esthetic or dermatological treatment.

While observing the skin under the magnifying lamp, make detailed, written notes of any problems and any discussion you have with the client. You should particularly note the following:

1. Number of lesions.
2. What type of lesions? Open comedones? Closed comedones? Papules? Pustules? Nodules? Cysts?
3. Chin breakouts, particularly if isolated to that area.
4. Breakout around the mouth, isolated to that area. (This could possibly be perioral dermatitis.)

5. Flaking in the hairline, sides of nose, eyebrows, and ear areas. (Possibly seborrhea.)
6. What is the thickness of the skin? Is it sensitive? Does it turn red easily?
7. Are the unaffected follicles clogged and enlarged? (An indication of generally oily skin.)
8. Large red pustules and surrounding redness in the nose area. (Possibly rosacea.)
9. Flat red lesions that look like scraped skin, sometimes with scabs. (Client is probably scraping with the fingernails.)
10. Scarring—make special notes of any existing scarring, icepick scars, raised (hypertrophic) scars, and any scars from cyst removal.
11. Macules, which are lesions that have healed but are still red or tan in color. They are flat and are most often found in the fleshy areas of the face, such as the cheeks.
12. Is there any surface flaking or dehydration? Is the skin tight or pliable?
13. What grade of acne exists?

The esthetician must check to see if any client with rosacea, seborrhea, perioral dermatitis, or cysts is seeing a dermatologist. These conditions are dermatologic, not esthetic. It is not the esthetician's place to diagnose or suggest these conditions to the client. Simply suggest that the client see a dermatologist. After the client sees the doctor, call the doctor and discuss esthetic concerns or arrange for the client to obtain a letter from the doctor.

Salon Treatments

Before discussing salon treatments, a few important procedures and precautions should be discussed:

1. Do not use any product or ingredient to which the client is allergic.
2. Extraction should never last more than 10 or 15 minutes in one session. If you are uncomfortable with extraction procedures, omit this step completely. Extraction is probably the most important part of esthetic salon treatment, but can also be the most harmful if done improperly. Never extract a lesion you are not sure about. Open and closed comedones and pustules are the only lesions that the esthetician should extract. Leave Papules, nodules, and cysts alone!
3. The esthetician should wear disposable latex gloves during the entire acne treatment.
4. If lancets are used they must be sterile and disposable.
5. Active acne should never be massaged. After the acne is completely cleared, then consider a light massage.
6. Clients should be told not to wear makeup for at least two hours after treatment.
7. Skin that has been exposed to Retin-A or other prescription peeling agents should not be exfoliated. Eliminate the use of all keratolytics, including benzoyl peroxide, salicylic acid, sulfur, resorcinol, or glycolic acid, for clients using Retin-A.
8. Be careful how much you extract on the first visit. As the client begins home care, the impactions will be much softer and easier to extract and a lot more comfortable for the client. Explain this so the client will understand that you will do more extraction on the second visit, when the client has been using the correct products for a week or two.

Basic Salon Acne Treatment

1. Thoroughly cleanse and analyze.
2. Re-cleanse with a foaming cleanser.
3. Apply a desincrusting pre-mask (see Chapter 10). Begin the steam treatment during the pre-mask. Allow to sit for eight minutes.
4. Remove the pre-mask. Proceed with galvanic desincrustation as normal, about five minutes in duration.
5. Begin extraction in the chin area first, moving up the face, finishing at the forehead. This will avoid contact with my blood or fluids. As previously mentioned, the esthetician should wear latex disposable gloves during extraction and throughout the remainder of treatment.
6. After extraction, apply a generous amount of antibacterial toner to the entire area extracted.
7. Unfold a 12-ply piece of gauze and place across the client's entire face. Avoiding the eye area, apply high-frequency current to the client's face (through the gauze) for about one to two minutes. Remove the gauze.
8. Apply a small amount of 5 percent benzoyl peroxide to the extracted areas.
9. Apply a drying mask with camphor. (For more severe conditions, you may use a sulfur drying mask or benzoyl peroxide mask.) Avoid the eye areas.
10. Allow the mask to sit for about 15 minutes. Wet the mask well with a cold spray solution of toner to loosen before removal. Remove with wet sponges or a soft cloth. Spray the face again with toner mixture to remove any excess mask.
11. Apply a small amount of sunscreen to finish the treatment.

Alternative Treatment #1 for Acne

This treatment is effective for thicker skin types with grades 2 and 3 acne.

1. Thoroughly cleanse and analyze.
2. Re-cleanse with an alkaline pre-mask or an alkaline rinseable cleanser.
3. Apply a soft-setting enzyme treatment to help dissolve surface cell buildup and dilate follicles. Begin the steam treatment during the enzyme treatment. Allow to sit for eight minutes.
4. Remove the enzyme treatment. Proceed with galvanic desincrustation as normal, about five minutes in duration.
5. If you are using a lancet, begin dilating the follicle openings of the closed comedones in the chin area, moving up the face to the cheeks and finishing on the forehead. Proceed with extraction. Gently dilate the top of any follicles with pustules with separate lancets. Extract pustules.
6. After extraction, apply a generous amount of antibacterial toner to the entire area extracted.
7. Unfold a 12-ply piece of gauze and place across the client's entire face. Avoiding the eye area, apply high-frequency current to the client's face (through the gauze) for about one to two minutes. Remove the gauze.
8. Apply a small amount of 5 percent benzoyl peroxide to extracted areas.

9. Apply a drying sulfur or benzoyl peroxide mask, avoiding the eye area. For more sensitive skins, apply a drying mask with camphor.
10. Allow the mask to sit for about 15 minutes. Wet the mask well with a cold spray solution of toner to loosen before removal. Removal with wet sponges or a soft cloth. Spray the face again with toner mixture to remove any excess mask.
11. Apply a small amount of sunscreen to finish the treatment.

Treatment for Clients Who Have Recently Begun Using Retin-A or Other Prescription Peeling Agents

1. Thoroughly cleanse and analyze, paying particular attention to any red or sensitive areas.
2. If the skin is red or sensitive, apply a light, noncomedogenic hydrating fluid. Proceed with steam for five to eight minutes. Be very careful not to get the skin hot from the steam. Cool steam, discussed in Chapter 6, is a good choice here. For skin that appears noninflamed, apply a disincrustant pre-mask instead of the dehydrating fluid.
3. Remove the pre-mask or hydrating fluid. Galvanic is best avoided on clients just beginning Retin-A treatment.
4. Begin extraction gently in the same chin to forehead pattern.
5. Apply a generous amount of antibacterial nonalcoholic toner on a cool, wet, cotton pad or soft cloth. Apply to all extracted areas. If you prefer, you may use a diluted cold spray toner solution.
6. Apply a noncomedogenic hydrating fluid. Cover with gauze and proceed with high frequency (mushroom attachment) for one to two minutes.
7. Apply a cool, soothing treatment with aloe, azulene, bisabolol, or chamomile. Gel masks are very beneficial and gentle, as long as they are free of alcohol and fragrance. For thicker skins, you may try a light application of light-setting, clay-based camphor mask.
8. Do not allow to sit for more than five to seven minutes. Remove the mask by thoroughly wetting it with cold spray, then gently wiping with cool, wet cotton or soft cloths.
9. Apply a light, noncomedogenic moisturizer with sunscreen.

Topics for Discussion

1. What is acne?
2. Trace the development of the comedo.
3. Explain how hormones affect acne.
4. Name some environmental factors influencing acne development.
5. Explain various cleansers, toners, and treatment creams and lotions available for acne and their action on the skin.
6. Discuss some acne-related conditions that should be referred to the dermatologist.
7. What are some questions that should be asked of the client during the first consultation?

Chapter 13

Comedogenicity

Objectives

Many ingredients used in cosmetics can make acne worse and can contribute to the development of comedones of all types.

Comedogenicity is the tendency of topical substances to cause the development of comedones, possibly leading to or worsening acne eruptions. Multiple comedones, both open and closed, can lead to the formation of inflammatory acne lesions. Dermatologists began scientific documentation in 1941 of topically induced acneiform eruptions in chlorinated hydrocarbons in occupational acne in workers handling certain chemicals.

Comedogenicity is a particularly important subject for the esthetician to understand, because the esthetics profession specializes in keeping skin healthy and clean and advising clients about cosmetic treatment preparations. It is a vital part of the esthetician's job to prevent potential reactions on their clients' skin and to educate clients about preventative treatment techniques, including avoiding treatments or products that may not be right for their skin.

In this chapter you will learn about these ingredients and how they affect the skin. You will learn how to check ingredient lists for possible comedogenic ingredients. You

Comedogenicity is the tendency of topical substances to cause the development of comedones, possibly leading to or worsening acne eruptions.

will also learn about the many products that are helpful for clog-prone, oily, and acne-prone skin.

BACKGROUND

For many years, dermatologists often told women who had acne or problem skin to avoid using makeup. Many doctors said this as a blanket statement and encouraged women with acne to avoid all cosmetics.

These doctors noticed that women often did not respond to traditional acne therapy. They also noticed that many of the women continued to use makeup and cosmetics on a regular basis.

These dermatologists did not know at the time specifically why the cosmetics caused acne to become worse or not to improve during treatment. Many thought that the cosmetics sat on the skin and occluded aeration of the follicles, not allowing oxygen to penetrate the follicles. Others were aware that many of the cosmetics had a high fat or oil content. It seemed to make sense that oily skin that developed acne lesions easily did not need additional oil from outside.

These theories made sense, and some studies touched on the subject of cosmetics and hair products aggravating acne, but it wasn't until the early 1970s that doctors published studies that showed increased retention hyperkeratosis or a buildup of cells within the follicle in patients using some types of cosmetics.

It was discovered that the use of certain ingredients within cosmetics was more likely to cause a pronounced buildup of cells within the follicle. This buildup lined the follicle walls, and when enough was accumulated, it began forming a microcomedo. The microcomedo eventually evolved into an open or closed comedone and then possibly into an inflammatory acne lesion, such as a papule or pustule.

The acne-prone women who used the cosmetics in question already had a predisposition to clog development. In other words, they already had a tendency to develop clogged pores from hereditary retention hyperkeratosis and oiliness.

Acne cosmetica is acne caused or worsened by the use of comedogenic or inflammatory cosmetics or skin care products.

Comedogenic means the tendency of a topical ingredient or product to increase the buildup of dead cells within the follicle, eventually causing comedone formation.

Noncomedogenic means that the ingredient or product does not cause excessive follicular hyperkeratosis, and therefore is unlikely to cause comedone development.

The doctors coined a term for this condition, **acne cosmetica**, meaning "cosmetic acne." They were able to correlate excessive buildup of dead cells within the follicles of patients using certain cosmetics. These cosmetics were said to be **comedogenic**. Comedogenic means the tendency of a topical ingredient or product to increase the buildup of dead cells within the follicle, eventually causing comedone formation. **Noncomedogenic** means that the ingredient or product does not cause excessive follicular hyperkeratosis, and therefore is unlikely to cause comedone development.

There are two basic types of reactions that are cosmetic-induced acne aggravators. First is true comedogenesis, which can take up to several months to occur, resulting in comedo formation. Comedogenic products essentially cause increased follicular hyperkeratosis, combining with sebaceous secretions and resulting in solidified plugs or comedones.

The second is a perifollicular irritation that can cause an acute eruption of papules or pustules in a very short period of time. Clients, from time to time, will experience an overnight flare of pimples when using a new cream, or even after a salon facial treatment. It is this irritant type of reaction that can cause overnight flares. The irritation from the chemical or product will cause follicular inflammation or swelling, creating a narrowing of the follicle thus creating an anaerobic pocket, which is ideal for acne bacteria to flourish. This is known as an **acnegenic** reaction. The product or ingredient causing the inflammation is known as an acnegenic ingredient or product. The term acnegenic is probably a more appropriate term than comedogenic, which can actually encompass both comedogenic and follicular irritant reactions.

Irritant reactions and true comedogenic reactions can be evaluated by microscopic examination of follicles exposed to the ingredients or of the finished product, and checking for inflammation, or thickening of the follicle wall.

The development of comedones through comedogenic product exposure can take months to occur. Acnegenic reactions due to perifollicular irritation can occur very quickly.

Acnegenic refers to the tendency of a topical substance, usually a cosmetic or skin care product, to cause inflammation or aggravate acne.

Analysis of Acne Cosmetica

Acne cosmetica is most often characterized by multiple open and closed comedones. These may be all over the face, or in isolated areas where a certain product is being used, or where the skin is oily and susceptible to comedo development.

Acne cosmetica often looks like bumpiness just under the surface of the skin. This can be particularly apparent in the chin or cheeks. You may also notice that the client wears a lot of makeup, very oily products, or tends to try many different skin-care and cosmetic products.

Ask the client the following questions:

1. Do you notice worsening of the acne after using certain products?
2. Do you notice excessive oiliness when using certain products?
3. Is one area more clogged than others?
4. Are there many clogged pores and comedones, or just papules without comedones?
5. Do pimples seem to flare during certain times of the month?
6. How long have you had this problem?

Here are some scenarios that may be helpful in determining causes of flares or comedones:

Clients reporting a recent worsening may be able to pinpoint a new or fairly new product as the culprit. Comedones can take up to 6 months to form, so you must help the client remember any product changes in the last 6 months. Sudden flares of papules are more likely to indicate acnegenicity or a follicle-irritating product. Follicle irritation can cause an overnight flare. This can be connected to a very recent product addition.

Flares of acne without comedones are **inflammatory acne**, and can result from hormonal flares or acnegenic products causing follicle irritation. Some medications may contribute to flares also.

Inflammatory acne are flares of acne without comedones, and can result from hormonal flares or acnegenic products causing follicle irritation.

Worsening of acne after using certain products also indicates that the products may be acnegenic. Excessive oiliness when using a particular product can indicate that an oily emollient is present in the products. This oiliness tends to worsen when the product has been worn for an hour or two, and body temperature has caused the product to feel more oily.

If one area is more clogged than another, this may indicate an isolated comedogenic product, or an area of the skin that is more prone to comedo development. **Blushline acne**, characterized by multiple closed comedones is a good example of acne in an isolated area.

When the rest of the face is clear, the clogged T-zone indicates a tendency of the skin to clog in this area. Careful monitoring of products applied to this area is needed.

Bumpiness in the skin of the forehead and around the hairline is known as **pomade acne**. This occurs when comedogenic or irritating hair products, usually styling gels, conditioners, scalp oils, or sprays, coat the surface of the skin around the hairline. Pomade acne is often seen in teenagers who use many hair gels, and on black clients, who often use scalp oils.

If the client reports worsening during certain times of the month, hormonal factors are likely playing a role in acne-prone skin. Sudden stimulation of the sebaceous glands from flares of male hormones produces sebum, irritating the follicle walls. Even though the client's acne flare may be hormonal, it is still important to make sure the client avoids comedogenic products.

TESTING FOR COMEDOGENICITY

Researchers have developed a test for comedogenicity using the inside of a rabbit's ear. Cosmetic or drug topical products were applied to the inside of the ear, because the follicles inside the rabbit ear develop comedones much faster than human skin. Within three weeks most cosmetics can be tested using the rabbit ear method.

The procedure for rabbit ear assays, as they are called by the scientific community, is really quite simple. A product is applied to the inside of one ear of a male albino rabbit at least 12 weeks old. The reason for the specific sex and age of the rabbit is due to the size of these particular animals' follicles, which are better for evaluation of comedo development.

The other ear of the rabbit is left alone, as a control. A *control* is an experimental factor that remains the same throughout the experiment. Scientists can compare the two ears at the end of the three-week period to determine the difference seen in the follicles of the skin of the two different ears of the rabbit model.

The product is applied to the test area daily for three weeks. Each day the ear is observed for obvious changes to the skin and checked carefully for comedo formation.

If after three weeks there are no comedones, the product testing is finished. However, to be absolutely sure there is no excessive follicular hyperkeratosis, small tissue samples are taken surgically from the skin of the ear and examined under a microscope. Any hyperkeratosis will be obvious as it lines the follicle walls. At the same time the follicle is examined for irritation that might cause immediate acne reactions due to follicle irritation. The test is not fully complete if this microscopic test is not run. This test is called a **histopathological** study (Figure 13–1).

Blushline acne is a type of acne cosmetica, with multiple closed comedones in the blushline; caused by comedogenic pressing agents and/or dyes in the blush.

Pomade acne is bumpiness in the skin of the forehead and around the hairline.

Histopathological refers to microscopic examination of tissue to determine causes of disease or abnormality.

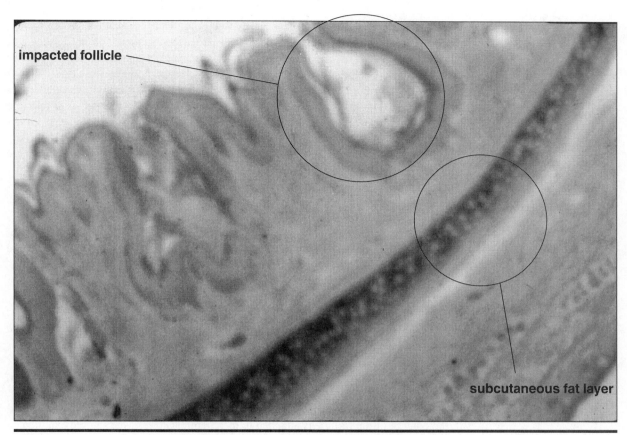

Figure 13–1   The microscopic view of retention hyperkeratosis shows excessive cell buildup and swelling. This slide represents a positive test for comedogenicity.

If comedo formation is detected, it is rated on a scale of 0 to 3. A score of 0 means that no comedones formed. A score of 3 means that the product or ingredient is comedogenic. Only products with overall scores of 0 on all rabbits tested are claimed to be noncomedogenic.

The hyperkeratosis and inflammation within the follicle found during the histopathological examination is also rated on the same scale. Although most follicles will develop a small amount of irritation and keratosis while being tested, large amounts of keratosis may indicate a delayed comedogenic reaction. In other words, a high test score in the histopathology report may indicate that longer exposure time to the product or ingredient may cause comedo development or that the test material causes sufficient irritation within the follicle to possibly promote sudden acne flares.

Materials that are found to be both noncomedogenic and show no significant irritancy or retention hyperkeratosis within the histopathological examination are said to be nonacnegenic.

A few scientists and physicians use a five-point scale. Both tests are run using scores of 0 to 5, rather than 0 to 3. If you look at various studies, you will notice that both scales are used, but the three-point scale is more often used and is the standard widely accepted by the cosmetic industry. If you look at comedogenicity studies or charts, you will notice that one rating number is followed by a slash mark and then a 3 or a 5. As an example you may see a rating of 2/3. This means that out of 3 possible points, the product or ingredient tested had a rating of 2, making it significantly comedogenic. Scores of 3/3, 4/5, or 5/5 indicate highly comedogenic materials or products.

A score of 1/3, 1/5, or 2/5 means that the product or material showed comedogenic results in the rabbit ear, but not as strong as a material with a higher score.

Remember, clients who are subject to easy development of clogged pores, comedones, and other acne lesions must first hereditarily develop retention hyperkeratosis. A client who does not develop clogged pores easily and has fairly oil-dry skin may show no reaction when treated with a product that has a low score of comedogenicity of approximately 1/3 or 2/5. Clients who easily develop acne flareups may be much more sensitive to even a mildly comedogenic material.

OTHER TESTS

Tests for comedogenicity can also be run on humans, most often human backs. The product or ingredient to be tested is applied and occluded with a patch or bandage. This is repeated on a daily basis for a specified amount of time. The skin is observed for comedo development by scientists or dermatologists. The skin can also be **biopsied**, which means a tissue sample is removed, using a **cyanoacrylate** biopsy. Cyanoacrylate, the main ingredient in powerful household glues, is applied to the skin. When peeled off, the content of the follicle is attached to the chemical. The tissue sample can then be examined under a microscope for follicular debris and hyperkeratosis.

Many scientists believe that the rabbit ear assay is a much more accurate test for determining comedogenicity. There are several reasons for this opinion. First, the rabbit ear forms comedones much faster than human skin, making the testing procedure much faster and therefore more economical. Second, rabbit ear skin is very sensitive to comedo development. Human skin develops clogged pores much more slowly. The skin on the back of a human may not necessarily develop retention hyperkeratosis hereditarily. Third, and probably most important, a rabbit can be easily controlled, and there are very few variables involved with testing. The rabbit is in a controlled environment, with a controlled diet and climate. Humans, on the other hand, are not confined, and you must consider literally hundreds of variables when you interpret test results. As examples, human models may have different diets, different environments, and different activities.

Because of these variables, many scientists believe that human studies are not as reliable or as accurate as rabbit ear studies.

The American Academy of Dermatology issued extensive guidelines for the scientific evaluation of products for comedogenicity and follicle irritancy. These tests involve applying finished products to skin and observing any comedo development, carefully

Biopsied refers to removal of a small sample of tissue for microscopic or other examination.

Cyanoacrylate is a synthetic polymer, commonly known as "super glue."

examining histological follicle biopsies for hyperkeratosis and perifollicular inflammation. The best confirmation of noncomedogenicity and nonirritancy is to have documentation by an independent test laboratory. Ask manufacturers how they determine if their products are noncomedogenic and nonirritating to follicles. Are the products tested by an independent laboratory, and what type of tests are run? Unfortunately, some companies make a noncomedogenic claim and have no tests to document their claim!

The bottom line of these guidelines is that for a true assessment of comedogenicity, the final skin-care or cosmetic product should be scientifically evaluated using this accepted protocol.

TYPES OF INGREDIENTS THAT ARE OFTEN COMEDOGENIC

The frequent culprit in the most comedogenic products is the spreading agent or vehicle. A good example of this would be a foundation or moisturizer with a comedogenic vehicle. These ingredients are used to apply the skin-care or cosmetic product to smooth, serve as an emollient or sebum replacement in alipidic (oil-dry) skin types, or add an elegant feel to the product. Oily skin areas are, of course, not alipidic. Because some of these emollients are designed to mimic human sebum, it is no wonder that some of these ingredients add to the problem of cell buildup and comedo development. Unfortunately, the vehicle often makes up the greatest part of the product, so when comedogenic ingredients are present in the vehicle, they can be present in fairly substantial quantities.

A second culprit is the emollient ingredient. Certain emollient fats, oils, waxes, fatty alcohols, fatty acids, and esters are the most common comedogenic ingredients, and many of these can be either vehicle or emollient ingredients. These ingredients often have waxy or sebum-like textures, and because of their oily and heavy texture are generally not appropriate for a skin that is already producing too much sebum.

Think of the dead corneum cells constantly shedding from the walls of the follicles as flakes of oatmeal lining a drinking glass. Because of the hereditary tendency to retain cells and because of this type of skin's oiliness, the flakes of dead cells naturally stick to the follicle walls.

Now imagine pouring oil down the sides of this glass filled with oatmeal. Imagine how oil would make the oatmeal sticky and clump together.

This may be a very rough metaphor, but it does illustrate the point. Many of the fats, oils, esters, and emollient ingredients used in cosmetics do penetrate the follicles of already clog-prone individuals, adding fatty substances to the follicles of the skin that is already burdened with too much sebum and cell buildup.

These ingredients are considered comedogenic. Their purpose in cosmetics is to lubricate or serve as a spreading agent. Although this may be helpful to truly dry skins that do not produce enough oil, it is bad for clog-prone skin. Unfortunately, not all comedogenic ingredients feel greasy or oily. In fact, some actually feel lightweight, confusing clients and estheticians alike. This is why it is so important that estheticians understand comedogenic and acnegenic principles, to prevent client use of the wrong products and to have available for purchase noncomedogenic and nonirritating formulations. Again, the bottom line is to make sure your products have been properly tested by an independent laboratory to ensure that they are truly noncomedogenic and nonacnegenic.

Emollients and Oils

Emollients that often clog pores are derived from fats or waxes of animal or vegetable origin. We will divide these substances into several categories.

Oils

Many vegetable and animal oils are comedogenic. Coconut oil, cocoa butter, peach kernel oil, linseed oil, grape seed oil, olive oil, and sesame oil are comedogenic oils. Less or noncomedogenic oils include avocado oil, safflower oil, castor oil, jojoba oil, and sunflower oil. Mineral oil is also noncomedogenic.

Other Waxes and Fats

Beeswax is noncomedogenic, particularly in small quantities of concentration, as it is often used. Emulsifying wax, carnauba wax, and candelilla wax, often used in lipstick, are noncomedogenic. Petrolatum is also noncomedogenic. However, because petrolatum is relatively greasy, it is not used often in cosmetics for oily and clog-prone skin, especially in large concentrations.

Fatty Acids

Probably the most comedogenic group of cosmetic chemicals are the fatty acids. Fatty acids, which are used to give cosmetics a creamy consistency, are often comedogenic. These substances are derived from animal and plant oils and include oleic acid, lauric acid, isostearic acid, palmitic acid, and myristic acid. Capric acid, caprylic acid, and behenic acid are less comedogenic, but still should not be used in large concentrations for oily, problem skin.

Esters

The fatty esters obtained from combining alcohols with fatty acids are also often comedogenic. As we learned in Chapter 8, these esters are often used in cosmetics because they feel less oily than raw fatty acids. However, their chemical alteration to an ester often renders them comedogenic. The esters that are comedogenic include isopropyl myristate, very well known as a highly comedogenic ingredient. Other comedogenic esters are isopropyl palmitate, octyl palmitate, isopropyl isostearate, decyl oleate, sorbitan oleate, isopropyl lanolate, iosopropyl linoleate, butyl stearate, and myristyl myristate.

Fatty Alcohols

Fatty alcohols are used in cosmetics as emollients. They are generally less comedogenic than their parent acids or esters. The comedogenic fatty alcohols include oleyl alcohol, isostearyl alcohol and octyldodecanol.

Lanolin

Lanolin is derived from sheep sebum. It is an excellent emollient, and in its purest form, in a small quantity, does not cause many problems for clog-prone skin. However, chemically altered lanolins, such as lanolic acid, isopropyl lanolate, and acetylated lanolin alcohol, are comedogenic.

Performance Agents

It is interesting that most extracts, pigments, humectants, and other performance agents are noncomedogenic ingredients. Emollients and fatty-type ingredients create the most problems. The other ingredients that create problems are inorganic pigments, specifically the red dyes.

Some ingredients, including some natural ingredients, may be irritating and still are not comedogenic, creating the possibility of an overnight type of acnegenic reaction.

The Red Dyes

Almost every red dye is comedogenic. This explains why you may often notice closed comedones on women's cheekbones. Red dyes are frequently used in blushes.

These dyes are derivatives of coal tar. Coal tar is extremely comedogenic. Red dyes are used in blush, lipsticks, powders, foundations, and skin-care products. They are not permitted to be used in eyeshadows. Coal tar is known to be a major eye irritant and is not safe for use in the eye area.

Unfortunately, many of the beautiful shades of blush or lipstick cannot be made without D & C red dyes. There is a red color in an organic pigment called carmine and in certain colors of iron oxide that are noncomedogenic. Carmine is more expensive to use than D & C red dyes and does not produce as vivid red colors.

Because of these facts, you may correctly assume that, in general, the more red a product is, the more likely it is to contain D & C red dyes and the more likely it is to be comedogenic. Again, these dyes do not produce problems for many clients who are not acne prone. However, they should be avoided in oily and acne-prone clients. Some cosmetics companies do manufacture blushes that are free of coal tar dyes.

CHEMISTRY BEHIND COMEDOGENICITY

The chemical reasons why certain cosmetic ingredients are comedogenic is not fully understood. It is certainly logical that the fats that simulate human sebum could potentially cause problems for oily, problem skin. It is believed that the size of the molecule has a great deal to do with comedogenic potential. The larger the molecule, the less likely it is to be comedogenic. This explains why some fatty acids become more or less comedogenic when they are altered chemically. When a large molecular structure is added to a fatty acid, it tends to become less comedogenic. When a fat is broken down to a smaller molecule, it is more comedogenic. This is theorized to be linked to the size of the molecule and its ability to penetrate the follicle. It makes sense that smaller fatty molecules penetrate more easily into the follicle and therefore may cause more problems.

Concentration of Comedogenic Ingredients

The amount of comedogenic ingredients used within a particular cosmetic formulation may also have an effect on the overall comedogenicity of the product. Moisturizers with large amounts of known comedogenic ingredients are more likely to be comedogenic than products with less concentration of comedogenic ingredients.

Controversy continues over the amount of comedogenic ingredients that should be used in cosmetics. Some scientists believe that as long as comedogenic ingredients make up less than 5 percent of the product, there will be no effect on the comedogenicity. The flaw in this idea is that neither the consumer nor the esthetician knows exactly how much comedogenic chemical is used in any particular product, because no cosmetic company publishes its percentages on the label. This makes this theory impossible to use practically.

The other argument against this theory is that known comedogenic ingredients should simply not be used in products that are designed for clog-prone, oily, or acne-prone skin. Again, the bottom line is to have the finished product tested. There are now many good noncomedogenic emollients and vehicle ingredients available.

Pressing Agents

Besides the problem with D & C red dyes, the other problem with blushes, as well as pressed powders, is the pressing agent. Emollients are added to talc and other products to create cake-type blush and powder. Pressed powder is an example. By mixing the powder with a sticky emollient, a pressed cake forms, which is usually marketed as a compact or powder blush.

If a comedogenic emollient is used to press the powder or blush, the product may indeed cause or increase comedone development. If a blush with D & C red dyes is pressed with a comedogenic agent, you get a "double-whammy" as far as comedogenicity is concerned!

Zinc stearate, octyldodecyl stearoyl stearate, and mineral oil are safe ingredients to use in pressing powders. They do not cause clogging and make good pressing agents.

The other problem with pressing agents is that they involve mixing a fat, which is liquid or semiliquid, with a nonsoluble powder. This means that, unlike moisturizers, which are usually water-based and always liquid, there are no liquid ingredients to "water down" the comedogenic effects of the emollient pressing agent.

Because of this, comedogenic powders tend to be very comedogenic because the skin is more directly exposed to the concentrated emollient.

Loose Powders

Loose powders are not immune from comedogenicity just because they are not in a cake form. Emollients are also added to loose powders to give them a silky texture and to help them adhere to the skin. Check powders carefully to make sure they are free of both comedogenic emollients and coal tar–derived D & C red dyes.

Skin-Care Products

Skin-care products are often comedogenic, particularly many types of moisturizers, lotions, fluids, and creams. They may be made with comedogenic emollients or other fatty ingredients. If you are treating a clog-prone client, check ingredients carefully (Figure 13–2).

The Controversy Over Ingredient Lists

Some scientists have objected to comedogenic ingredient lists (like the one included here). Their objection is based on the theory that mixtures of ingredients may not be as harmful as the individual ingredient's test score indicates.

While it is true that the bottom line is to have the final product tested, many companies do not test their products or publish the results of testing.

Testing for comedogenicity can be expensive and time-consuming. This is an additional expense for the company. Theoretically, claims testing should always be performed by an independent testing firm. By having testing performed outside the cosmetic company, the test results will be more likely to be accurate, reliable, and nonbiased. The reason lists like this one exist is so that estheticians and consumers can check the labels of their skin-care products and cosmetics for comedogenic ingredients. Even though this may not always be the most scientific or accurate method of determining potential comedogenicity, it is certainly the most practical for helping clients choose the right products.

COMEDOGENIC PRODUCT ANALYSIS

When you consult with a client who has acne or develops clogged pores easily, ask the client to bring in the products being used currently, so that you may check them for comedogenic ingredients.

Consumers today have heard the word *noncomedogenic,* but they generally are not aware of the variety of cosmetic ingredients that are comedogenic. One of the most important duties of the esthetician is to educate consumers about cosmetic chemistry. Although your clients do not need to know everything in this chapter, they will appreciate your knowledge about comedogenic ingredients and products, as well as the advice you can give about eliminating comedogenic products from home skin-care and cosmetic routines.

Although you cannot run a comedogenicity test on every product that your client might bring in, you can check the products for comedogenic ingredients content. Check each ingredient against charts like the one here. Companies that produce noncomedogenic cosmetics often have charts available that list ingredients and their comedogenic levels. On request, many of these same companies will be glad to share their comedogenic studies on their own products with you.

Returning to your product analysis, check with your clients to see what products they are routinely using. Clients will often bring in products that they are not actually using. It is important that your client is honest with you regarding daily habits.

Common Comedogenic Ingredients

Highly Comedogenic (4-5/5 or 5/3)

Linseed Oil
Olive Oil
Cocoa Butter
Oleic Acid
Coal Tar
Isopropyl Isostearate
Squalene
Isopropyl Myristate
Myristyl Myristate
Acetylated Lanolin
Isopropyl Palmitate
Isopropyl Linoleate
Oleyl Alcohol
Octyl Palmitate
Isostearic Acid
Myreth 3 Myristate
Butyl Stearate
Lanolic Acid

Moderately Comedogenic (3-4/5 or 2/3)

Decyl Oleate
Sorbitan Oleate
Myristyl Lactate
Coconut Oil
Grape Seed Oil
Sesame Oil
Hexylene Glycol
Tocopherol
Isostearyl Neopentanoate
Most D & C Red Pigments
Octyldodecanol
Peanut Oil
Lauric Acid
Mink Oil

Mildly Comedogenic (2-3/5 or 1/3)

Corn Oil
Safflower Oil
Lauryl Alcohol
Lanolin Alcohol
Glyceryl Stearate
Lanolin
Sunflower Oil
Avocado Oil
Mineral Oil
(Please note that mildly comedogenic ingredients are generally not a problem when used in diluted concentrations. Check to see their ranking of concentration on the ingredient label.)

Noncomedogenic

Glycerin
Squalane
Sorbitol
Sodium PCA
Zinc Stearate
Octyldodecyl Stearate
SD Alcohol
Propylene Glycol
Allantoin
Panthenol
Water
Iron Oxides
Dimethicone
Cyclomethicone
Polysorbates
Cetyl Palmitate
Propylene Glycol Dicaprate/Dicaprylate
Jojoba Oil
Isopropyl Alcohol
Sodium Hyaluronate
Octylmethoxycinnimate
Oxybenzone
Petrolatum
Butylene Glycol
Tridecyl Stearate
Tridecyl Trimellitate
Octyldodecyl Stearoyl Stearate
Phenyl Trimethicone

Figure 13-2   Chart of common comedogenic ingredients

Begin by checking your client's moisturizers and treatment preparations. The most important products to observe are products that remain on clog-prone areas of the face for prolonged periods of time. These include day creams, night treatment creams, moisturizers, hydrators, sunscreens, foundations, powders, blushes, and any other specialty products that the client uses that stay on the face for long periods of time.

Cleansers and toners should also be noncomedogenic, but these products do not stay on the face for eight hours at a time. Cleansers should be very easily rinseable and should not leave residues on the face. Superfatted soaps, for example, tend to leave a film on the face. Often the fat added to these soaps is comedogenic. Toner can also be made with fats, particularly if they are designed for extra dry, alipidic skin.

A good noncomedogenic cleanser should be made with noncomedogenic emulsifiers. Many contain a detergent. They may vary in strength, but many will be on the stronger side, because most skin types that develop clogs easily are also predominantly oily, making thorough cleansing a necessity. These detergent cleansers will do a good job of cleansing surface oil and debris. The cleansers may be too strong for very dry skin, but most alipidic skins do not clog easily.

A foaming cleanser is often used. These cleansers are extremely rinseable and leave the skin feeling very clean, a feeling clients often describe as "squeaky." There is nothing wrong with this feeling, as long as the cleanser does not have a high pH, stripping off too much oil and creating impaired barrier function. Most oily clients like to feel superclean. They enjoy and will use a foaming-type cleanser, particularly if they use soap on a regular basis. In short, foaming cleansers give the client the feeling of using soap without the undesirable effects of some soaps. Foaming cleansers are also convenient and can be used in the shower or bath easily.

Toners should be, as previously discussed, free of fats. They should have moderately strong astringent action, helping to remove excess oils and cell buildup. Some may contain an antibacterial, and some of the stronger ones for oily skin may contain a mild peeling agent like salicylic acid. Cleansing milk can be used for makeup removal, but should be easily removed and should not leave a residue on the skin. For oilier skin, clients may want to use a foaming cleanser after removal of makeup with a cleansing milk. Cold cream type of cleansers should not be used for clog-prone skin because they leave too much of a residue and do not remove enough oil from the surface.

Sunscreens and Day Creams

When most people think of sunscreens, they imagine greasy, coconut-fragranced oils and creams worn at the beach. Obviously, many of these oily products are comedogenic, and many clients may associate them with a previous acnegenic experience.

Sunscreens are now made for daily use, and are much more lightweight than the beach products many of us remember. Still, it is important to check to make sure that the sunscreens you are using and selling to acne-prone clients are truly noncomedogenic, and are also lightweight in texture for those clients with oily and combination skin.

Sunscreens for oily skin are usually in a light lotion, blended with hydrators and/or silicones like dimethicone to help prevent dehydration. Like all sunscreens, they should be broad spectrum, screening both UVA and UVB light. It cannot be stressed enough that day sunscreens be very comfortable for the user. They cannot be sticky, and they must perform well under makeup.

Night Treatments

There are two basic types of night treatments for clogged and problem skin, hydrators and exfoliating products.

Hydrating creams or fluids are made for skin that is clogged or acne prone but still dehydrated—in other words, skin that really needs hydration but also breaks out easily. These fluids are water-based, very light in texture, noncomedogenic, free of the offending ingredients we have discussed, and contain hydrating agents that will not clog, such as sodium PCA, glycerin, sorbitol, or hyaluronic acid. These agents hydrate without causing clog development and may be used in products without high levels of fatty emollients. Exfoliating treatment products and fluids are designed to help exfoliate excess dead cell buildup to break loose impactions. These products contain peeling agents such as benzoyl peroxide, salicylic acid, glycolic acid, resorcinol, sulfur, or a combination of these. They should be used in a lightweight vehicle base that is noncomedogenic. For more information on how to use these acne treatments, please see Chapter 12.

Foundations for Clog-Prone Skin

Foundation makeup for clogged and acne-prone skin must be noncomedogenic, preferably in a "fat-free," water-based liquid. As a general rule, liquid foundations are the only appropriate type of foundation for clogged and acne-prone skin. The foundation should be completely free of comedogenic ingredients and should be very lightweight. Coverage can still be attained if you look for foundations that contain a lot of talc and pigment. Many of these foundations contain some sort of evaporating agent, like witch hazel, to help control surface oiliness. These foundations often dry to a matte finish, a good characteristic for oily skin. Some of the newer foundations contain silicones like cyclomethicone as a spreading agent. These foundations are good for older clients with acne problems, because they do not dry as matte.

Mineral makeup, another term for loose powder makeup foundation, largely comprises earth-based ingredients. This product contains coverage pigments like zinc oxide and titanium dioxide, both of which are also physical sunscreens.

Recently, loose powder makeup foundation, also known as **mineral makeup**, has been developed. Called mineral makeup because it largely comprises earth-based ingredients, this product contains coverage pigments like zinc oxide and titanium dioxide, both also physical sunscreens.

The powder is often blended with some sort to binder, usually a fatty substance, to help it adhere to the skin. Mineral makeup provides good coverage, but it should be checked for comedogenic binders that may serve as spreading agents to help the powder adhere to the skin.

Other Products That May Be Comedogenic

Hair products and many kinds of face creams may contain comedogenic agents. The purposes of these creams, or claims, may vary greatly. They may not fall into the categories just mentioned. Check all products that come in contact with clog-prone areas.

Some items such as lipstick, eyeshadows, and other products need not be noncomedogenic because they are not being used in clog- or acne-prone areas. The only reason you may want to check these is if the client has an isolated clogged area, such as the lipline (you should check her lipstick or lip conditioner), or if the client is using the product in an area for which it was not intended (i.e., using a hair conditioner on the face). Hair conditioners and styling products often contain fats, oils, and other comedogenic ingredients. They are not designed to be used on the face.

Eye creams or concealers can be a factor in cosmetic acne. Because of gravity, these products may "drift" on to the upper cheeks while being worn. If comedogenic, they could cause problems for acne-prone areas.

Comedogenic ingredients are also sometimes used in ointments and prescription topical drugs. Although you should never tell a client to discontinue the use of a prescribed drug, you should be aware that some topical medications can be comedogenic.

DEHYDRATED, CLOGGED SKIN

Many women, particularly mature women, suffer from dehydrated skin that is also clogged. This is caused by the client mistaking dehydrated skin for dry skin. In other words, the client actually has dehydrated (water-dry) skin, but mistakenly uses products designed for dry (oil-dry) skin. These products designed for mature alipidic skin are often full of fatty acids, esters, waxes, oils, and fats. In the attempt to treat their dehydrated skin or wrinkles, they expose oily areas to the excessive fats and oils present in these emollient products.

Unfortunately, these clients have often been misdiagnosed by a cosmetic salesperson, or more unfortunately, a poorly educated esthetician. Many woman have a fear of "dry skin," because they fear aging and associate "dry skin" with aging. They do not understand that aging is not caused by "dryness" but by hereditary factors and sun damage. They attempt to treat aging with oils.

It is very important to educate this client about dehydration versus oil dryness. Explain to clients that dehydration makes the skin look dry and flaky, but this does not mean that they need oil; they need water!

Hydration can be achieved in one of two ways. Hydrating active agents can be used to increase the water level of the surface cells, easing dehydration and flaking, and making the skin look smoother, softer, and feel better.

Adding oily products to this type of skin keeps the skin from further dehydration, but it does not necessarily add significant water to the surface cells. Fatty, oily products often contain comedogenic ingredients. While these clients attempt to "moisturize," they actually cause clogged pores to form, possibly developing into acne, and are not best treating their dehydrated skin.

Almost all hydrating active agents are noncomedogenic. Many emollient-active agents for oil-dry skin are comedogenic. Retrain clients to use noncomedogenic products with noncomedogenic emollient ingredients, and use good noncomedogenic hydrating agents such as sorbitol, sodium PCA, glycerin, or hyaluronic acid. Make sure you check the vehicle ingredients for comedogenic ingredients. Most often the spreading agents are comedogenic.

Avoid using overdrying peeling agents on these clients. Psychologically they will feel that their skin is even more dry, particularly in the first few days of treatment. It is important to make sure that the client is comfortable to ensure compliance with the new program.

Heavy Creams

Many heavy creams can make acne-prone or oily clog-prone skin worse. Some of these creams are not actually comedogenic, but they contain large amounts of oils or petrolatum. They are simply too heavy for these oily-skinned clients. Although neither petrolatum or mineral oil is particularly comedogenic, they are not appropriate in large concentrations for oily, clogged, or acne-prone skin.

Oil-Free and Water-Based

These two claims are often made for products supposedly designed for oily skin. Neither of these two terms mean the same thing as *noncomedogenic*. *Oil-free* means, technically, that there are no oils in the product. That doesn't mean that there are no fatty esters, fatty acids, or other comedogenic ingredients.

Water-based simply means that the main ingredient is water, which might be mixed with comedogenic ingredients. The bottom line is, check the product carefully for comedogenic ingredients.

CLINICAL COMEDOGENICS

Some clients will have a sudden acne flareup when introduced to certain new products. Although there can be many reasons for this reaction, occasionally even a noncomedogenic product can cause an acne flareup due to irritation of the follicles. If your client reports such a flareup, advise your client to try the cream again after a short time. If the reaction continues, the client should discontinue use of the product.

Checklist of Products

The following products should be checked during a comedogenic analysis:

- Cleansers, washes, and soaps
- Toners, fresheners, and astringents
- Day creams, moisturizers, and sunscreens
- Night fluids, creams, specialty products, and ampoules
- Foundation makeup
- Blush
- Any other product that is being used over a clog-prone area of the face for a prolonged period of time

Checklist of Analysis Procedures

1. Analyze the skin and the areas that have comedones, clogged pores, sebaceous filaments, or other acne lesions.
2. Check the client's current products for comedogenic ingredients.
3. Are the products the client is using really correct for the skin type, or is the client using products for oil-dry skin when the skin is actually dehydrated?
4. Is the client using fluids and lotions or creams?
5. Are the products the client is using simply too heavy for the skin?
6. Is the client skipping steps that should be done?
7. If the products the client uses contain comedogenic ingredients, are they high or low on the ingredient list? If the client has a minimal number of clogged pores, it may not be caused by the products. Remember, in order to have a comedogenic reaction, you must have comedogenic products and a skin type that tends to clog due to hereditary oiliness and hyperkeratosis.

CLIENT PRODUCT ANALYSIS

As we have previously discussed, you should ask a client who is clog prone to bring in all products for analysis on the first visit. First, check the products with the checklist for analysis.

After checking the products for correct skin type, and so forth, begin checking the products for comedogenic ingredients. Let's look at a typical label. You have already established that the client is definitely clog prone. Here are the products the client is using:

Product: Cleansing Cream. Ingredients: Mineral oil, purified water, beeswax, sodium borate, isopropyl palmitate, petrolatum, stearyl alcohol, lanolin alcohol, ceteareth-20, magnesium aluminum silicate, sodium dehydroacetate, methyl paraben, propyl paraben, D & C red # 6.

Analysis: More than comedogenic, this cleansing cream is simply much too greasy and heavy for oily, clog-prone skin. It contains isopropyl palmitate, a known comedogenic ingredient. However, the ingredient is fairly low on the ingredient list. It also contains D & C red # 6, which is not very comedogenic compared to other D & C red dyes and is present in a fairly small quantity. The biggest problem with this cleanser is that it is oil based, very heavy, and is probably not being rinsed off well, which can be a real problem for oily, clog-prone skin. This cleanser is a good cleanser for drier skin types or for those who wear heavy or theatrical makeup and need a thorough oil-based cleanser. It should be replaced for your client with a rinseable foaming cleanser and/or a non-greasy cleansing milk.

Product: Day Protectant. Ingredients: Water, isopropyl palmitate, isopropyl myristate, mineral oil, propylene glycol, proplyene glycol stearate, stearic acid, magnesium aluminum silicate, oleic acid, cellulose gum, methyl paraben, propyl paraben, fragrance.

Analysis: This day cream is loaded with potentially comedogenic ingredients. Isopropyl myristate, isopropyl palmitate, and oleic acid are all comedogenic chemicals.

Isopropyl myristate and isopropyl palmitate are extremely high on the ingredient list, indicating a fairly large concentration of these problem agents. This cream is left on the face all day, creating a true exposure time. This day cream should only be used on skin types that are not clog prone. Your client should discontinue this product.

Product: Liquid makeup. Ingredients: Water, propylene glycol, SD alcohol 40, titanium dioxide, talc, witch hazel extract, zinc oxide, magnesium aluminum silicate, methyl paraben, propyl paraben; may contain iron oxides, ultramarine blue.

Analysis: This is an excellent example of a noncomedogenic product. It contains no comedogenic ingredients and no real emollient fats. It contains witch hazel and SD alcohol as mild drying agents—a plus for oily skins. This makeup is safe enough to be used on acne. Your client made a good choice here and should continue to use this product.

Product: Loose powder. Ingredients: talc, myristyl myristate, zinc stearate, fragrance, methyl paraben, propyl paraben, iron oxides, fragrance.

Analysis: This product would be acceptable if it did not have myristyl myristate as a pressing agent. It should not be used on oily, acne, or clogged skin.

These are only a few examples of how to do a comedogenic analysis. Use your head and the facts you have been taught. The bottom line of all of this testing and analysis is: Is your client's skin developing clogged pores? If it is, something is not working correctly!

You should of course have available to your clients an entire range of noncomedogenic products. When purchasing products for your salon, remember to check carefully for the ingredients and testing procedures we have discussed throughout this chapter.

Topics for Discussion

1. Discuss testing for comedogenicity.
2. Discuss the difference between noncomedogenic and nonacnegenic products.
3. Discuss the concentration of possible comedogenic ingredients in a product and how this may affect comedogenicity.
4. Why are comedogenic ingredient lists controversial?
5. Discuss the various types of products for clog-prone skin. What should you look for in a day cream? Night treatment? Foundation?
6. Discuss treatment of adult, mature, clogged, and dehydrated skin.
7. Why is it important to test the final product for comedogenicity and irritancy?

Chapter

14

Extraction

Objectives

Extraction is an extremely important part of the esthetician's skills, and it is a difficult process to master.

With proper hands-on supervision, this chapter will help the esthetician learn about extraction procedures for many different types of follicle impactions. Different methods of extraction will be discussed as well as specific unusual problems that may be encountered during extraction.

Extraction refers to the removal of dead cells, sebum, bacteria, and other debris from the skin's follicles. This expulsion technique is probably the most important function of a facial treatment. The solid mass of sebum, dead cells, and other matter stuck in the follicles are both an esthetic and a physiological problem. Besides being unsightly, failure to treat these lesions may lead to more serious acne and health problems, not to mention permanent scarring.

Extraction techniques cannot be learned by simply studying a book. You must have hands-on training in all areas of extraction, taught by a well-qualified instructor. Do not attempt any of the procedures outlined in this chapter without the supervision and hands-on demonstration of a qualified, licensed instructor.

Extraction refers to the removal of dead cells, sebum, bacteria, and other debris from the skin's follicles.

Extraction is a very important part of the esthetics profession and is possibly the most important service that estheticians perform. It can also be an uncomfortable and unsafe procedure if performed incorrectly.

Some states do not allow the use of lancets for extraction. Check with your esthetics instructor or school for laws governing the use of lancets by estheticians in your state.

ANALYSIS OF THE NEED FOR EXTRACTION

Almost every skin that you will see under the magnifying lamp will need at least some extraction. Even dry, older skin will be likely to have some clogged follicles in the nose area. Observe your client's skin closely under a magnifying lamp. Check all areas of the face well, including behind and in front of the ears, the neck, and the jawline.

Understanding Clogged Pores

All clogged pores (follicles) and comedones have several developmental factors.

Retention hyperkeratosis refers to an overabundance of sebum that often begins at the time teenagers begin producing larger amounts of sex hormones.

Retention hyperkeratosis, a hereditary factor, refers to the tendency of dead skin cells (corneocytes) not to shed in a regular and uniform manner. These dead cells accumulate inside the follicle, lining the walls.

Sebum production levels are also hereditary, and in clog-prone individuals, overactive glands secrete excess sebum, coating the buildup of cells. As sebum becomes exposed to air (oxygen), the sebum oxidizes and forms a semisolid mass; any sebum exposed to the oxygen turns dark, creating the black part of the "blackhead."

Sebum is basically a complex of fatty materials and can solidify similarly to the way chicken fat turns solid when refrigerated. It is this solidification that helps form the impaction in the follicle.

Sebaceous filaments are small impacted follicles on the nose and other facial areas caused by oxidized, solidified sebum.

Sebaceous filaments are the small clogged pores many clients have on their noses. These are not classic comedones, mostly just oxidized sebum and very little cell buildup. This explains their frequent occurrence and presence on many clients' skin.

Open comedones are noninflammatory acne lesions usually called blackheads.

Open comedones are classic "blackheads," with a distinctly dilated follicle opening. They contain a mix of keratinized cells and solidified sebum.

Closed comedones are noninflammatory acne lesions called whiteheads.

Closed comedones appear as small bumps just underneath the skin. They are frequently found in the cheekbone area, especially in the blushline. They are often associated with comedogenic skin-care and makeup products, hence their frequent appearance in the blushline from blushes pressed with comedogenic fats or use of coal tar–derived red dyes. They are frequently found just under the corners of the mouth. The difference between closed and open comedones is that in the closed comedo, the follicle is not uniformly dilated. The follicle opening, or **ostium**, is barely visible, even when examining the skin with a magnifying lamp.

Ostium is the opening in follicles.

Analysis

After thoroughly removing all makeup using a light, nonfragranced cleansing milk, examine the skin carefully using a magnifying lamp. Do not tone the skin before analysis, because this will make the pores look smaller and will also constrict them for proper extraction. Spread the skin taut between your fingers and observe all areas, moving down the face and continuing the spreading movement and observation. Look for clogged pores (follicles), small white bumps just under the skin (closed comedones), large dilated open comedones, papules, and pustules. Carefully note the size of the pores and the location. This pattern will determine the type of skin (oily, combination, etc.). Clogged pores are rarely found on a truly dry or **alipidic** (does not produce enough sebum) skin. Because oil-dry skin does not produce much sebum and therefore has very small pores, it is very unlikely to suffer from comedones or clogged pores.

Alipidic means "lack of lipids." These skin types do not produce enough lipids.

On combination skin you will likely see small clogged pores through the T-zone area and scattered larger clogged pores or blackheads. In any area you may see small white bumps or closed comedones, milia (whiteheads), pustules, and papules associated with acne. The width of the T-zone will determine the oiliness of the area and therefore the number of clogged pores. Clogged pores are always a sign of an oily area (Figure 14–1).

The perimeter of the face is an ideal place for clogged pores and acne lesions to form. These are areas your clients often miss while cleansing. You can think of these areas as "cobwebs" in the corner of a room! (See Figure 14–2.)

Figure 14–1   T-zone of clogged pores

Think about your client doing at-home cleaning. The client is not a skin-care specialist and probably does not take the time or care cleaning as you would cleaning your own face. The client applies the cleanser and massages it but does not notice the remnants of cleanser or makeup left in front of the ears, in the hairline, and under the jawline. The client may also omit toner as a follow-up in these areas.

Failure to remove makeup and cleanser in these areas means that dead cells build up here as well as emollients and ingredients left from the cleanser. Clogs will inevitably form.

The first thing you should do when you encounter "perimeter acne" is to gently make the client aware of it and why it is probably there. Instruct your client to pay extra attention to cleaning these areas and to use toner after cleansing. You may also suggest that a foaming cleanser be used as a second cleanser after makeup removal. This not only helps remove any emollients left from a cleansing milk, but the foam itself is very obvious when it is still on the face or in one of those hidden corners! Your client will see the foam and rinse off the area.

Continuing the Analysis . . .

Gently spread the skin with your thumb and forefinger. Move the fingers across the face, constantly spreading the skin gently. Observe if there are any small white bumps that are only visible when the skin is pulled taut. These are often closed comedones and can be seen on any area of the face, but especially can be hidden in the chin area, just under the lower lip, and under the chin and jawline.

Examination Procedures for Extraction

1. Cleanse the skin well.
2. Using a magnifying lamp, examine the skin observing areas with enlarged pores, noting areas with smaller and larger pores.
3. Combination skin—Note enlarged pores through the T-zone indicating oilier skin, smaller pores around the edges of the face, indicating less oil production. The width of the oily T-zone determines whether the skin is oily-combination or dry-combination. The wider the visible enlarged pore structure, the oilier the skin is.
4. Clogged pores, comedones, closed comedones, papules, and pustules are more likely to be seen in the oilier areas.
5. The small clogged pores in the nose are usually sebaceous filaments, not open comedones; they are simply follicles filled with oxidized sebum.
6. IN THE OILY AREAS . . . Pull the skin taut with the thumb and forefinger and observe any small white bumps under the skin. These are closed comedones.
7. Check the perimeter of the face well, including the chin, jawline, the neck, and in front of and behind the ears.

Figure 14–2 Examination procedures

Check the skin for sebaceous filaments, which are not really open comedones. They are what most clients refer to as "clogged pores." These are follicles that have filled with sebum, sometimes over a very short period of time. They are most noticeable on the nose, but can appear in any area. On very oily skin, they can literally seem to be in every single area (Plates 24a, 24b).

Sebaceous filaments indicate an oily area. They are not nearly as large or dilated as an open comedo, but they are basically the same type of lesion. The only real difference is that a sebaceous filament is mostly sebum, whereas a real open comedo is dilated, is much larger, and is filled with many dead cells. An open comedo may take weeks to form, but sebaceous filaments may form in just a few days. The debris extracted from a sebaceous filament will be much smaller than that of an open comedo, and you will also notice that the plug is not as deep or as solid (Plate 25).

OPEN COMEDONES

Open comedones may appear anywhere on the face. They are most noticeable in acne conditions and in clients who have neglected their skin for a long time. They are also frequently observed in young adolescents who have a budding adolescent acne problem, but may not be cleaning well and have not taken a true interest in their personal appearance yet.

Open comedones can certainly appear in any skin type, but they are more prevalent in the above-mentioned situations. Clients who are very conscientious will be aware of these lesions and will either have them extracted or attempt to do so themselves. Open comedones are often about the size of a pinhead. They have a large black top, hence the term *blackhead.* Open comedones are the easiest lesions to extract.

PRESOFTENING BEFORE EXTRACTION

The procedure you follow before extraction will significantly help loosen follicle impactions, making extractions less difficult for the esthetician and less uncomfortable for the client. The skin must be pretreated before extraction. This pretreatment will help soften the accumulations in the follicles as well as the surface of the skin, making the skin more soft and flexible during the extraction procedure.

Desincrustation

Desincrustation refers to the process of softening the skin and sebaceous impaction by applying a chemical that helps liquify the sebum, reducing hard, solid plugs to a softer consistency. This technique softens clogs significantly. The chemical used for this procedure is usually an anionic surfactant. Thus, desincrustation solutions usually have a higher, or more alkaline, pH.

Desincrustation refers to the process of softening the skin and sebaceous impaction by applying a chemical that helps liquify the sebum, reducing hard, solid plugs to a softer consistency.

Desincrustation solutions are usually either liquids or a soft gel-cream consistency, often referred to as a pre-mask.

The liquid is applied to the affected areas of the face after preliminary cleansing or is sometimes poured onto cotton compresses and then applied to the face.

The "pre-masks" can be applied to the face either with a brush or your hands. Pre-masks have a thicker consistency than liquid solutions. They can be seen on the skin, whereas liquids cannot. Being careful to follow manufacturer's instructions, allow the solution or pre-mask to sit on the face for 5 to 10 minutes. Steam treatment is frequently used at the same time. Steaming does not "open the pores"; however, it does hydrate the surface, helping to make the skin considerably more flexible for extraction. Galvanic desincrustation may be applied over the pre-mask or liquid, depending on the manufacturer's instructions. Galvanic treatment with a desincrustant chemical provides for better penetration of the product and better reduction of the plug due to chemical reactions produced by the electricity within the follicle. (See *Milady's Standard Textbook for Professional Estheticians* for further explanation and instructions for use of galvanic current.)

The oilier and more impacted the skin, the better it is to use galvanic treatment. Some clients who have a minimal number of clogged follicles and more dehydrated skin may find galvanic treatment to be too drying. It is a good idea to use galvanic treatment routinely on acne conditions, provided there are no medical contraindications for use.

After the "soak" period with desincrustation solution or pre-mask or galvanic treatment is completed, remove the desincrustant product well and proceed with extraction.

Desincrustant chemicals are often slippery and must be removed thoroughly before extraction. Otherwise the skin will be too slippery for extraction procedures.

OTHER PRE-EXTRACTION PROCEDURES

The use of a brushing machine may help loosen dead cells, particularly on skin that is both dehydrated and clogged.

The electric rotating brush should be gently applied after steaming. The brush should be used over a layer of emulsion-type cleanser to prevent too much scratching of the face during the brushing procedure. Do not use the brush on acne, couperose, or sensitive skin. (For further instruction on brushing, see *Milady's Standard Textbook for Professional Estheticians.*)

Suction, or vacuuming, may be performed with a skin suction machine after desincrustation or steaming. Suction may help to further loosen impactions that have already been loosened with desincrustation. Suction removes very little debris from the follicle, but the procedure feels good to the client and has a nice psychological effect. Again, suction should not be used on sensitive or couperose skin or acne. See *Milady's Standard Textbook for Professional Estheticians* for instruction on suction machines.

Enzyme Treatments and Peels

Light peeling treatments performed with enzymes or alphahydroxy acids can help loosen clogged pores and impaction significantly. The light exfoliating effects help remove dead cells from the skin's surface and helps loosen and slightly dilate the follicle openings. This makes extraction easier. Clients who are both dehydrated and clogged may particularly benefit from an enzyme pore treatment.

Enzymes are normally applied during the steam treatment for an 8- to 12-minute period of time. For further information on how to use enzymes, see Chapter 18, Chemical Peeling and Exfoliation Procedures.

HYGIENE AND EXTRACTION

It is very important to always wear gloves during extraction. It is generally good practice to wear gloves throughout the treatment, especially if there are any acne lesions present. Please review Chapter 4 before beginning extraction.

EXTRACTION OF OPEN COMEDONES

After presoftening the accumulations, remove all products from the skin, leaving the face moist but not wet. Wet skin or skin that still has product on it is impossible to extract. Take two cotton swabs. Hold them as you would hold two pencils. It is best to use the type of swab that has a soft, flexible plastic stick. These plastic cotton swabs are much easier to work with and will snap if too much pressure is applied, a built-in safety feature (Plate 26).

Place a swab on each side of the open comedo. Gently press down on the swabs and then gently move the swabs closer together, with the tips touching the skin. This will have a lifting effect on the solid plug. Keep applying gentle pressure until you see the plug come out of the follicle. If the plug does not come out easily, move the swabs to another angle around the sides of the comedo and repeat the procedure. Once the plug is out, continue to press gently on the sides of the follicle to make sure all of the debris has been removed.

Finger Technique

Wrap your gloved forefingers in damp cotton. Using the same gentle downward and inward pressure technique, attempt to extract the comedo. Work your fingers all around the comedo with the same pressure technique.

Cotton swabs are easier for many people because they are smaller than fingers. It is the consensus of clients that the cotton swab technique is more comfortable and more efficient.

Extractor Technique

Comedo extractors are best to use on non-fleshy parts of the face, such as the forehead or cheekbones, or on clients whose skin does not have a fleshy thickness that can be physically manipulated. Comedo extractors should never be used on thin, fragile, sensitive, or couperose skin.

Place the extractor over the open comedo, with the hole in the extractor directly over the comedo. It is very important that the lesion be smaller than the hole in the metal extractor. If the lesion is wider than the hole in the extractor, do not use the extractor. Either try a large extractor or try the cotton swab method.

Assuming that the comedo can easily fit into the hole in the extractor, gently press straight down on the extractor, using the leverage of the handle end to exert pressure. The plug should come out of the follicle and be noticeable inside the hole of the extractor. It is a good idea to follow this extraction procedure with another gentle expression of the follicle with the cotton swabs to check for any further debris that might be trapped in the follicle.

Remember when using a metal extractor that the extractor is metal and is not flexible. The use of a comedo extractor can be very painful for the client, particularly if used over the entire face. They should be reserved for use on bony areas or non-fleshy skin. In general, comedone extractors are more uncomfortable than using finger or cotton swab extraction techniques.

Comedo extractors are available in a variety of sizes. Some are made with a slight bend for better leverage. Some are made with a round hole, and some with an oval or rectangular hole. You should have some of each type available, and you will, over time, develop a feel for which is appropriate to use. Comedo extractors must be sterilized after each client. Plastic disposable extractors are breakable and are generally not advised. See Chapter 4 for sterile and aseptic procedure.

CLOSED COMEDONES

Closed comedones appear as small bumps just underneath the surface of the skin. They can be found on any area of the face, but are frequently found on the cheeks, jawline, and chin. Often you will see a large number of closed comedones on the cheekbones of female clients. These are often caused by a comedogenic reaction to a blush. (See Chapter 13.) The closed comedo is just beneath the skin and normally has a very small follicle opening. If you look carefully through a magnifying lamp, you may detect a very small opening in the top of the closed comedo. Often, these follicles must be dilated with a lancet before extraction.

EXTRACTION OF CLOSED COMEDONES

Closed comedones are the most difficult of any lesion to extract, because they are just beneath the surface of the skin, have a very small pore opening, and may vary greatly in size. If you can see the opening of the follicle well and the white area surrounding the opening does not appear to be very large, you may attempt to extract the area by using the cotton swab technique. Make sure you have softened the area well with a desincrustant. Place the tip of the cotton swabs on either side of the closed comedo, being careful to make sure you are clear about the border of the lesion. In other words, make sure you have the entire comedo within the placement of your swabs. Failure to do so may result in extracting only part of the comedo. Gently press down on the swabs and then gently turn them inward while pulling the skin taut with the outside fingers. A solid white stream of sebaceous material will emerge from the comedo. Continue to gently press the area until no more material emerges.

In many closed comedones, follicle dilation is necessary. This procedure is performed for three reasons. Dilation of the follicle allows more room for the sebaceous material to emerge. Secondly, dilation of the closed comedo relieves pressure on the follicle walls, helping to avoid follicle wall rupture during extraction. Finally, relieving the pressure on the lesion by lancet dilation makes the extraction procedure much more comfortable for the client.

To dilate the follicle, find the small opening in the top of the closed comedo. Using a sterile, disposable lancet, gently dilate this follicle opening by gently pressing the tip of the lancet through the follicle opening. DO NOT attempt to force the lancet into the follicle (Figure 14–3 and Plate 27).

After the follicle is dilated, extract the comedo using the cotton swab technique. Waiting a few seconds after lancet dilation sometimes helps to expel the debris. Relief of the pressure accomplished by dilation will often cause some "self-expelling" action. This will help make the extraction process easier. It is not advisable to use comedo extractors on closed comedones. Closed comedones are often found in fleshy areas of the face, making use of an extractor cumbersome and difficult. Second, closed comedones often have a larger diameter than that of the opening in a comedo extractor, making the use of the extractor unsafe and inappropriate.

Figure 14–3 Dilation using a lancet

EXTRACTION OF PUSTULES

Pustules are raised, inflammatory acne lesions. They have a "head" that is filled with pus. Most of the pustule and its contents are above the surface of the skin.

To extract a pustule, gently place the tip of a sterile disposable lancet against the side of the pustule. Bracing the outside of your hand against the face, gently "lift" the very top of the pustule away with the lancet. This procedure is similar to removing a splinter from your finger, except that the lesion is above the skin. Because you are strictly removing dead cells from the top of the pustule, this procedure should not be very uncomfortable to the client.

When the top of this dead cell layer has been removed, the pus will begin to emerge from the follicle opening. Placing two cotton swabs on the sides of the lesion, gently press downward and inward on the swabs, being careful to hold the area taut with the outside fingers. The rest of the impaction should emerge from the follicle. Following the pus will be the emergence of the actual comedo, often referred to as the "core." This part of the extracted material will look much like the debris extracted from an open or closed comedo, except that these impactions will be slightly harder and more dense.

It is not unusual for a small amount of bleeding to occur while extracting pustules. Remember, the follicle wall has ruptured in a pustule, allowing blood to come into the follicle. A slight amount of red blood appearing after extracting a pustule indicates that there is no more debris or sebum present in the follicle. Papules, nodules, and cysts are deep inflammatory lesions and are the domain of the dermatologist. Do not attempt to extract these lesions. Although papules will often develop into pustules or dissipate without treatment, cysts and nodules should be referred to the dermatologist for treatment.

FACIAL TREATMENT BEFORE AND AFTER EXTRACTION

We have discussed the actual extraction procedures used in removing debris from the follicles. Treatment before and after extraction is very important, to help ease the extraction process by softening the follicle accumulations, to treat the area after extraction to prevent infection, and help further dry the lesions. The following is a suggested treatment in which extraction takes place. This treatment is known in the esthetics industry as "deep-pore cleansing."

1. Completely remove all the makeup from the face with a liquid cleanser.
2. Analyze the skin under the magnifying lamp. Check all areas of the face for clogged pores (sebaceous filaments), open and closed comedones, milia, and pustules. At the same time, of course, check for other disorders of the skin.
3. Apply steam treatment to the face with a vapor machine in the usual manner. Apply a desincrustant pre-mask, desincrustation lotion compresses, or enzyme treatment to the skin.
4. Remove the desincrustant treatment or enzyme treatment after allowing the treatment to sit on the face for about eight to ten minutes, or the time prescribed by the product manufacturer.

5. Galvanic desincrustation treatment may be used to further loosen the debris in the follicle, especially in cases of multiple impactions or acne.

6. Suction may be used, providing that there are no contraindications, as previously discussed.

7. Begin extraction in the chin and jawline area first, working upward on the face. This order of extraction helps the esthetician avoid contaminating the hands or other areas of the face from debris extracted from the lower part of the face. It is the most hygienic and aseptic pattern of treatment.

8. After extraction is completed, apply an antiseptic toner to the face with damp sponges or cotton pads. This will help kill any bacteria on the surface of the skin. It will also lower the pH from the use of the alkaline desincrustant treatment.

9. Apply the appropriate treatment for the particular skin type. An ampoule or antiseptic lotion may be appropriate. Benzoyl peroxide or salicylic acid can be used on oilier and acne-prone skin.

10. Apply high frequency over the face. This also further helps kill surface bacteria. Using a piece of gauze over the face while extracting helps intensify the frequency treatment and helps the electrode move easily across the skin.

11. Apply a drying clay-based mask to the area that was extracted. A mask containing sulfur, salicylic acid, or benzoyl peroxide may be used for acne. A bentonite-based mask with camphor may be more appropriate for oily or more sensitive clogged areas. The mask should be allowed to dry completely, usually for about 15 to 20 minutes.

12. Remove the mask with damp, soft cloths, sponges, or cotton pads. Apply more toner after mask removal.

13. Apply a noncomedogenic hydrating sunscreen.

It is strongly advised that clients not wear makeup for about two hours after extraction. Extraction can be slightly irritating, and application of makeup to freshly extracted areas may be more irritating.

EXTRACTION OF MILIA

Milia are small deposits of sebum between the follicle and the corneum (Figure 14–4). A milium is not the same as a comedo. The sebaceous material is trapped above the skin's surface, covered with a layer of dead cells. Milia may occur for several reasons. Milia is frequently seen on older, mature skin (Plate 28). This may be associated with the use of heavy creams loaded with emollients for treating dry, dehydrated skin. Injuries to the skin sometimes also cause milia to develop. Dermabrasion by a plastic surgeon is often followed by a large number of milia forming. This will be discussed more in detail in Chapter 19, Treating the Plastic Surgery Patient.

To extract a milium, make sure that it is large enough to be extracted. Milia are almost always perfectly round in shape and are found on any area of the face, but especially the cheeks and the forehead. A milium must be large enough to easily lift off the

Milia are small deposits of sebum between the follicle and the corneum.

Some General Rules for Extraction

1. Always wear disposable latex or vinyl gloves during extraction and throughout the remainder of the treatment.
2. Do not extract for over ten minutes in any single treatment. More than ten minutes of extraction is too stimulating for most skin types and can be very uncomfortable.
3. Reduce discomfort of the client by keeping the skin pulled taut during extraction, and only extracting very small areas at a time.
4. Never attempt extraction if you have not had hands-on experience with a qualified instructor.
5. The biggest mistake made in extraction is failure to properly presoften impactions. Make sure you are using the correct products for this important phase of the treatment.
6. Always use an antiseptic, low pH toner, or special after-extraction product after completing your extraction procedures. This is important to reduce the chance of infection, soothe the skin, reduce redness, and reestablish the proper pH.
7. Do not use any alphahydroxy or beta hydroxy acid products immediately after treatment, especially salon concentrations. Clients may use a low percentage AHA that evening, if recommended.

top with a lancet. This is about the size of the heads of two pins. Make sure that you are absolutely positive that the lesion is a milium. Other types of skin lesions look like milia, including some types of skin growths. Check the shape carefully. The milium should not have any capillaries running through it. If the lesion has a capillary associated with it, leave it alone. Also, if the milium seems to give you any resistance while using the lancet, leave it alone. The dead cell layer on the top of a milium is very thin. Milia are easily treated with a lancet and should not give any resistance to pressure from the lancet.

Gently spread the skin taut around the milium with your fingertips. Using a sterile disposable lancet, gently lift off the top cell layers from the milium. Gently place the lancet against the side of the top of the milium. The lancet should slide easily into the top. These are all dead cells in the elevated part of the milium, so the client should barely feel the lancet at all.

You should barely see the opening you have created in the top of the milium. Sometimes a very small amount of sebaceous material will emerge from the side of the milium where you have lifted the dead skin. After the lancet procedure is complete, place a cotton swab on both sides of the milium and gently press and lift on the milium. You may find it helpful to put slightly more pressure on the "unopened" side of the milium. This pressure will help the sebaceous material exit the follicle easier.

Horny zone of epidermis grown over follicle opening

Trapped sebum, keratin and bacteria

Dead cells, sebum, and bacteria

Figure 14–4   Milia

If the milium does not extract easily, you may try lifting more dead cells with the lancet. Sometimes when the milium is small enough, it is easier to use a comedo extractor, particularly on non-fleshy areas of the face such as the forehead. Place the comedo extractor over the milium. Gently press down on the unopened side of the milium, moving the extractor very slowly toward the open side of the milium. You should see the emerging sebaceous material.

If the milium does not respond to treatment, do not continue attempting to extract it! You must have lots of experience to extract milia! Do not extract milia until you have been given hands-on instruction by a qualified licensed instructor.

LESIONS AROUND THE EYES

Many clients will complain of small milia-like lesions around the eye area. Some of these lesions are milia. Some are other types of skin growth or lesions called xanthalasmas. **Xanthalasmas** are much larger and flatter than milia, have a yellowish appearance, are below the skin's surface, and may have irregular shape. They are rarely round like a milium. These lesions should be referred to a dermatologist—they are not in the domain of the esthetician. Xanthalasmas can sometimes be indicative of other diseases

Xanthalasmas are much flatter than milia, have a yellowish appearance, are below the skin's surface, and may have irregular shape.

or disorders, such as high cholesterol. Refer the client to a dermatologist for treatment and follow-up (Plate 29).

Syringomas are small pinpoint lesions that occur under the eyes. These are actually small cysts on the sudoriferous glands. They may look like very small milia and are usually in multiple numbers. They are thought to be hereditary, or possibly caused by sun damage. They are generally not extractable, and should be referred to a dermatologist or an ophthalmologist for treatment.

Other small milia in the eye area are often associated with the use of heavy eye creams, concealers, and other eye cosmetics that are thick, heavy, and loaded with fatty emollients. This can cause a buildup of dead cells in the area. Advise the client to switch to a lighter eye cream or a gel-type treatment. These have fewer or lesser concentrations of emollients.

Improper cleansing has also been associated with milia development around the eyes. Clients who do not remove their eye makeup well on a nightly basis have a tendency to develop milia. These clients leave traces of makeup or do not remove the eye makeup at all. Instruct the client about the correct procedure to remove eye makeup and make sure she is using a proper eye makeup remover.

Clients who are very rough in removing their eye makeup may also suffer from milia development around the eyes. Injuries and excessive manipulation of the eyelid tissue have been associated with milia development.

Do not attempt to remove milia found on the eyelids. This tissue is extremely difficult to handle properly and is extremely fragile. Refer this client to an opthalmologist or dermatologist and give proper home care advice. Sometimes milia will disappear after the adjustment of proper home care.

TREATING CLOGGED AND DEHYDRATED SKIN

Skin that is both clogged and dehydrated is extremely difficult to treat. The client's skin will feel dry, but is actually oily and dehydrated. The follicle will become "crimped shut" from the tightness of the surface dehydration, making extraction difficult, if not impossible.

You should avoid heavily drying products. Products that are made with high levels of humectants and low levels of emollients are appropriate for this skin problem. The hydrating agents will help hydrate the skin's surface, making it less dry feeling and more pliable so that extraction is more easily accomplished.

To treat this type of skin, apply a hydrating fluid during salon steam treatment. Allow to steam with the humectant-based hydrating fluid for eight to ten minutes. This water from the steam and the humectant will help soften the skin, hydrate the surface, and reduce the "crimped" effect on the follicles.

After this procedure, proceed with extraction. Follow extraction with a toner and then apply hydrating fluid to the skin before applying a gentle, clay-based drying mask. Applying a drying clay-based mask without applying a hydration fluid can be over-drying to this type of skin problem. Clients should be instructed to use the hydrating treatment with the mask at home too. Twice-a-week application will help clear the clogged pores.

The client with both dehydrated skin and clogged pores are often middle aged, trying desperately to "fight aging" through the use of heavy moisturizing, and believing that he or she is "drying up" with age. These heavier, and often comedogenic, cosmetics (see Chapter 13) clog the skin while the client attempts to treat the wrinkles and lines associated with aging, dehydrating, and sun damage.

This client needs lots of education about the aging process, sun damage, and comedogenic cosmetics. It is up to the esthetician to provide this education and help the client find a product program that helps dehydration but will not be clogging to this clog-prone skin condition.

SOLAR BLACKHEADS

In older clients, often men, you will find a concentration of large open comedones around the eye area. Although the development of these huge blackheads is similar to acne-related blackheads, these lesions are caused by excessive long-term sun exposure. This condition is called Favre-Racouchot syndrome. More on this condition will be discussed in Chapter 16, Sun and Sun Damage (Plate 30).

Extraction of solar comedones must be done very gently. This type of skin often has extremely fragile capillaries, also associated with excessive sun exposure and damage. This sun-damaged skin bruises easily, and it is easy to cause redness that lasts for days after treatment. You must be extremely gentle while treating this fragile skin.

Begin by cleansing or steaming the skin. Applying a fluid hydrating agent while steaming will help loosen the impactions and make the skin more pliable. Very gently extract the lesions with the cotton swab technique. Do not attempt to remove every single clog in one session. Advise the client to have weekly treatments in the salon until the problem is clear, and then regular monthly treatments to prevent or control their return. Favre-Racouchot is a chronic problem, and this client will often have other sun-related skin problems. There are medical treatments for Favre-Racouchot syndrome and other sun-damage conditions.

DURATION OF EXTRACTION

Extraction should not be performed for more than 10 to 15 minutes on any client during one treatment visit. Extraction that is longer than this can be painful and traumatic to both the client and the skin. You will, of course, have to assess the needs and the duration for each client as an individual.

Clogged skin should never be massaged, at least not for prolonged periods of time. Avoid massage on excessively clogged skin, until such time that the skin is almost completely clear of clogged pores and any other type of acne lesion. As a general rule, if you take 10 minutes or more for extraction on a client, that client should not be massaged.

Massaging of the clogged skin will simply stimulate more oil production and apply pressure to clogs, forcing them to become more impacted in the skin.

Topics for Discussion

1. Discuss extraction—can any skin type need extractions?
2. Why is it important to presoften the skin before extraction? What are some techniques used to presoften the skin for extraction?
3. Describe the extraction process for closed comedones. When is follicle dilation necessary? Describe the extraction procedure for pustules.
4. Describe the order of facial treatment procedures involved in a deep cleansing treatment.
5. Discuss problem impactions around the eyes. Which should be referred to the dermatologist?
6. What are some special procedures used for treating clogged skin that is also dehydrated?

Chapter 15

The Intrinsic Aging Process

Objectives

Aging is a process that almost every person fears. Some changes in the skin inevitably happen as years pass. In this chapter we will discuss the way the skin changes as it becomes older, and some of the ways we can manipulate these changes to make the skin look better.

It is the natural order of life that matter changes as it ages. Skin is not immune to this natural law.

We must take a minute to differentiate between two major types of factors that contribute to aging skin. **Extrinsic** aging factors are the effect of outside influences on the skin's health. The very best example here is sun exposure, known to be the major factor in premature skin aging, as well as skin cancer development. Many medical and cosmetic scientists now believe that 85 percent of the aging process is due to extrinsic factors.

Intrinsic aging is the part of the aging process that is due to the actual passing of the years, wearing out of the body, and hereditary factors. Expression lines are an example of intrinsic facial aging. Regardless of our sun protection habits, we still "fold" our

Extrinsic aging factors are the effect of outside influences on the skin's health.

Intrinsic aging is the part of the aging process that is due to the actual passing of the years, wearing out of the body, and hereditary factors.

faces in expression, and this eventually leads to wrinkles in the skin due to repetitive movement of the skin in the same way.

It is important to separate between the two types of aging factors when analyzing and treating aging skin, so we may determine which symptoms are caused by intrinsic or extrinsic factors. There is also, inevitably, some overlap of the two. This chapter will mostly deal with intrinsic aging factors but will mention some symptoms, normally associated by the consumer with passing of the years, that are actually extrinsic and preventable!

A human baby has beautiful, supple, smooth skin that is all one color. As skin is exposed to the environment, defends itself against disease, and is affected by nutrition, health habits, exposure, and time, it begins to change.

Scrapes and accidents we receive as children inevitably leave scar tissue, which develops from injuries. At puberty, the hormonal system begins functioning in a new way. Suddenly pores begin to enlarge, skin becomes oilier, apocrine glands start functioning differently, and the skin's appearance changes. Pimples form from impacted follicles and sometimes leave scars, particularly from the more severe forms of acne. Body hair begins growing, and skin texture changes as well.

Most teenagers are more concerned with the zit on their cheek than with how they will look at age 35 or 55. Many take their good skin for granted.

During the early 20s is when most people notice the beginnings of changes associated with aging skin. They begin to notice small lines and wrinkles around the eyes and sometimes other areas.

If you look closely and carefully at a square inch of skin on a baby's face and compare it with a square inch of skin on the face of someone in their 20s, you will notice many differences. The skin will look rougher; the texture will be coarser to the touch. The skin will no longer be all one color, but multicolored due to melanin deposits.

If you again compare this square inch of skin with that of someone in their 40s or 50s, you will notice even more dramatic changes. Many of these changes are due to sun exposure, which we will discuss much more completely in Chapter 16, Sun and Sun Damage.

However, some of these changes happen naturally as years go by. The natural aging process of the skin is called intrinsic aging. In other words, these changes happen within the body and are not directly associated with external factors such as sun or weather (Plates 31a–h).

HEREDITY

Some intrinsic aging factors are hereditary. Family history and ethnic background do govern skin aging. For example, red-headed, thin-skinned, and fair-skinned individuals develop the skin characteristics of aging much more rapidly than thicker, darker skin, such as black or Hispanic skin. Although it is true that darker skins produce more melanin and therefore ward off more solar damage, the skin itself is very different between different ethnic groups.

In general, the darker the skin, the less visible aging will take place, depending on the amount of sun exposure an individual experiences. Thicker skin does not show signs of aging as fast as thinner, fragile skin types.

This is certainly not to say that dark skin types cannot or do not age. It is just that they are less likely to look aged as fast. A lot of this depends on how the skin is cared for.

WHAT CAUSES AGING?

We will discuss several factors that influence aging. Gravity is certainly a factor. The gravity of the earth constantly pulls on our bodies, including the facial skin. This gravity is one factor that causes skin and muscle to sag. Even an individual who takes immaculate care of both skin and body will have some sagging of the face over a period of years. Even persons who have never exposed their faces to the sun will have some sagging. This sagging is referred to clinically as **elastosis**, which means loss of elasticity. Although facial treatments and good products can help the surface appearance temporarily, the appearance of sagging skin is best corrected on a long-term basis by plastic surgery.

Elastosis means loss of elasticity of the skin.

Let's look at an example of elastosis. If you purchase a new pair of underwear, it has an elastic waistband. If you wear this underwear many, many times, the elastic will begin to wear out. At some point the elastic waistband will no longer "snap back" the way it did when the underwear was brand new. Skin is the same way—aging causes a wearing down of the elastin fibrils in the dermis that give skin its elasticity. If you pinch the skin of a 50-year-old's cheek, it will not "snap back" as fast as that of a 20 year old.

Gravity also causes the nose to droop downwards and the ears to become larger over a period of years. In addition, cartilage in both the nose and ears can grow after age 40, making the nose and ears larger.

Expression Lines

Expression lines are another symptom of intrinsic aging. Individuals will develop lines from consistent and repetitive facial movements. "Smile" lines occur in the nasolabial area. "Frown" lines may also occur in the forehead, eye, and chin areas. Any repetitive movement of a facial expression such as raising the eyebrows, frowning, smiling, scowling, or any other facial movement will eventually cause a crease to occur, just as pants will wrinkle more the more you wear them. "Eye smilers" smile and squint at the same time, creating additional eyelines. Squint lines also occur around the eyes from squinting due to sun exposure, light exposure, or facial expression. It is important to wear ultraviolet protective sunglasses while outside to provide protection against both ultraviolet light exposure and the tendency to squint when exposed to light.

Smokers will inevitably get "smoker's lines" around the mouth and eyes from continually moving these areas during smoking activities. Smoking also causes thousands of free radicals to invade the body, and is known to interfere with proper collagen production.

Sleep habits, such as sleeping on one side or directly on the face, will eventually create lines and elasticity problems. Advise clients to sleep on their backs as much as possible, helping to avoid "sleep creases," which when they happen repetitively have a strong effect on the aging symptoms of the face.

The "Wearing-Out" of the Foundation

As time progresses, the muscles, fat, and skin on our faces undergo structural changes. The amount of fat in the subcutaneous layer decreases with age, providing less cushion and plumpness to the skin, resulting in less support. People who are overweight often do not have as many noticeable wrinkles on the face as thin people or people of normal weight. This does not mean that the skin has not aged; it simply means that there is more fat to "plump out" the skin, creating a smoother looking appearance. The skin is stretched back and forth over a lifetime, causing an "enlarging" of the skin, and gravity pulls down on the skin. The muscles have partially receded, causing the effect of more elastosis.

PREVENTION OF AGING SKIN

Each year we learn more and more about prevention of aging of both the body and the skin. One of the newest theories is that the symptoms that we think of as "aging" are actually only an accumulation of tissue damage that has occurred over a number of years. In other words, the signs of aging may be a lot more related to damage of tissue than the actual passing of the years.

Although there is really very little anyone can do to completely prevent inevitable intrinsic aging of the skin, one can develop certain health habits that will help delay the onset and possibly lessen the severity of intrinsic aging symptoms. Prevention of sun exposure is the biggest preventable factor. Sun exposure is, of course, an example of extrinsic aging, which will be covered in great detail in Chapter 16, Sun and Sun Damage.

Diet and Exercise

Again, this will not prevent all of intrinsic aging, but good health habits will help the body nourish the skin better and therefore help to fight aging. Avoiding excessive alcohol will also help the body function better. A regular aerobic exercise program and a well-balanced, healthy diet can certainly help an individual live longer and better, as well as helping the skin function in a more healthy manner.

Many scientists believe that a diet rich in antioxidant foods, or use of antioxidant supplements such as vitamins C and E, and grapeseed and green tea extracts, may help protect body tissues, including the skin, from free radical damage, reducing the signs of aging. Smoking is known to severely affect health and function of all cells within the body. Smoking and exposure to second-hand smoke should be avoided for a healthy body or skin.

We learn more and more each day about nutrition and its relation to health. Although we will not focus on nutrition in this book, many estheticians find it helpful to receive a good nutrition education. Although it is not the role of the esthetician to give nutritional advice and counseling (this is the role of the physician and registered dietician), the esthetician should have a working knowledge of the elements of nutrition in order to better understand skin function and health and be able to refer clients with nutritional or eating disorders to the proper qualified professionals. Investigate taking courses in nutrition and wellness through the departments of health or home economics at your local community college or university.

Good Skin Care

Using good skin-care products and developing a routine facial skin-care program will obviously help the skin look better. As the skin ages, production of intercellular cement decreases, which decreases the skin's ability to hold water. This is **dehydration**, and it results in a rough-textured appearance. Many theories support the use of hydrating agents in lessening the signs of aging. Many researchers believe that good skin care with proper conditioners, free-radical scavengers, stimulating chemicals, hydrating agents, and sunscreens may help lessen the physical aging of the skin. It is obvious that many of these conditioning treatment agents help the skin look better, regardless of any long-term positive effects. Research continues in the use of these many agents to help lessen the symptoms of skin aging.

Dehydration is the decreasing ability of the skin to hold water.

Plenty of Sleep

This is another good health habit, giving the body time to regenerate its tissues and repair damaged cells. Lack of sleep can cause eye circles, puffiness, and contribute to stress that can have a debilitating effect on both the mind and the body.

Stress

Each day medical researchers are learning more and more about stress and its effect on health, nutrition, and aging. Avoiding high amounts of stress certainly will help avoid premature aging signs of not only the skin, but of the other organs of the body.

Many resort spas, as well as day spas, now offer stress management, yoga, and other body treatments designed to reduce and manage stress. Massage services, aromatherapy services, and a soothing environment within the spa can help reduce daily services for you and your clients! Again, although estheticians cannot permanently change their clients' lifestyles, they should be abreast of the newest research regarding stress and health in order to help give their clients the best esthetic care possible and be aware of referral services to qualified professionals who handle stress, such as psychologists.

THE BEGINNING OF AGING

Many clients will notice signs of aging and occasionally "freak out" at the first wrinkle. Be understanding and give them the best advice you can, teaching them realistic preventative techniques. The word *realistic* should be emphasized, because ethical estheticians do not endorse "miracle" treatments, but rather advise clients about the best proper realistic skin-care program.

The key word here is program. Treatment of the aging skin must address the many factors of aging. One cannot apply a hydrator and expect to revive 40 years of sun damage and bad habits.

Good skin-care habits are most effective if started early in life to prevent problems, but realistically many clients do not start using proper home care or develop good skin-care habits until they notice the first signs of aging.

A combination of good skin-care products, including daily-use sunscreens, hydrators, topical antioxidants, lipids, and alphahydroxy acids, along with regular salon treatments and alphahydroxy acid treatments can help the client manage and significantly reduce the visible signs of aging.

We will discuss sun damage and sunscreen usage more in detail in another chapter, but it certainly cannot be repeated enough that daily use of broad-spectrum sunscreen is by far the most effective method for prevention of premature aging.

Hydrators help add water to the skin surface, cosmetically smoothing the surface of the aging skin. Hydration ingredients include sodium PCA, sorbitol, glycerin, hyaluronic acid, or sodium hyaluronate.

Decrease in cell turnover occurs as the skin ages, results in uneven skin texture and a dull look to the skin. The decrease in cell turnover also results in a decrease of lipid production by the epidermal cells, decreasing barrier function and resulting in an uneven skin surface, making the skin look dull and rough textured. Lack of intercellular lipids causes the skin to become dehydrated, causing the skin to look less smooth and less firm, as well as interfering with other cellular functions.

Regular use of exfoliants such as alphahydroxy acids remove dried-out, dead, dull, crusty cells, helping the skin surface look much smoother. Mild daily exfoliation helps to stimulate the cell renewal process, increasing lipid production, relayering surface cells, and improving hydration as well as cellular and barrier function. Long-term results are a much younger and healthier-looking skin.

Use of mechanical exfoliants at home several times a week can also help remove dead cells loosened by daily use of alphahydroxy acids. Mechanical exfoliating ingredients include polyethylene granules, corn meal, ground almonds, or hydrogenated jojoba oil beads. These products literally "bump off" dead cells and can produce a boost to the look of tired or neglected skin.

Enzymes such as bromelain, papain, or pancreatin, or professional alphahydroxy acid products can be used in the salon to freshen dull-looking, aging skin.

Be careful, as with all skins, not to overexfoliate, which can be very irritating and damaging to the skin. Aging skin may be more vulnerable to mechanical or chemical damage because it is thinner or may have impaired barrier function. For more information, see Chapter 17, The New Science of Aging Skin Treatment, and Chapter 18, Chemical Peeling and Exfoliation Procedures.

DERMAL AND EPIDERMAL STRUCTURAL CHANGES

Several histological changes take place within the dermis and the epidermis as the skin ages. These changes are often associated with sun damage and chronic sun exposure, but some of this occurs through the natural intrinsic aging process.

The epidermis slowly becomes thinner with age, and the dermis increases in thickness. Breakdown of the network of collagen and elastin fibrils within the dermis also occurs. Blood vessels tend to fragment, causing redness—telangiectasias, known to many estheticians as couperose. Because of this fragmented blood vessel formation the blood supply is also fragmented, resulting in poorer blood distribution than in younger skin.

Older skin, as we previously discussed, tends to be thinner than younger skin. Clients must be careful not to overexfoliate, use harsh abrasives, or use too much pressure. Hot water and extremely cold water should be avoided on skin with couperose or capillary fragility. Avoid using hot masks or steaming the face too closely. Clients who have extreme redness should be told to avoid alcoholic beverages, tobacco, and spicy foods, because all of these are **vasodilators**, which means they cause dilation of the blood vessels and sudden surges of blood flow in the already fragile vessels.

Vasodilators dilate the blood vessels, making more blood flow through the arterial system.

"AGE SPOTS"

Hyperpigmentation, or dark splotching, is one of the first signs of what we think of as aging. Sun-induced skin discoloration begins in the late teens and early 20s and gets continually worse. The main noticeable difference between teenage skin and skin in the early 20s is the discoloration caused by deposits of melanin. If you look carefully at makeover pictures, one of the biggest differences between the "before and after" photographs is the even coloring of the individual in the "after" picture. Hormones can also play a significant role in hyperpigmentation.

Hyperpigmentation refers to any condition that has more than a normal amount of melanin.

Almost completely caused by long-term sun exposure, **chloasma**, also known as "liver spots," have nothing to do with the liver and everything to do with cumulative sun exposure. These dark brown patches primarily on the face and hands are areas of concentrated pigment. You may notice that many clients do not exhibit hyperpigmentation on the body as they do on the face and hands. Although there are exceptions to this rule, the face, hands, and arms are areas that have been chronically exposed to the sun for many years. Hence the pigmentation is much worse in these areas (Plates 32a, 32b).

Chloasma, commonly known as liver spots, are lesions of hyperpigmentation generally caused by long-term sun exposure.

Hyperpigmentation is treated by having the client apply a solution containing a **melanin suppressant**. These agents stop the chemical reactions occurring in the melanocytes at the basal cell level that lead to hyperpigmentation. **Hydroquinone** is the best known of these agents, and the only one officially recognized by the FDA. Other unrecognized yet effective melanin suppressive ingredients include **kojic acid**, **magnesium ascorbyl phosphate** (also an antioxidant), **arbutin**, **bearberry extract**, and **azelaic acid**.

Melanin suppressant is a topical substance that interferes with the melanocyte's production of melanin.

Hydroquinone is a melanin suppressant drug available to the esthetician in concentrations of up to 2%. Physicians prescribe concentrations up to 6%.

Clients being treated for any form of hyperpigmentation must agree to avoid sun exposure, which is what causes more hyperpigmentation. Even hyperpigmentation caused by hormonal imbalances can be made worse by sun exposure.

Kojic acid is a skin-lightening agent.

Explain to clients that wherever they have a hyperpigmented area, there is a concentration of active melanocytes in the lower epidermis and upper dermis, producing melanin and depositing it in epidermal cells that are drifting toward the corneum. This is the "factory" where the pigmentation is produced. The melanin is the "product." Melanin suppressors, like the ones mentioned above, work by interfering with chemical reactions that cause production of the melanin. They do not actually stop the "factory";

Magnesium ascorbyl phosphate is a vitamin C ester, antioxidant, and a melanin suppressant.

Arbutin is a melanin suppressant.

Bearberry extract is a melanin suppressant.

Azelaic acid has skin-lightening effects.

they just interfere with production. Because of this fact, the "factory"—the melanocytes—are still active, even when the hyperpigmentation has faded. This is why it is so important for the client to avoid the controllable factor that stimulates the melanocytes, namely sun exposure. As long as the client continues to expose herself or himself to the sun and not use a daily broad-spectrum sunscreen, melanin production will continue.

Many clients concerned with hyperpigmentation are or have been active sun worshippers. It must be explained to these clients that sun exposure is likely what caused the pigmentation problem in the first place, and they must change this factor of their lifestyle to achieve the change in their skin.

PSYCHOLOGICAL EFFECTS OF AGING

Clients may experience psychological effects when they realize that the aging process has begun. They may seek "immediate result" treatments, which do not exist. Work with these clients to establish a good, solid home care program, coupled with good salon treatments. The more often the client comes into the salon, the better the program will be, because this client needs lots of encouragement and "coaching."

Try to steer the client away from unrealistic "nonsurgical face-lift" approaches to skin care. Stress using sunscreens, avoiding sun exposure, using good hydrators designed for the client's skin type, and using specialty products, such as conditioners containing glycolic acid.

This type of client will also sometimes have a tendency to "drown" in heavy moisturizers, often causing comedogenic or acnegenic results. Explain to the client that aging is not a lack of oil. Only clients who are truly alipidic (oil-dry) need to be using heavy oily products, and then they need to contain the right kind of emollient.

HOME CARE FOR THE AGING CLIENT

Home care should be adapted to help the client's aging signs, whatever their severity. Begin by thoroughly analyzing the skin. Always adapt the entire program to the skin type. Treatment conditioners for aging skin will not be useful if they are for the wrong skin type. Aging clients will still be predominantly dry or oily. For oily clients, stick to noncomedogenic fluids, lotions, or gels. For more oil-dry skin, you can use heavier emollients.

Stick to very gentle cleansers with little or no detergents. Remember, the aging skin already has fewer intercellular lipids. You do not want to strip these essential lipids by using too aggressive a cleanser. Low-foaming washes and cleansing milks are best to use for the aging skin.

Toners should be alcohol-free and should contain a humectant such as propylene glycol or glycerin. Toners should not have a strong astringent action.

Specialty products for aging skin may include alphahydroxy gels or creams, antioxidant serums, and lipid-based serums. These are special functional products that help protect the skin from free-radical damage, and help exfoliate or hydrate the skin. These serum-type products are often layered under or over other products.

Day creams should contain a broad-spectrum sunscreen and a sealant agent such as dimethicone, mineral oil, or cyclomethicone. These agents will help the skin retain water better in the surface layers. The consistency of the day cream will vary depending on the oiliness or dryness of the skin. "Poreless" skin with poor sebum production will need more emollients, and the cream should generally be heavier. Oily skin should be treated with a noncomedogenic day cream containing less emollient and more hydration agents.

Night treatment will vary, again depending on the skin type. Hydrators such as lecithin (liposomes), sorbitol, sodium PCA, glycerin, and hyaluronic acid are appropriate.

Special treatment products for the eye and neck areas are very helpful to the aging skin. The skin of the eyes and the neck is much thinner than the rest of the facial skin, and is therefore very likely to show signs of aging. Heavier emollients are often used for these areas, with the exception of some of the newer liposome gels. The client should use eye and neck care products 24 hours a day for best results.

Many estheticians vary the night treatment for clients, alternating different types of night treatments. The theory here is that the change in night treatment will help stimulate sluggish skin.

FACIAL TREATMENTS FOR AGING SKIN

Salon facial treatments for aging skin must be administered frequently. You should begin by treating the skin weekly or biweekly for 6 to 12 treatments, slowly decreasing to once every two to four weeks. Although it is normal to administer salon treatments monthly, aging skin often needs treatment more often. It is certainly advisable to perform facial treatments weekly or biweekly on drier, aging skin, if this is affordable for the client.

You should always design the facial based on skin type and conditions. Aging skin often will be thin, so be careful with harsh exfoliants, brushing, and suction machines. As skin gets older, it tends to become more oil-dry, particularly after age 50. Keep this in mind when treating the skin. Occasionally, you will see an oily or, more often, a combination aging skin. Because many treatment products designed for aging skin contain larger percentages of emollients and fats, be careful not to use creams that are too oily or heavy for combination and oily skin types.

Exfoliation

Mild exfoliation is good for aging skin. It gently stimulates the skin and removes dead, dry cells on the surface, helping the skin look and feel smoother and softer, and also helping to minimize the appearance of rough textures and wrinkles. Mild enzyme peeling treatments are effective in helping to remove this dead cell buildup. Mild alphahydroxy acid exfoliation treatments also are very helpful in improving aging skin symptoms. For more information on peeling treatments, see Chapter 18, Chemical Peeling and Exfoliation Procedures.

Massage helps to soothe and hydrate aging skin, stimulating blood flow. Be careful not to overmassage or use rough massage techniques on fragile, thin, aging skin with distended capillaries.

Treatment for Aging Skin

1. Remove makeup by gently massaging a cleansing milk into the skin and then removing the makeup and cleanser with damp, soft, facial cloths, sponges, or cotton pads. Follow with gentle toner on cool wet pads or a soft cloth.

2. After cleansing and toning, carefully examine the skin for elasticity, dryness, dehydration, couperose or distended capillaries, hyperpigmentation, and sun damage symptoms (see Chapter 16, Sun and Sun Damage).

3. Apply a very lightweight hydrating fluid during steam treatment. Steam the skin at a distance of 14 to 20 inches with the hydrating fluid on the skin. This will help soften the skin and attract the steam. Do not use oil-based fluid or heavier creams. This will repel water instead of attracting it. As an alternative treatment a gentle enzyme mask may be applied during steam instead of a hydrating fluid.

4. If the skin is not too fragile, you may use the brushing machine over a thick coat of hydrating fluid. (Do not use the brushing machine after enzyme or alphahydroxy acid treatment.) Avoid brushing if the skin is thin, red, or couperose.

5. Gently extract any clogged pores or comedones.

6. Use cold spray with a mild toner solution after extraction.

7. Apply a hydrating fluid, ampoule, or cream to the skin, designed for both the aging skin and the individual skin type. Gently massage the skin. Massage should last about ten minutes. If using an ampoule, you may want to use electrical treatment before continuing massage.

8. Apply high frequency at a low setting or ionization rollers over the ampoule, hydrating fluid, or specialty cream. Make sure to check all health precautions and contraindications before using electrical therapy.

9. Apply masks appropriate for the particular skin types. Most masks for aging skin are creamy and soft setting, or are the gel variety. Clay masks may be used on oily or clogged areas.

10. Allow the mask to sit for 15 to 20 minutes. For extra dry skin, you may apply extra hydrating fluid or cream in lieu of a mask.

11. After 15 to 20 minutes, spray the mask with an atomized cold spray of diluted toner or conditioning water. This will help soften and loosen the mask. Apply strips of cool, wet cotton or soft facial cloths in a compress technique, gently molding the compresses to the face. Remove the strips one at a time, wiping the mask off the skin as you remove the compress.

12. Finish by applying an appropriate day cream with sunscreen.

Aging skin can be stimulated, cleansed, softened, firmed, and hydrated. With careful management, aging skin can be made to look much softer and smoother. However, no one can actually turn back the clock. Avoid using "miraculous" "anti-aging" treatments. Explain sensible care to your client, emphasizing the importance of careful, consistent, diligent care both in the salon and at home.

Topics for Discussion

1. What changes occur in the skin from birth, to the 20s, to the 40s and 50s?
2. Discuss hereditary characteristics and aging.
3. What is the difference between intrinsic and extrinsic aging?
4. Discuss other factors related to aging.
5. Discuss home care procedures for aging skin.
6. Discuss salon treatment for aging skin.

Chapter 16

Sun and Sun Damage

Objectives

The sun is a phenomenal structure that helps plants convert carbon dioxide to pure oxygen. We cannot live without oxygen, and we cannot live without sun. Yet the sun is, by far, the worst enemy of the skin. The sun creates free radicals, which cause cell damage. Cell damage eventually results in the destruction of collagen and elastin and possibly alters the DNA, eventually resulting in skin cancers. Repetitive exposure to the sun causes severe skin damage, premature aging, and skin cancer. In this chapter we will learn all about the way the sun affects the skin, in both the long and short term. We will learn about the best ways to prevent sun damage and skin cancer, as well as how to detect skin cancer.

Over 93 million miles away, the sun is a source of energy for the earth and our ecosystems. It is a vitally important part of human life.

It is also the worst enemy of the skin. It is the number one cause of premature aging and skin cancer. Yet many people continue to bask in the sun's rays, achieving a golden tan, but also accumulating terrible damage to the skin.

The sun projects three basic kinds of **ultraviolet rays**, or UV rays (Figure 16–1). UVC rays are short rays that are blocked by the ozone layer. They have germicidal properties, and in large doses are deadly to live creatures.

Ultraviolet B rays (UVB) are the next longest ultraviolet ray. UVB rays cause most skin cancers and are responsible for sunburns. They penetrate the epidermis to the basal layer. Some UVB rays penetrate the dermis, but most stop at the basal layer. UVB are much stronger than UVA rays, even though UVA rays are longer and penetrate the dermis.

Within the basal layer and upper dermis are the **melanocytes**, the pigment-producing cells. These cells are stimulated by exposure to ultraviolet rays and manufacture **melanin**, the skin pigment that is the body's natural sunscreen. Although many people think a tan is healthy, a tan is actually a chemical reaction of the body defending itself from the damaging rays of the sun! A tan is actually the body and the skin saying "don't do this to me"—just like a warrior picking up a shield to ward off an enemy!

Again, UVA rays are longer rays, penetrating the dermis and the precious collagen and elastin fibrils. UVA only burns in large doses and is therefore the type of UV ray used in most tanning beds and booths. Although the tanning bed is unlikely to burn the skin, the damaging UVA rays penetrate the dermis, affecting the supportive structure of the collagen and elastin fibrils and causing other detrimental changes to the skin.

Ultraviolet rays are short rays that are blocked by the ozone layer.

Melanocytes are cells that are "pigment factories" for the skin.

Melanin is the pigment of the skin.

SHORT-TERM SUN PROBLEMS

Most of know that long-term sun exposure causes skin aging and skin cancer, but very few people are aware of the short-term damaging effects of ultraviolet and sun exposure. Sun exposure causes a variety of short-term skin and esthetic problems. These may affect both beauty and health.

Sunburns happen very frequently, especially in the summer months. They can be mild to severe. The skin becomes very red, sore, and sensitive to the touch, caused by dilation of blood vessels and stimulation of nerve endings in the skin. The skin will eventually peel due to the extreme dryness associated with the sunburn. The skin literally

Figure 16–1   Dispersion of light rays by a prism

bakes to a very dehydrated condition, just as cookies will burn and become dry if cooked too long in the oven. Many of these sunburns happen because people are ignorant about sun protection. Whereas Floridians and Californians are very familiar with sun protection, tourists from areas where sunbathing is not popular due to the climate are especially vulnerable to sunburn. It is important that estheticians be very familiar with sun protection methods to help their clients protect themselves from sunburn as well as from long- and short-term sun damage.

A variety of remedies can ease the pain of a minor sunburn. These include cool baths with vinegar added to cool water, applying cool packs, applying plain yogurt to the area, and using local spray anesthetics. The latter must be used with caution. Although the spray anesthetics can provide temporary pain relief to the sunburned area, many people have allergies to localized skin anesthetics. Advise clients to be very careful if using these products. Sunburn is actually a medical condition and therefore is in the domain of the physician, not the esthetician. Severe sunburns can cause shock, fever, nausea, and even death. Any "bubbling" of the skin or severe blistering should always be referred to a medical doctor.

After the initial burn is relieved, your client may ask you for help with the remaining esthetic skin problems associated with a sunburn. The skin may be extremely dehydrated, flaking, and peeling. Occasionally, these discolorations may be long term. First and most important, strongly advise the client no to expose him- or herself to any more sun until all the symptoms of the sunburn are completely gone, especially peeling of the skin. Further sun exposure during the peeling process following a sunburn often results in further long-term skin damage and permanent solar lentigenes (freckles induced by the sun) and other skin discolorations.

You should not attempt to treat sunburned skin that is still red or sensitive. If the skin is no longer red or sensitive, you may use very gentle techniques to hydrate the skin. Use cool steam, fragrance-free hydrating fluids and lotions, nonhardening nonstimulating masks, and other products designed for super-sensitive skin. Avoid exfoliating or stimulating treatments, including brushing, galvanic desincrustation, or heavy massage. Advice the client to use similar procedures at home until all symptoms subside. Give the client good instruction about the proper use of sunscreens to avoid a reoccurrence of the situation.

Other Short-Term Sun-Related Problems

Hyperpigmentation refers to any condition that has more than a normal amount of melanin.

Hyperpigmentation is both a long- and short-term cosmetic problem caused by the sun. Hyperpigmentation literally means overpigmented. Skin that has been repeatedly burned or has not healed from the sun before additional sun exposure is especially vulnerable. If you look at the skin of a 15 year old and compare it to that of a 25 year old, the biggest difference you will notice is in the skin pigmentation. Hyperpigmentation occurs in many patterns and is also associated with hormone fluctuations and pregnancy. (See Chapter 5.) Hyperpigmentation can usually be treated, as we will learn in Chapter 17, The New Science of Aging Skin Treatment.

Hyperpigmentation may appear suddenly, especially in women, after years of sun exposure. It may first appear as subtle splotching that you may notice when examining the skin under a magnifying lamp or especially a wood's lamp. From this relatively mild splotching, darker, larger splotches may develop. The best treatment for hyperpigmentation is, of course, prevention by using an SPF-15 or higher broad-spectrum sunscreen on a daily basis.

Tinea veriscolor is what many refer to as sun "spots" or sun "fungus." These white splotches, which usually appear on the chest and back of avid sunbathers, are actually a fungal condition. The fungus interferes with the melanocytes' ability to make melanin, which causes the white splotches to appear when the body is tanned. If you have a client with this condition, refer the client to a dermatologist for treatment (Plate 33).

Tinea versicolor is what many refer to as sun "spots" or sun "fungus." These white splotches are a fungal condition.

The Real Damage from the Sun

Continual exposure to sun results in the formation of more and more damaging free radicals. Although not visible at first, or even for years, the routine damage to the cells eventually accumulates, resulting in wrinkles, hyperpigmentation, elastosis, and rough-textured skin.

As we have previously discussed, the sun-exposed skin falls victim to the inflammation cascade, resulting in breakdown of collagen and elastin due to self-destruct enzymes manufactured through the immune system's defense against the sun exposure and damage to the cells of the skin. When enough damage occurs, it becomes visible in the skin's appearance.

What You Don't Know About Short-Term Sun Exposure

We now know that sun exposure may actually suppress the immune functions of the skin. Exposure to sunlight "chases off" your protective macrophage "guard cells," allowing substances and organisms to enter the skin, increasing the chance of infection. A good example of this immune suppression is the flares of herpes simplex that occur in some individuals when they are exposed to sun. Many cases of lupus, an autoimmune disease, are diagnosed after a sunburn, when the immune system has overreacted to the injury.

It is so important that we teach young children to use sunscreen daily. We receive about 80 percent of the sun's damage to the skin before the age of 18. Sun freckles appearing on teenagers' faces represent problem areas in the future. Most sun exposure is not from sunbathing but from day-to-day exposure. Think about how many children play outdoors. Everytime they go outside, they expose themselves to harmful ultraviolet rays. That's why every time they go outdoors, they should be protected with a good sunscreen! We tend to think about sunscreens during the summer months, but it should be a year-round consideration.

LONG-TERM PHOTO DAMAGE

Almost every symptom we think of as aging is directly related to sun exposure. Even intrinsic aging symptoms, such as facial expression lines, are made worse because of sun damage. Hyperpigmentation, leathery texture, roughness, wrinkles, some forms of hypopigmentation, severe elastosis (sagging of the skin), chest and cleavage wrinkling, splotchiness, couperose and telangiectasias, flare of rosacea, neck texture problems, severe dehydration, and barrier function problems are all directly related to sun exposure.

Dermatoheliosis is the medical term coined to describe long-term damage to the skin caused by sun exposure. The skin is severely affected by long-term exposure.

Collagen and elastin fibrils in the dermis begin a process called **cross-linking**. In essence, collagen and elastin fibrils collapse due to cumulative effects of cell damage from repeated sun exposure, causing the support system for the skin also to collapse. Esthetically, this results in deep wrinkling of the skin, sagging, and elastosis.

Sun-damaged skin appears much more severely aged than skin that has aged solely from intrinsic factors. The wrinkling does not only appear in expression lines. Many, many lines develop, in all areas and in all directions. Wrinkles may be both horizontal and vertical. Normal expression lines are much deeper in sun-damaged skin.

The abnormal structure of the dermis and the epidermis give the skin a "leathery" appearance and feel. This type of skin is also severely discolored due to melanin deposits and hyperpigmentation.

The skin of a sun-damaged person is very rough to the touch, and the surface is actually uneven. This is caused by damage to the cells, which causes the corneum and other epidermal cells not to shed in a normal, even manner. This is due to the altering of the DNA from chronic sun exposure. The cells become "confused," divide unevenly, and no longer retain their normal shape. If you look at a cross-section of normal skin, you will notice that the cells in the epidermis form layers that look like layers of brick in a brick wall. In sun-damaged skin, the same structure looks like a brick wall that is collapsing, made with uneven bricks that are poorly made!

The epidermis of sun-damaged skin becomes progressively thinner, and the dermis slowly begins to atrophy, or collapse, and fall apart. This is how the sun eventually "zaps" the skin and destroys it!

Your sun-damaged client will have multiple wrinkles, not just around the eyes and neck, but all over the face. There will be many more pronounced wrinkles than in other clients. Their skin is literally a multitude of uneven colors, very freckled. This skin will have a leathery feel and look. There may be patches of dryness frequently, and clients may often complain about how "dry" their skin is. The truth is that as the skin cells become disfigured, they also fail to produce sufficient amounts of intercellular cement causing an impaired barrier function and making proper hydration of the skin practically impossible.

Use of lipid replacement ingredients such as ceramides, cholesterol, and phospholipids, along with the routine use of an 8 to 10 percent, pH 3.5 alphahydroxy acid serum or cream and the use of a good hydrator like hyaluronic acid, glycerin, or sodium PCA can help this damaged skin retain more moisture.

Sun-damaged skin may also have many telangiectasias or couperose areas. Sun damage also causes collapse of some of the blood vessels and decreased blood flow. The small capillaries look like tributaries of a river. These vessels may be very fragile, and bruises may appear easily. You may notice how easily some of your older clients bruise. Although this may be due to many medical factors, sun-damaged skin bruises

Dermatoheliosis is the medical term coined to describe long-term damage to the skin caused by sun exposure.

Cross-linking is a process in which collagen and elastin fibrils in the dermis collapse, causing the support system for the skin also to collapse.

much more easily than normal, healthy, nondamaged skin. You will also notice that these clients who bruise easily have very thin-looking, dry, hyperpigmented skin. This is because the skin is almost always severely sun damaged.

SKIN CANCERS AND OTHER SUN-RELATED SKIN GROWTHS

Skin cancer is caused by the damage to the DNA that we have been discussing. The cells begin dividing unevenly and rapidly, but the genetic material in the DNA is damaged from the sun. This rapid dividing of the cells may take the form of small tumors, which we know as skin cancer.

There are three major kinds of skin cancer. **Basal cell carcinomas** are the most common. They are almost always found on the sun-exposed areas, typically on the face, hands, legs, back, and chest. They look like small pearls. Sometimes they have a small blood vessel running through them. They are not usually perfectly round like a milium. On older hyperpigmented skin, they may be hard to differentiate from milia. You must look carefully to tell the difference (Plate 34).

Basal cell carcinomas are the most common forms of skin cancer; lesions have a pearl-like appearance with small blood vessels running through.

Estheticians are not in the business of diagnosing skin cancer. However, you should know the signs of the major forms of skin cancer and be able to refer suspicious-looking lesions and areas to a dermatologist.

Basal cell carcinomas are very often curable. In fact, 95 percent of these cancers are cured. They rarely spread to the internal parts of the body, but can grow, and if they are not treated they can affect large areas of the skin. Basal cell carcinomas are sometimes removed surgically, sometimes frozen, and sometimes treated with an electric needle called a **hyfrecator**.

Squamous cell carcinomas are the second most frequently diagnosed form of skin cancer. They may look like red or pink solid bumps on the skin. They may appear as open sores or ulcers that do not seem to heal. They may look crusty, or the client may notice a crusty area that bleeds easily (Plate 35). Many clients notice this when washing or cleansing the face. Again, these lesions appear on chronically sun-exposed areas. Treatment is similar to treatment for basal cell carcinoma, but squamous cell carcinoma may sometimes spread to other areas of the body.

Hyfrecator, or an electric needle, is an electrical device used by dermatologists to remove certain lesions from the skin.

Squamous cell carcinomas is a common form of skin cancer characterized by unexplained skin bleeding or a small red or pink, sometimes ulcerated, lesion.

The least frequently seen form of the three major kinds of skin cancer is also the most deadly. **Melanoma** is characterized by moles or mole-like lesions that are dark in color. The Skin Cancer Foundation has coined an expression that is easy to remember when looking at suspicious lesions. They call this the "ABCDs of Melanoma." "A" stands for asymmetric. The melanoma lesion is usually growing to one side of the lesion and is uneven. "B" stands for border. The borders of melanomas are uneven and not smooth. "C" is for color. Melanomas often have dark brown and black colors and are usually splotchy and not all one color. "D" stands for diameter. Melanomas are usually at least the size of a pencil eraser or bigger. Regular moles are usually smaller than this.

Melanoma is characterized by moles or mole-like lesions that are dark in color.

Melanomas can be found on any area of the body, but are most likely, again, to be found on areas that have had repeated sun exposure. They are most typically found on individuals with a history of sunburn and light-skinned individuals.

Other Sun-Related Growths

Actinic keratoses are rough areas of sun-damaged skin, indicated by dysplastic cell growth. **Dysplastic** means abnormal growth. Actinic keratoses are frequently found on the faces of individuals who have had chronic sun exposure. They are also prevalent in light-skinned individuals. They are rough patches of skin and can be crusty, scaly, and rough to the touch. Sometimes they feel like small needles or splinters sticking out of the skin when they are touched with the fingers. They frequently occur in small groups or patches. Because they are dysplastic cells, they can become cancerous, and are often referred to as **pre-cancers** (Plates 36a, 36b).

Actinic keratoses may be treated surgically, with **cryosurgery** (freezing with liquid nitrogen), or with chemical therapy with a chemical called **fluorouracil** (also commercially known as Efudex®).

Unusual looking moles or moles that are changing should be checked by a dermatologist. If you or your client notices changes in a wart or mole, refer the client to a dermatologist for diagnosis and treatment.

Sebaceous hyperplasias are small, donut-shaped lesions that look like large, open comedones surrounded by a ridge of skin. Sebaceous hyperplasia actually means "overgrown oil glands." They are frequently seen on oily skins that have had repeated sun exposure, but they can appear on any skin, usually in someone 25 years old and older. You will frequently find them on the forehead and temples, although they may appear anywhere on the face (Plate 37). Sebaceous hyperplasias are benign lesions that rarely cause any problems, except esthetically. They are rarely removed surgically, because the scar from excision is usually worse than the appearance of the lesion. Sebaceous hyperplasia can be treated with electrodessication with an electric needle or sometimes, cryosurgery. This helps flatten the lesion, but may need to be re-treated periodically, because the oil glands are deep within the skin and can still keep growing. Sebaceous hyperplasias are seen very frequently by estheticians, and clients are often concerned about them. Clients who have them also may have other symptoms of sun damage.

Seborrheic keratoses are large, flat, crusty-looking, brown, black, yellowish, or gray lesions that are often found on the faces of older, sun-damaged clients. They are frequently found on the temples or cheekbones, although they can appear anywhere on the skin. They look almost like a scab, and clients will sometimes pick at them, which they obviously should not do. They are usually harmless growths, but can occasionally turn into other more serious lesions, such as basal cell carcinomas. They are treated by the dermatologist, usually by curettage, in which a curette, a small, scoop-like instrument, is used to "scoop" the lesion off the face. Seborrheic keratoses are more of a cosmetic nuisance than anything in most cases. Nevertheless, they should be referred to a dermatologist for treatment. Also, they may indicate other areas or other forms of sun damage that may require treatment.

After a dermatologist treats skin cancer, the doctor may suggest that the client not have skin-care treatments until the lesion is healed completely. As a general rule, clients should not have facial treatment if there are still **sutures**, or "stitches," present in a treated lesion. Clients treated with fluorouracil should not have facial treatment until the

---

Actinic keratoses, or pre-cancers, are rough areas of sun-damaged skin, indicating dysplastic cell growth.

Dysplastic means abnormal growth.

Pre-cancers are conditions in cells that may become cancerous.

Cryosurgery is the dermatological removal of lesions by freezing, usually with liquid nitrogen.

Fluorouracil is a topical prescription drug used to remove multiple actinic keratoses.

Sebaceous hyperplasias are small, donut-shaped lesions that look like large, open comedones surrounded by a ridge of skin.

Seborrheic keratoses are large, flat, crusty-looking, brown, black, yellowish, or gray lesions that are often found on the faces of older, sun-damaged clients.

Sutures are materials used in reconnecting areas of surgical incisions.

therapy is completed, unless approved by the dermatologist, who may occasionally refer such a client for help with side effects. Make sure you have been properly trained by the doctor before treating these clients.

Other forms of growth treatment, such as electrosurgery or cryosurgery generally do not cause any problem for treatment, except that facial treatment should not be performed until the lesion is healed or unless the doctor advises otherwise. Avoid these areas completely, and simply treat the rest of the untreated areas of the face. If you have any questions, contact the dermatologist, and remember always—when it doubt, don't!

Solar freckles, also known as "liver spots," are clumps of hyperpigmentation caused by sun exposure. They can appear on any area, but frequently appear on the face and hands. These can be treated by the esthetician, and more severe cases can be treated by the dermatologist. More on treating hyperpigmentation will be covered in Chapter 17, The New Science of Aging Skin Treatment.

> **Solar freckles** also known as "liver spots," are clumps of hyperpigmentation caused by sun exposure.

PREVENTION OF SUN DAMAGE

Without question, the most effective treatment for sun damage is prevention. This involves routine use of sunscreen products. Sunscreen products are designed to filter, reflect, or absorb UVA and/or UVB rays emitted by the sun. Sunscreen products are regulated as over-the-counter drugs by the FDA. There are sunscreen ingredients that absorb and neutralize ultraviolet light, and there are materials that reflect ultraviolet light.

Chemical absorbing sunscreen ingredients include the most popular sunscreen ingredient, octyl methoxycinnimate, and benzophenone-3, octyl salicylate, para-aminobenzoic acid (PABA), padimate O, padimate A, methyl salicylate, oxybenzone, and avobenzone, also known as Parsol 1789. These ingredients chemically neutralize ultraviolet light. They are often used in combination: as methoxycinnimate and octyl salicylate, they screen parts of the UVB spectrum; whereas as benzophenone-3 and avobenzone, they screen more of the UVA rays. Combining two or three of these sunscreen active ingredients help screen larger spectrums of light and produce what is known as **broad-spectrum sunscreens**.

> **Chemical absorbing sunscreen** contains ingredients that absorb and neutralize ultraviolet rays.

The advantages of the absorbing sunscreen ingredients are that they cannot be seen when worn, and are easier to formulate in higher SPFs. Their main disadvantage is that they are more reactive with the skin, particularly sensitive skin. Absorbing sunscreens are one of the primary causes of skin allergy and irritation.

> **Broad-spectrum sunscreens** protect against both ultraviolet A and B rays.

Physical sunscreen ingredients work by reflecting the light off the skin. There are only two approved for use by the FDA: titanium dioxide and zinc oxide. Physical sunscreens are sometimes referred to as sunblocks. They are excellent sunscreens, blocking out large portions of both UVB and UVA light. For many years, these took the form of opaque creams, such as the white cream that surfers wore on their noses (some still do). Micronized versions are now available, which are less noticeable. Unfortunately, the micronization process still leaves particles big enough to see, particularly on dark skin. These finely ground minerals sit on the skin, and literally bounce the light off. Physical sunscreens are much less likely to react with the skin than the absorbing screens, making them good choices for sensitive or allergy-prone skin. In high SPF numbers, however,

> **Physical sunscreen** contains an ingredient that works by reflecting ultraviolet rays off the skin.

they are hard to formulate without looking white or pasty on the skin or being sticky. Just like the absorbing screens can be combined to provide a broader spectrum of protection, the physical screens can also be mixed with the absorbing sunscreen agents. This works very well in many cases, producing cosmetically acceptable, higher SPF sunscreens, with broad-spectrum protection.

Because sunscreen is so important in skin treatment and sun damage prevention, broad-spectrum sunscreens are now included in most better day creams, along with moisturizing, conditioning, and other functional cosmetic ingredients. Sunscreens can be mixed into lotion or cream forms, with different weights and different amounts of emollient for different skin types.

SPF stands for **sun protection factor**. SPF is a number that represents how long a person can stay out in the sun without burning while using the product. It is a measurement of the **minimal erythemal dose (MED)**, which means how much time passes without the skin turning red from irritation. If a person normally burns in one hour without sunscreen, an SPF-2 sunscreen theoretically will allow the person to stay out in the sun two times as long, or two hours, without burning. An SPF-4 would allow the skin to be exposed four times as long, or four hours without burning. SPFs are really designed to prevent sunburns. They do not measure how much light is actually being blocked from the skin or how much UVA and UVB rays are being screened, which is actually more important in terms of sun damage prevention. An SPF-15 sunscreen blocks about 94 percent of UVB light, whereas an SPF-30 blocks about 98 percent. However, for sensitive skin, the higher the SPF, the more potentially irritating sunscreen chemical is used.

As a general rule, most dermatologists, pharmacists, and estheticians consider an SPF 15 sunscreen product to be a good protection against sun damage. It does not guarantee no sun damage. It simply means that an SPF 15 screen provides a fairly high amount of protection. Results will vary depending on the individual's heredity, method of application, frequency of application, his or her own skin, weather and climate conditions, and other factors.

Sun protection factor (SPF) is a number that represents how long a person can stay out in the sun without burning while using the product.

Minimal erythemal dose (MED) means how much time passes without the skin turning red from irritation.

SUN SKIN TYPES

There is a universal system of classifying skin types when discussing sun exposure. This typing system is generally accepted by the scientific community, and is referred to as **Fitzpatrick Skin Typing**, named after its originator, Dr. Thomas Fitzpatrick. The following is an excerpt from a brochure provided by the Skin Cancer Foundation.

Fitzpatrick Skin Typing is a way of classifying skin by its tendency to sunburn or tan; indicates how susceptible a person is to sun damage and erythema.

- Type 1: Always burns; never tans. Very fair, with red or blond hair and freckles.
- Type 2: Burns easily; tans minimally. Usually fair skinned.
- Type 3: Sometimes burns; gradually tans.
- Type 4: Minimum burning; always tans. Usually white with medium pigmentation.
- Type 5: Very seldom burns; always tans. Medium to heavy pigmentation.
- Type 6: Never burns, but tans darkly. Blacks as well as others with heavy pigmentation.

As you can see, the scale has a lot to do with hereditary and genetic skin characteristics. According to the Skin Cancer Foundation, your choice, or your client's choice, of a sunscreen should be based on the sun skin type, the amount of time you plan to spend in the sun, the intensity of the sun in your geographic region, and the preference of the formulation.

The geographic location does affect the intensity of the sun. As a general rule, the closer to the equator you live, the more intense the sun's rays.

TYPES OF SUNSCREENS

Water-resistant screens are designed for individuals who participate in water sports, or who are outdoors in hot environments, or who plan on staying out in the sun for long periods of time. These products are often used by fishermen, athletes, and people who work outdoors. They usually contain a fairly large amount of oil, petrolatum, or fat, which makes them highly water-resistant. These products sometimes cause problems for oily-skinned individuals, and often the water-proofing ingredients are also comedogenic or acnegenic.

Sunscreens that are made for oily skin are often in an alcohol gel. They are lighter weight and generally noncomedogenic. Unfortunately, they are also usually not very water-resistant, and therefore should be applied more frequently.

Sunscreens are also available in oils, creams, and lotions. These are choices that are really a matter of personal preference and individualized skin type. Many cosmetics companies make a variety of products that vary in SPF strength, vehicles, and usage directions.

TIME OF DAY AND THE SUN

Because the earth revolves, during certain times of the day the sun is closer and more intense, and more ultraviolet rays reach the earth's surface. Most estheticians and dermatologists agree that the sun is at its most powerful between 10 A.M. and 3 P.M. Advise your clients not to go in the sun during these hours.

FREQUENT MISCONCEPTIONS ABOUT SUN DAMAGE AND SUNBATHING

Consumers have many misconceptions about sunbathing and the way the sun damages the skin. It is the duty of the esthetician to dispel these wrong ideas. Some of these misconceptions are:

1. *You cannot tan or burn if the weather is cloudy or rainy.* This, of course, is completely false. Clouds do filter a small amount of UV light, but not enough to affect damage to the skin. It is certainly possible to tan or burn even in cloudy, overcast weather, particularly without using sunscreen.
2. *You cannot burn if you are in the water.* This too is false. Water may feel cool to hot skin that has been basking in the sun, but it has no effect on the sun's burning and damage potential. The heat from the sun is caused by infrared rays, not ultraviolet rays. Swimming and going into the pool or ocean may indeed remove some or a

large amount of the sunscreen applied earlier. If your client plans on swimming or participating in water sports, advise him or her to use a water-resistant sunscreen product. Sunscreens should be reapplied when swimming every time the client gets out of the water, or about once an hour.

3. *Umbrellas or large hats will prevent sun damage.* The real truth is that although these are a help, they do not prevent much sun from reaching the fragile skin and certainly do not replace a good sunscreen. They primarily cut down on glare so that the person does not squint as much, helping to prevent worsening of the expression lines. It's a good idea to wear lightweight but sun-resistant clothes, which also help filter light, but ultraviolet rays can burn the skin right through a lightweight shirt. Advise your clients to wear a hat, proper attire, and sit in the shade as much as possible, but to still wear a good sunscreen.

4. *Baby or mineral oil accelerates tanning.* This is simply not true. In fact, because these do not contain sunscreen, they may accelerate burning, and they do not provide protection against sun damage.

5. *Applying moisturizer after sunbathing will prevent peeling.* This is completely false! If the skin has burned, it will peel no matter what is done to the skin. Applying moisturizer to well-protected skin may help replace some of the water in the dehydrated, exposed skin, or may lubricate peeling areas, making the skin look better, but it will not stop the sun-damaged skin from peeling.

6. *Applying lots of moisturizer will counter the damage the sun causes.* False again. Hydrating fluids do help replace some of the water that is also being robbed from the surface cells during sun exposure, but ultraviolet rays cut right through the skin. Remember, the UVA rays penetrate right through the dermis, destroying collagen and elastin fibrils, not to mention causing dysplastic cell growth and other horrifying effects we have already discussed. Esthetically, you should administer good, soothing, hydrating facial treatments to your sun-worshipping clients, but this will not treat or prevent the damage the sun causes to these clients.

7. *Wearing sunglasses helps prevent sun damage.* True, only if the sunglasses contain UV filters, and only if they are worn constantly while out. When purchasing sunglasses, make sure to check if the glasses contain UV filters. The larger the glasses, the more area they will help protect.

THE QUEST FOR THE GOLDEN TAN

In medieval and Elizabethan times, a suntan was considered a sign of poverty. A suntan meant that the person worked outdoors on a farm or less prestigious job. White skin was considered fashionable and a mark of success and sophistication.

However, in the 20th century, as leisure time increased, many people considered a tan a mark of success, because the person was successful enough to afford leisure time spent in the sun. Some clients will always value this "beautiful tan." Unfortunately, golden brown skin at age 20 translates to wrinkled, leathery, ugly, splotchy, old-looking skin at age 40 or 50. Although some clients will never listen to reason about tanning, you should always make an effort to inform, educate, and save them from the ugly, long-term ravages of sun exposure!

Tell your clients that:

1. Sun exposure is the number one cause of premature aging and skin cancer. The best way to prevent sun damage is to stay out of the sun.
2. They should wear sunscreen every day, not just when sunbathing. We do not spend the majority of time at the beach. Hour for hour, most people receive more sun damage going to work, walking outside, and sitting by a window than we do basking in the sun. Sunbathing certainly makes the damage worse, but clients should use a good sunscreen moisturizer, for their skin type, daily.
3. As we discussed before, it is best not to go in the sun between 10 A.M. and 3 P.M.
4. Sunscreen should be applied 30 minutes before sun exposure. This provides better protection and allows the product to distribute itself more evenly.
5. Reapply sunscreen often if you are in direct light. Although sunscreen applications are not cumulative (two applications of SPF-15 sunscreen do not make an SPF-30 sunscreen), they are at least reapplying protection to these areas where the screen may have rinsed off due to sweating or water exposure.
6. Consider using self-tanning milk instead of sunbathing. These new products cause surface tanning. Used on a regular basis, they can produce a beautiful golden color. Two words of caution: Self-tanning products generally work better and more evenly on the body than on the face. A "tan" produced by a self-tanning product provides no additional resistance to sunburning!
7. A tanning booth is not a safe alternative. These machines still use rays that promote long-term damage, which can cause premature aging!

The sun is the number one enemy of the skin. Educate, teach, and warn your clients about its effects!

Self-Tanning Products

Self-tanning lotions are becoming more and more popular. These safe alternatives to the tanning impart a tan color without exposure to the sun. These products contain **dihydroxyacetone (DHA)**, a chemical derived from sugar cane or beets that turns brown when exposed to alkaline environments. Self-tanning products stain the very surface cells in the stratum corneum, and therefore shed in a few days to a few weeks. A darker color can be obtained by more frequent applications. Products containing more DHA will produce a darker tan (Plate 38).

Dihydroxyacetone (DHA) is an ingredient used in self-tanning agents that causes keratin to turn brown when applied.

Self-tanning lotions will provide the best results when applied to healthy hydrated skin. Skin that needs exfoliating or is very dehydrated will tend to "grab" the lotion, producing a splotchy result.

Some tips for good results with self-tanning are:

1. Carefully follow the manufacturer's directions. Self-tanning products do vary in spreading agent or DHA concentration.

2. Exfoliate with a mechanical scrub product before using the products. Loofahs tend to leave uneven texture, creating streaking. Continue to exfoliate at least twice a week.
3. Daily moisturization will help the self-tan look better.
4. Even application is extremely important. Uneven application will produce a muddy, splotchy result.
5. Make sure to wash your hands well immediately after application. Otherwise, your palms will turn dark, especially in the crevices between your fingers.
6. Make sure your feet are well exfoliated for an even application.
7. Do not shave immediately prior to application.
8. Generally speaking, self-tanning produces better results on the legs and arms than on the face. Facial skin renews faster and is therefore more likely to look splotchy or muddy.

Most importantly, make sure your clients understand that this is a fake tan. Many people have made the mistake of going to the beach, thinking they are "tan" and not using sunscreen! The result—a terrible, painful, and damaging sunburn!

Tanning "Pills"

There is a chemical called canthaxanthin that appears on the "health food" market every few years as a "tanning pill." What this chemical does is accumulate in the skin *and the eyes,* turning them a yellowish-brown color. This product has not been proven safe. Avoid any pill that promotes tanning!

Topics for Discussion

1. Why is the sun the worst enemy of the skin?
2. Discuss what happens to the skin histologically after long-term sun exposure.
3. Discuss esthetic problems caused by long-term sun damage.
4. What are the ABCDs of melanoma?
5. Discuss some rules for sun exposure and some common misconceptions about sun exposure.
6. What are UVA and UVB rays? What are the differences?
7. Explain what SPF means. What is broad-spectrum and why is it important?
8. What are some precautions for using self-tanning lotions?

Chapter

17

The New Science of Aging Skin Treatment

Objectives

Until recently there was relatively little that could be done to help the appearance of sun-damaged skin. In this chapter you will learn about some new developments in the treatment of photo-damaged skin and techniques the esthetician can use to help improve the appearance of sun-damaged, prematurely aging skin.

PHOTO DAMAGE

As we have previously discussed, aging skin does not look like it does because of the passing of years. The skin looks bad because of accumulated damage, most of which is from sun exposure, also known as photoaging or photo damage.

We have already touched on the long-term damage that cumulative sun exposure does to the skin. We have also already defined the difference between intrinsic aging, or aging of the skin that appears normally over time, and extrinsic aging, aging of the skin that occurs from induced or environmental causes, such as sun damage from exposure. These signs of aging skin from extrinsic sources do not show up for years.

Sun-damaged skin is significantly more leathery, with deeper and more numerous wrinkles and severe loss of elasticity. Sun-damaged skin also has significant discolorations, splotching, and hyperpigmentation. Intrinsically aged skin does not have nearly as great a problem with hyperpigmentation and demarcation, nor does it have as many wrinkles or as pronounced elastosis.

Histologically, sun-damaged skin shows very large differences from normally aging skin. The epidermis of photoaged skin is remarkably thicker. There is a large increase in elastic tissue in sun-damaged skin, but it takes on the form of a disorganized "blob," with little apparent organized structure. The fibroblasts in the thickened dermis of sun-damaged skin are considerably more numerous and are overactive, producing more collagen, but obviously in a disorganized fashion. There are also significant decreases in the vascular system of sun-damaged skin, which carries much-needed blood to various areas of the skin.

In short, the skin has obviously desperately tried to repair itself, producing an overabundance of tissue fibrils, but in a panicked and dysfunctional manner.

THE NEW SCIENCE OF AGING SKIN TREATMENT

Only in the last few years have we understood more about photo damage and discovered methods of effective treatment for photoaging. Although prevention and daily use of broad-spectrum sunscreens are still the best treatment, we now have at our disposal new and promising techniques and ingredients to help reduce the esthetic effects of photo damage, and to help protect and maintain healthy skin.

Although the esthetician primarily treats the appearance of the skin, there is mounting scientific evidence that many of the new techniques and ingredients likely have a positive effect on skin health as well as sun-damage prevention.

ANALYSIS OF PHOTOAGING SKIN

You will notice many symptoms of photoaging skin. Some of these symptoms may show up as early as the 20s. Severely sun-damaged skin will appear thick, leathery, rough to the touch, and will have many wrinkles, which may be both vertical and horizontal. Severe and multiple wrinkling in the nonintrinsic aging areas may be present. In other words, wrinkles around the eyes and nasolabial folds is normal, intrinsic skin aging. Severe wrinkling and surface roughness in the neck, cheek, chest, and other areas are usually not the result of intrinsic aging. These areas show cumulative effects of repeated sun exposure. Severe telangiectasias (couperose) are also often present. The skin is muddy looking, with diverse dark coloration, lentigines, and general brown splotchiness.

The treatment of the photo-damaged or photoaging skin is a program, not a magic bullet. There are many treatment methods that contribute to a successful age-/sun-damage management program. This combination topical skin-care program for photo-damaged skin can be summarized into five basic concepts:

- Prevention, using daily sunscreen protection
- Use of topical alphahydroxy acid (AHA) or other exfoliating agents
- Daily use of topical antioxidants
- Use of lipid-based products to repair or improve barrier function in ultradry skin
- Regular use of hydrators that help attract and bind essential moisture to the skin

---

Redness on the sides of the neck in a horseshoe pattern may be a definite sign of photoaging. These red areas may be accompanied by hyperpigmentation and telangiectasias. This is known as **poikiloderma of cevattes**.

In younger clients, you may notice all of the above symptoms in lesser amounts. The first sign may be hyperpigmentation, or dark blotchiness of the skin. Other signs might include rough, patchy skin, and the beginning of "chicken neck," in which the skin of the neck has constant "goose pimples," which is reflected by small, pinpoint, noncolored elevation of the follicles on the sides of the neck, like a plucked chicken. Wrinkles around the eyes and mouth may be especially severe for the client's age. However, brown splotchiness is the most evident sign of premature aging due to sun damage. The use of a Wood's lamp will indicate even more hyperpigmentation beneath the skin's surface. Lack of pigmentation will also be observable.

Poikiloderma of cevattes is a condition in sun-damaged skin resulting in horseshoe-shaped pigment and red splotching on the neck.

THE TREATMENT OF PHOTOAGING SKIN

Prevention—No Sun!

Daily use of broad-spectrum sunscreen is the very first step in photo-damage treatment. Even if the skin is already severely sun damaged, daily application of sunscreen will not only prevent more damage, but will allow the skin to have a better chance for good effects from other topical treatments.

The use of sunscreen on a *daily* basis cannot be emphasized enough! Many clients erroneously only worry about sunburn. They think of sun damage occurring only from visible sunburn and irritation. They are often likely to apply sunscreen only when they know they will be exposed to direct sunlight for several hours.

The truth is that the majority of our sun damage occurs from day-to-day exposure. Driving to work, going to the mailbox, playing with our children, and taking a walk are examples of everyday sun exposure that becomes cumulative. Even sitting by a window exposes us to deep-penetrating (and aging) UVA rays, which go right through glass!

This is why it is *so* important that we help our clients by advising a good sunscreen to be used daily.

Remember from Chapter 16 that broad-spectrum sunscreens are important to shield the skin from UVA and UVB rays. Look for active ingredient lists with ingredients that protect against both forms of UV light. Effective combinations include octyl methoxycinnimate with titanium dioxide or zinc oxide, or combinations of absorbing octyl methoxycinnimate, benzophenone-3, octyl salicylate, or avobenzone.

In most cases, clients can wear a day cream with built-in sunscreen. Most scientists and dermatologists recommend an SPF-15 or higher with broad-spectrum protection. It is usually not necessary to wear a separate moisturizer cream, except in extremely dry skin, or extremely cold, dry climates. Good day sunscreens are now available in a variety of weights, in lotion, gel, or cream forms, so they can be selected for the right skin type. Many contain hydrators like glycerin or hyaluronic acid, soothing ingredients like green tea extract, and other conditioners for specific skin types.

Having this variety of daily-use sunscreens available helps with client compliance in using a sunscreen everyday. Clients will use a product that is comfortable and meets their individual needs, such as a lightweight product, a product that works well under makeup, or one that is also a moisturizer.

The very first treatment should be a thorough discussion with the client of the harmful effects of sun. This author recommends a no-holds-barred lecture (in a friendly way!) about the ravages of cumulative sun damage. Emphasis should be placed on the cumulative nature of sun damage. Many clients will say, "I haven't had any sun in months!" The truth is that most of the sun damage you will see is from sunbathing that occurred twenty years ago, and years of daily exposure.

Unless the client implements good sun habits, or better yet, stays out of the sun altogether, improvement will be minimal, if any improvement occurs. The first need of sun-damaged skin is to remove the source of damage.

Exfoliation

The cell "turnover rate" slows down with aging anyway, but even more so in sun-damaged skin. Not only is the rate often slower, the cells are disorganized and are not in even layers. You must remember that sun damage causes abnormal cell growth and generally disorganizes normal cell patterns. This, of course, also affects the epidermis, piling dead cells on top of the skin in uneven patterns as they accumulate. Microscopic cross-section photographs of sun-damaged skin show severe disfigurations of the normal growth patterns of the strata of the epidermis. This can be both a medical and a cosmetic concern. Dysplastic cell growth can eventually cause skin cancer but esthetically causes a rough, dry, scaly appearance on the skin's surface as well as contributing to the appearance of wrinkles.

Production of intercellular lipids is diminished, interfering with barrier function, and reducing the ability of the skin to hold essential moisture. Clients who have this type of sun-damaged skin have a great deal of difficulty keeping their skin moisturized. Hydrators attract water to the skin, but there is not enough lipid to bind the moisture. By removing this conglomeration of dry, dead cells, the surface of the skin appears much smoother, and wrinkles appear less deep. Hydrators applied over the alphahydroxy treatments perform better because they do not have to moisturize the dead cell buildup. Instead they work to hydrate the skin more evenly, which results in a much smoother appearance of the skin.

Imagine a thick layer of cells lying on top of the skin. These cells are all dried up, like a thick layer of dust lying on top of a piece of furniture. This cell buildup makes the skin's surface look dull and flat, just as dust prevents light from reflecting from a piece of furniture. Surface mechanical exfoliation, which we have already discussed, helps to remove some of the "dust." Alphahydroxy acids, however, work by loosening the "glue" of lipids that hold the cells together, helping to continually shed off this sheath of cells. This removal of dead cells is also beneficial to acne-prone skin, helping to loosen both surface cell buildup and impacted dead cells inside the follicle, which, as we have previously discussed, can lead to comedones and, possibly, acne.

Use of a daily chemical exfoliant helps to rid skin of thick epidermal corneum that makes skin look dull. Cell buildup can make wrinkles look worse, dryness more uncomfortable, and splotchiness and hyperpigmentation more apparent. Daily use of an alphahydroxy and/or beta hydroxy acid treatment product can significantly improve skin texture, color evenness, depth of surface wrinkles, and smoothness.

More importantly, regular use of AHAs helps to "re-layer" the epidermal cells, improving barrier function, hydration, and intercellular lipid production. All of these changes not only help the appearance, but also result in healthier skin. Using chemical exfoliants like AHAs, BHAs, or retinoids make the daily use of broad-spectrum sunscreen even more important!

Retinoids

The first real science that showed that topical agents could be used to improve photodamaged skin was performed in the 1980s. Women who had been using the prescription drug Retin-A for their acne noticed that their wrinkles were less noticeable and that their treated skin looked smoother. Studies of this drug followed for the treatment of photoaging skin. Retinoids are vitamin A-based chemicals that include prescription tretinoin or retinoic acid, better known as Retin-A or Renova®.

These remarkable prescription drug chemicals have been shown to reduce wrinkles, roughness, solar freckles, and hyperpigmentation, and generally improve the skin's appearance. Renova®, a more moisturizing version of tretinoin, is the first prescription drug ever approved to treat the symptoms of sun damage.

Histologically, tretinoin has been shown to "reorganize" the skin, reestablishing a more normal epidermis, increasing blood vessel formation, increasing collagen production, and generally improving the damaged skin.

With these positive changes, there are some side effects, including redness, irritation, flaking, dryness, and severe dehydration. Sun exposure should be avoided, because the drug makes the skin more sun sensitive. A broad-spectrum sunscreen, as with any skin, is even more important for the tretinoin patient.

Nonprescription retinoids used in skin-care products include retinol and retinyl palmitate, which are other forms of vitamin A. These are good antioxidant ingredients, but do not work by the same mechanism or show the same results as tretinoin. Retinol, combined or used with alphahydroxy acid, has been shown to improve sun-damaged skin.

Alphahydroxy Acids

Alphahydroxy acid treatment is probably the most effective tool that the esthetician has to treat the photoaging skin. We have already discussed how alphahydroxy acids affect the skin. (See Chapter 9 to review information.) Alphahydroxy as well as beta hydroxy acids have a remarkable effect on photoaging. They are an integral part of any program for treating photoaged skin.

Rules for the Tretinoin Client

1. Tretinoin is a prescription drug. It is important to follow the advice of your dermatologist regarding usage procedures.
2. Cosmetic and skin-care product use may be affected by the use of tretinoin. Clients may find that they must change moisturizers, and that they may be more sensitive to products that they normally use. The esthetician can help the client choose the right new products for the tretinoin patient.
3. Facial treatments may need to be adapted for the tretinoin patient. This includes discontinuing the use of any exfoliation treatment, the use of gentle, fragrance-free hydrators, and avoidance of heat and any alcoholic or stimulating products.
4. Redness and peeling are normal transitional side effects when beginning tretinoin therapy. These can be minimized with good hydrators and being careful not to use too much tretinoin. Some clients may find it helpful to "phase in" to using tretinoin, using it every other night and slowly switching to every night use.
5. Sun should be completely avoided when using tretinoin. Deliberate sun exposure is contraindicated, and is counterproductive to any therapy for the improvement of photoaged skin.
6. Scented and fragranced products, alcohol-based lotions, stripping products, abrasive scrubs, alphahydroxy or beta hydroxy acids, benzoyl peroxide, sulfur-resorcinol, and other exfoliating agents should be avoided on skin using tretinoin.
7. DO NOT WAX AREAS BEING TREATED WITH TRETINOIN! Electrolysis is usually acceptable after the transitional side effects have passed.

The terms alphahydroxy acid and glycolic acid are often used interchangeably. However, technically, glycolic acid is an alphahydroxy acid, and treatments may involve both alphahydroxy and beta hydroxy acids.

Alphahydroxy acids include glycolic acid, lactic acid, tartaric acid, and malic acid. These functional agents can be used in products as an individual acid, or in special AHA blends. Although very different from tretinoin, these agents also help to "reorganize" the epidermis. Regular use of an 8 to 10 percent alphahydroxy treatment product, with a pH of no less than 3.5, can reduce the appearance of wrinkles, smooth the skin surface, reduce uneven coloring, and improve hydration and firmness. It cannot completely rid the skin of sun-damage symptoms, especially advanced sun damage and elastosis, but it certainly improves the appearance of almost all sun-damage symptoms.

Long-term use of alphahydroxy acids helps to replenish intercellular lipids that decrease with age and sun damage. The intercellular lipids, as discussed in previous chapters, make up the barrier function and are responsible for epidermal hydration.

Besides typical aging and wrinkles, alphahydroxy acids can help improve hand and foot calluses, general dry and dehydrated skin, and dry body skin.

Stimulation

The circulation of sun-damaged skin is impaired by the malformation of blood vessels due to the sun damage. Therefore, the skin is not nourished properly through normal blood flow. The use of good but gentle massage techniques is helpful in improving the circulation.

Be careful when massaging skin that is being treated with a keratolytic such as glycolic acid or Retin-A. This skin can be treated, but be careful not to overstimulate.

Alphahydroxy Home Treatments

Different products are formulated differently with different vehicle ingredients, release symptoms, and different concentrations of alphahydroxy acid, depending on the type of problem treated. Preparations for acne, oily, and problem skin are usually in a gel form, so designed to combat oily skin. They are very helpful when used in conjunction with other acne treatments. As a word of caution, be careful when combining peeling agents. Combining glycolic acid with benzoyl peroxide, salicylic acid, resorcinol, sulfur, or retinoic acid must be done very carefully, if at all. Check the manufacturer's instructions well before combining home keratolytic treatments. The alphahydroxy solution for oily and acne-prone skin should be applied to the face, usually twice daily, under a protective sunscreen moisturizer, or coupled with a light, noncomedogenic hydrating product at night. Some companies suggest treatments only once a day at home. Always check the manufacturer's instructions!

Alphahydroxy products for the body are usually made in lotion form, to be applied like a body lotion. These are almost always oil-in-water emulsions and sometimes are not designed for facial use. Again, check the instructions.

Alphahydroxy products for fading hyperpigmentation are in a gel or lotion form. The glycolic acid is mixed in the solution with a bleaching agent, hydroquinone or another melanin suppressant such as magnesium ascorbyl phosphate, licorice extract, kojic acid, bearberry extract, or arbutin. Alphahydroxy acid helps remove the buildup of dead cells, which helps the bleaching agent work better and faster. Age spots, sun freckles, pregnancy masks, and hyperpigmented areas from acne all can be helped with such a solution. As with any bleaching solution, the client should be instructed to use a good sunscreen and avoid sun exposure, which, of course, can result in recurrence of the hyperpigmentation.

In the treatment of wrinkles and the appearance of sun damage, alphahydroxy acid loosens the dead cell buildup, again helping make the skin look smoother and softer. The appearance of wrinkles can be greatly improved with continued use. The products available to help the appearance of aging skin are usually in a cream or lotion form. The cream form is for alipidic, dry, dehydrated, aging skin. Lotions are more appropriate for combination skin showing signs of aging including wrinkles, leathery texture, dull appearance, and uneven surfaces. The cream or lotion is applied under the moisturizer or sunscreen and under the night treatment. Most companies recommend twice daily application.

Recommending Alphahydroxy Home Care

First, as always, carefully evaluate the appearance of the client's skin. You must also assess the client's current home care. If he or she is currently using home care that is inappropriate, such as strong soap for aging skin, this must first be corrected. Alphahydroxy treatment is most effective when used with a well-planned general home care program, designed for the skin type and conditions.

Explain how alphahydroxy acid works on aging skin and the importance of the "program." Best results cannot be expected if the client is using a hodgepodge of products along with the alphahydroxy acid. Be careful to find out if the client is using other peeling-type products or drugs. Heavily scented products or products that are extremely stimulating should also be avoided when alphahydroxy acid is being used. The client should also be instructed in the importance of regular use. No product will work if it is sitting in the medicine cabinet! Other problems such as hyperpigmented skin or problem oily areas should be addressed separately.

Alphahydroxy acid often produces a mild-to-moderate tingling sensation when applied to the skin. Usually the tingling feeling lasts only 10 or 20 seconds. The client should wait for a short amount of time (a few minutes) before applying other hydrating or conditioning products. When a client first starts using alphahydroxy acid, some slight cosmetic side effects might be experienced. In the case of dry or aging skin, the skin may show some flaking, which the client may misunderstand as dehydration. Explain that this is the dead cell layer coming off the surface, is a normal occurrence, and can be controlled by using the appropriate products along with the alphahydroxy acid cream. This is another reason why the "surrounding" products are so important. If the client uses the wrong treatment cream or a cleanser that is too harsh, side effects will be more intense. The client's skin may feel "crunchy," as if it is peeling. Again, this feeling can be alleviated by using a good hydrating fluid. In the case of clog-prone or combination skin, make sure that you recommend a moisturizer that is noncomedogenic.

If the client experiences severe peeling, tell the client to call you. Instruct the client to discontinue using the alphahydroxy solution temporarily until the peeling subsides. Then phase in the alphahydroxy product, starting once a day, and eventually working back into twice daily application.

Some clients with extremely thin skin may have problems with waxing. This is unusual, but it does occur sometimes. Waxing in these clients, or any other procedure that involves removing cells, should be discontinued. Allergic reactions to alphahydroxy acid are rare, but like with any other cosmetic ingredient, allergic reaction is possible. Allergic symptoms are the same as for any other reaction. These may include redness, itching, and general irritation. The client should, of course, discontinue the treatment.

Treatments with glycolic acid are also performed in the salon. For more information, please see Chapter 18, Chemical Peeling and Exfoliation Procedures.

Antioxidant Therapy

There is growing evidence that the use of topical antioxidants helps reduce the visual signs of aging, and may make the skin behave in a healthier way. Vitamin C, in the forms of both l-ascorbic acid and magnesium ascorbyl phosphates, and liposomed vitamin E (tocopherol) and tocopheryl acetate (vitamin E acetate), are well-known topical antioxidants. Natural extracts, such as grapeseed extracts and green tea, are loaded with antioxidant chemicals. Grapeseed extract is known to be 50 times as strong an antioxidant as vitamin C.

No one knows at the time of this writing exactly how the antioxidants work to improve skin, but it is theorized by many skin scientists that antioxidants interfere with the inflammation cascade, reducing the production of damaging enzymes that can injure or dissolve the collagen and elastin fibrils that keep the skin smooth and elastic. There is certainly growing evidence the topical antioxidants are very helpful in the prevention and treatment of sun-damaged skin.

It is not enough to simply include these ingredients in a treatment product. Be careful when purchasing antioxidant products to sell or use in your practice. Antioxidant ingredients are often very unstable, and must be protected until they come in contact with the skin. One sign of an unstable product is that the product turns brown quickly upon exposure to air, specifically oxygen.

The protection of these fragile antioxidants in products is accomplished with the use of microencapsulated delivery systems such as liposomes. The use of lipid-based encapsulation mechanisms helps protect the antioxidants from oxidizing, and the lipids help the agents to penetrate into the epidermal layers easier.

Antioxidants are often in serum form and are designed to be applied under an alphahydroxy acid treatment product, sunscreen, or hydrator.

Use of Lipid Products and Hydrators

Hydration is very important in improving the appearance of photo-damaged skin. Sun damage results in the skin losing its ability to hold water. Lipid ingredients, as previously discussed, are helpful in "patching" the "mortar" between the cells, helping to boost hydration, firmness, smoothness, and to reduce inflammation potential. These lipids include phospholipids, sphingolipids or gycosphingolipids (also known as ceramides), cholesterol, and fatty acids.

These lipid complexes can be included in sunscreens, hydrators, specialty creams, masks, or serums. They are extremely effective as a treatment for dry, alipidic, or extremely dry skin. The lipids work by helping hold essential hydration in the epidermis. They should be used with a hydrator to attract water to the skin.

Hydration ingredients include butylene glycol, hyaluronic acid or sodium hyaluronate, glycerin, sodium PCA, or sorbitol. These ingredients are also blended into the same products for sun-damaged skin as mentioned above.

Be careful to remember the skin type when you are choosing a hydrator or other cream. Aging oily or combination skin can become impacted and comedonal from exposure to too many fatty emollients. Gels, liquids, and lotions that are especially designed for oily or acne-prone oily skin should be recommended.

Avoidance of Irritation

The symptoms of what we think of as aging is an accumulation of damage to skin tissue caused by chronic irritations, such as sun exposure. All clients should avoid irritating the skin at any age, but especially in the already photo-damaged skin.

A Typical Home Care Program for Photoaging Skin

Clients with photoaging skin should have the entire skin-care program explained to them in detail. It is important that they understand the function of all products prescribed, and why each has importance in the success of their program. It should be

---

The Basics of Treating Sun-Damaged Skin

- Sun exposure must be carefully avoided, especially during the hours of 10 A.M. and 3 P.M.
- An SPF-15 broad-spectrum sunscreen should be worn on a *daily* basis, incorporated into a day cream or fluid.
- An 8 to 10 percent alphahydroxy acid product, with a pH no less than 3.5 should be used regularly.
- A daily stabilized antioxidant serum applied to the skin may help the skin against free radicals that can damage cells, resulting in wrinkles and elastosis.
- Avoid all irritation to the skin.
- Hydration helps improve moisture content in the skin, improving smoothness and elasticity.
- Lipid-based products are especially effective for dehydrated sun-damaged skin. Lipid products help improve hydration and barrier function.

emphasized that the client must be diligent about home care use for a successful program. Provide them with a step-by-step home care instruction sheet to follow, and use it to describe each step during the consultation.

Clients who are not used to a several-step program may wish to "phase in" to the program. This sometimes is helpful in getting clients used to a home regimen, but you should insist to the client that the whole program must be followed for results they are expecting. In other words, be understanding of their need for simplicity, but also make them understand that all the products must be used to see the results they want.

Cleansing should be gentle and thorough, and the client must avoid any harsh cleanser, including bar soaps, which can be stripping and damaging to the barrier function. Cleansing milk or light rinseable liquid cleanser is advised. This should be followed by a mild nonalcoholic toner, which helps to remove cleanser residue and also lower the pH of the skin.

After cleansing and toning, apply your antioxidant serum. It is important to follow manufacturers' instructions because products do vary in ingredients and product form, such as a serum versus a lotion.

Apply the alphahydroxy product, which could be a gel, lotion, or cream, depending on the skin type. During the day, this will be followed by an SPF-15 or higher broad-spectrum sunscreen, with built-in hydrator. For drier skin, make sure the sunscreen contains lipids to help support the barrier function and protect against daytime moisture loss. In the evening, the same basic steps are followed, but this may vary depending on the client's specific needs or differences in product type. For example, some clients may only be able to use an AHA once a day, depending on climate, skin thinness, or genetic characteristics. Some companies may prefer that the client use an AHA at night and an antioxidant during the day. Again, follow the instructions of your product manufacturer. In the evening, use a hydrating cream instead of sunscreen.

Supplemental products, such as eye creams, or specialty serums, such as a concentrated lipid serum, may be also advisable depending on the skin type. Concentrated lipid serums are very helpful for very dry, wrinkled skin, or areas of extreme damage like the neck or wrinkles around the mouth or eyes. Lipid serum is applied after all other products, including sunscreen, but before makeup application.

Salon Treatment Program

Begin by treating the skin with regular clinical facial treatments, emphasizing moisturization and light stimulation through massage techniques. Design the treatment for the skin type (oily, dry, etc.) and, if necessary, perform deep cleansing with extraction to any sun-damaged skin that is also oily or comedonal.

AHA exfoliations are extremely helpful in treating the sun-damaged skin. After the client has been using 8 to 10 percent AHA home care treatment for at least two weeks, administer 30 percent AHA applications in the salon, twice a week for three weeks; follow with weekly treatments if necessary. Discontinue or temporarily delay any treatment that is irritating or produces lasting redness. Long-term, regular monthly or twice-monthly AHA exfoliation treatments are advisable, alternating with hydrating facial treatments.

Hyperpigmentation Treatment

One of the main symptoms of photoaging is hyperpigmentation. It is also one of the main concerns of sun-damaged clients, and one of the most difficult disorders to manage. We have already discussed in previous chapters how hyperpigmentation occurs during sun exposure. Long-term sun exposure, as well as hormonal activity, particularly in female clients, results in overproductive melanocytes in the skin.

The melanocytes, which are the cells that produce the melanin, are in the lower epidermis and upper dermis. They produce melanin when they are stimulated by sun exposure, but also can be stimulated by hormones, exposure to some chemicals (including overstimulating skin-care products), injuries to the skin (including laser surgery or some forms of chemical peeling), and many forms of inflammation. In some clients, melanocytes may actually be present in lower areas of the dermis. These clients will rarely be responsive to treatment.

When stimulated, the melanocytes produce melanin as a protective mechanism. Melanocytes have dendrites, which are small branches on the cells containing the melanin. The dendrites are "embraced" by the skin cells, which absorb the melanin, before they drift toward the surface of the skin. This process gives the cell a characteristic melanin color, which is seen as hyperpigmentation when concentrated areas of cells contain melanin.

There are three types of products and therapy that are effective in reducing skin pigment: chemical exfoliation, melanin suppressive agents, and sunscreens. Normally, all three are used in treating hyperpigmented photo-damaged skin.

Chemical exfoliants include alphahydroxy acid (usually glycolic or a blend), beta hydroxy acid (salicylic acid), *or* tretinoin (Retin-A or Renova®). Use of both is not advised because this may produce unnecessary irritation. Chemical exfoliants remove cells containing melanin, helping to fade the skin. They also clear hyperkeratinized areas of cell buildup on the skin surface, enabling better treatment of the skin.

Melanin suppressive agents interfere with the chemical process of melanin production. Many inhibit tyrosinase, an enzyme used to convert the amino acid tyrosine, very instrumental in the production of melanin. The only FDA-approved skin-lightening agent at the time of this writing is hydroquinone, available in over-the-counter products at 2 percent and 4 percent prescription strengths. Other nonapproved so-called "brightening" ingredients, which are all basically melanin suppressants, include kojic acid, arbutin, asafetida extract, bearberry extract, magnesium ascorbyl phosphate (also an antioxidant), and azelaic acid. There are two drawbacks to melanin suppressants, particularly hydroquinone. Many clients are allergic to hydroquinone, and it is a strong oxidant, which means it neutralizes and turns darker fairly quickly on exposure to air (oxygen). It is best to patch test clients for hydroquinone use before dispensing the product. It is also advisable to explain that hydroquinone solutions are fairly easily ruined and should be kept in a cool, dark place; and they should always be securely closed after each use.

Broad-spectrum sunscreens, used daily (as all sunscreens really should be), and avoidance of sun exposure are imperative if the hyperpigmented client wants to see results. Unfortunately, many of these clients are "sun addicted" and it is hard for them to give up tanning. Nevertheless, the esthetician should insist that for any pigment-evening treatment to work, sun must be avoided.

It should be mentioned here that hyperactive melanocytes do not just react to ultraviolet rays. They also react to heat from the infrared rays from the sun. There is no sunscreen available, or none on the immediate forefront, that blocks infrared heat. So, the bottom line is that sun and heat must be avoided for these clients. A very thorough consultation with each client explaining all the facts about hyperpigmentation treatment as well as a handout is advisable.

Most companies recommend that an AHA product be used before application of melanin suppressant, then followed by sunscreen, or night hydrator. Some companies recommend AHA during the day, and the melanin suppressant at night. It is best to check with the individual manufacturer, and to remember that clients' skin types vary, and twice-a-day application of both treatments may be too much for some.

PREVENTION IS STILL THE BEST TREATMENT

Avoiding sun exposure and using sunscreens are still the best and most viable treatments for sun damage. Clients should always be instructed in the proper use of sunscreens to help prevent this terrible insult to the skin.

Topics for Discussion

1. What are some signs of the beginning of sun damage?
2. Discuss the research on the use of retinoids for photoaging skin.
3. What would you say when discussing sun damage with a client?
4. What precautions would you take to avoid overstimulating photoaged skin?
5. Discuss alphahydroxy acids and their effect on the appearance of photoaged skin.
6. How does alphahydroxy acid improve the surface of aging skin?
7. Explain the treatment for hyperpigmentation, and why it is important to have a thorough consultation with the client who is hyperpigmented.

Chapter

18

Chemical Peeling and Exfoliation Procedures

Objectives

Many different types of peeling and exfoliation treatments are available, ranging from brushing treatment and light enzyme peels to strong surgical peels that are administered by dermatologists and plastic surgeons. This chapter discusses the various types of peeling treatments, both cosmetic and medical, and the various conditions that can benefit from different types of peeling treatments. This chapter is not a substitute for hands-on training in the use of superficial salon chemical peelings. The esthetician should always receive hands-on training before attempting any of the procedures discussed in this chapter.

The process of peeling the surface of the skin dates back to the 19th century in Europe. Chemical peeling was actually brought to America by a young esthetician, the daughter of a European doctor, who immigrated to America. The process of peeling the skin can take place in varying degrees, ranging from scrubs to salicylic creams to surgical-level phenol peeling. Removing cell layers from the surface of the skin can be used to treat a variety of both cosmetic and medical problems.

The esthetician's domain is the superficial epidermis. It is important to note that the esthetician should not perform treatments that involve live layers of the skin. This is medical peeling and is the domain of the dermatologist or plastic surgeon. Removal of dead cells by chemical means is chemical or esthetic exfoliation. It is preferred terminology that estheticians perform exfoliation treatments rather than "peels." However, we must be realistic and say that both estheticians and consumers alike use the terms interchangeably.

SURFACE EXFOLIATION

There are basically two types of exfoliation treatments. Mechanical exfoliation uses some method of physical contact to literally scrape or bump cells off the skin. Granular scrubs, such as honey and almond scrubs, preparations with polyethylene granules or jojoba beads, or the use of a brushing machine are all examples of mechanical peeling treatments. When the granules of these products or the bristles of a brushing machine come in contact with the surface corneum cells, the movement of the product or the brush literally "bumps off" cells from the surface of the corneum.

Many skin-care companies include brushing as a standard part of their salon treatments. The brushing machine is used over a layer of cleanser or moisturizer, which helps to buffer contact with the skin. The skin should be thoroughly cleansed, toned, and steamed before the brushing machine is used. Applying a noncomedogenic hydrating fluid before steaming the face is helpful in hydrating the dry surface cells, also helping to loosen dead cell buildup on the surface. This makes removal of the dead cells much easier, and gentler pressure can be used.

Removing the surface cells help the skin in the following ways:

1. The procedure helps remove uneven buildup of dead cells, so the skin appears much smoother.
2. It helps clear away dead cells and debris from the pore openings, making extraction and other treatment of clogged pores much easier.
3. By removing the dead cell layer, the lower-level cells are moved to the surface more quickly, improving the moisture content of the surface.
4. Mechanical treatment stimulates blood flow to the surface of the skin.
5. Removing the dry, dead cell buildup helps deliver moisturizers and other treatment deeper into the epidermis.

All of these advantages generally help to smooth the skin's surface, which makes makeup apply more evenly. The dead cells will eventually build back up on the surface, making this procedure only a temporary appearance change. However, regular use of mechanical exfoliators such as granular scrubs or alphahydroxy acid home treatment products helps maintain this appearance. Granular scrubs for normal to dry skin are usually recommended two to three times per week.

Disadvantages of Mechanical Treatment

There are many circumstances when mechanical treatment is not appropriate. Do not use brushing machines, microdermabrasion, or any harsh mechanical peeling techniques on the following skin types and conditions:

1. Couperose skin, or telangiectatic skin, with many visible capillaries and blood vessels. The blood vessels in these skin types are very fragile and should not be subject to brushing treatment.
2. Fragile, thin skin that reddens easily. The epidermis of this skin is considerably thinner than other skin types. Brushing or abrasive treatment may redden and irritate this skin easily.
3. Older skin that is thin and bruises easily.
4. Severely sun-damaged skin. This skin also will often have many distended capillaries and redness.
5. Skin that is being medically treated with tretinoin (retinoic acid or Retin-A), azelaic acid, adapalene (Differin®), alphahydroxy acid, or fluorouracil. (See Chapter 17, The New Science of Aging Skin Treatment.)
6. Acne-prone skin types, particularly those with inflamed acne, papules, and pustules.
7. Accutane® patients.
8. Any skin that is red, irritated, thin, or extremely fair.
9. Skin that has a history of being easily irritated.

Other Mechanical Exfoliation Techniques

As an alternative to using a brushing machine, you may choose to use a granular scrub, such as honey and almond scrub, after steaming. Apply the scrub with your fingertips and gently massage in upward, outward circular movements. Do not scrub the face for more than 1 or 2 minutes. Be extremely gentle with the pressure you apply. For thinner skin types, you may dilute the scrub with cleanser or moisturizer before applying the preparation. This dilution helps to provide a buffer between the skin's surface and the scrub, which cuts down on irritation potential.

For oilier skins, you may apply a granular scrub made with fine polyethylene beads or granules. These preparations often contain a small amount of sulfur or salicylic acid as additional chemical exfoliators and antiseptics. These scrubs are generally excellent for oily, problem skin and will help clear the surface of dead cells and other debris, making extraction easier.

One of the most recent techniques in mechanical exfoliation is the technique known as microdermabrasion. This process involves "shooting" aluminum oxide (corundum) crystals at the skin with a special apparatus. The crystals, after hitting the skin and exfoliating dead cells, are then picked up by a vacuum attached to the same handheld apparatus. This technique must be learned hands-on, under the supervision of an expert in the procedure.

Microdermabrasion is used to treat superficial symptoms of aging, similar to those treated with an alphahydroxy acid product and salon exfoliations. It is generally administered in a series of treatments.

Microdermabrasion is favored by many estheticians because it shows fairly quick results in improving skin texture. There are no long-term studies to measure long-term improvement, as there are for alphahydroxy and glycolic acids. Microdermabrasion should be used with extreme care, especially in clients prone to hyperpigmentation. Overuse can cause increased pigmentation in some clients.

It would appear that even though alphahydroxy treatments do produce visible improvements in skin texture, the ongoing and long-range improvements in skin moisture, lipid content, and barrier function are likely due to daily applications of AHAs, which does not happen with microdermabrasion. Microdermabrasion should not be performed with alphahydroxy treatments, unless the two treatments are spaced well apart. Most estheticians recommend that clients not use AHA home products for up to two weeks after having had a microdermabrasion treatment.

Home Care Using Mechanical Exfoliation

For dry to normal skin, recommend a light scrub such as honey and almond scrub two or three times per week. The client should apply the scrub after cleansing with a milk-type cleanser. Instruct the client to be very gentle with the scrub. Home care scrubs should not be recommended for extremely thin skin or skin that is being treated with the therapies already listed in the precautions.

For oily and problem skin, granular scrubs are sometimes recommended on a daily or twice daily basis. This, of course, will depend on the skin type, contraindications previously discussed, and what other drug or esthetic therapies are being used to treat this skin type. Exfoliation and removal of dead cells is usually very helpful in treating problem oily and clog-prone skin.

SALON EXFOLIATION TREATMENTS

These treatments are actually a type of chemical exfoliation, but they are extremely gentle. They are sometimes appropriate to use when mechanical exfoliation is not appropriate. These procedures involve the use of enzymes, specifically proteolytic enzymes. *Proteolytic* means "protein dissolving." The enzymes work to destroy the keratin in the dead cells on the surface of the skin. These are often referred to as enzyme peeling or enzyme treatments.

One enzyme often used in these treatments is papain, which is derived from the papaya fruit. Papain is also used in meat tenderizer for its ability to soften tissue and dissolve protein. In Europe, this type of treatment is known as a lysing or lysis. Another biological enzyme often used is pancreatin, which is derived from beef by-products.

There are two basic types of proteolytic enzyme peeling. One is a cream that is applied to the skin after steaming and initial preparation. This cream contains paraffin, which dries and forms a hardened crust. The cream dries in about 10 minutes, and then is massaged or "rolled" off the skin. Treatments of this type are often called "vegetal" or "vegetable" peelings. This treatment is actually a combination of enzyme and mechanical peeling. The "rolling" provides friction that physically removes dead cells. The flakes coming off the skin are not dead cells but dried paraffin. The actual dead cells removed are not visible without a microscope. They can also be irritating for the skin types listed previously.

The second, and probably more popular, type of enzyme treatment uses a powdered form of enzyme. Mixed with warm water immediately before application, this treatment stays soft during application and does not dry. It is easily removed because it is soft and moist. This type of enzyme treatment generally produces a more even peeling of the cell buildup and helps to slightly dilate the follicle openings, which makes extraction much easier. Brushing the skin may miss some of the cells while this type of enzyme treatment works evenly across the surface of the skin. Enzyme peelings are often available in varying strengths and suitable for the following conditions:

1. Oily, clogged skin with open and closed comedones and minor acne breakouts.
2. Dry or dehydrated skin with cell buildup, flaking, and tight dry surface.
3. Dull, lifeless looking skin. This skin condition actually has a tremendous buildup of dead cells that produces a slight gray color on the surface of the skin.
4. Skin with multiple milia.
5. Clients who desire a smoother appearance to their skin and a more even surface for makeup application.

Enzyme treatments are generally gentle enough to repeat even on an every-two-week schedule, although most clients have them with their regular monthly facial treatments. Most clients notice immediate softening of the skin after the very first application of the enzyme. Because enzyme treatment slightly dilates the pore openings, which helps with extraction, clients notice that extraction is more comfortable and that gentler pressure may be used to facilitate extraction of the clogged pores, comedones, and other impactions.

Procedure for Enzyme Treatment

Caution: Always follow manufacturer's directions for using particular peeling treatments! The following is an example of typical treatment with enzymes, but these directions may vary with the manufacturer.

1. Remove all makeup and cleanse the skin well, using a milk cleanser appropriate for the skin type.
2. Apply a pre-peel lotion, usually furnished by the manufacturer. This solution is applied in a similar method as a toner. This solution is normally slightly alkaline, which helps remove excess oils on the surface of the skin, making the enzyme come in better contact with the dead surface dells.
3. Choose the appropriate strength of enzyme preparation for the particular skin type, thickness, and condition. Most companies make at least two strengths or furnish formulas to dilute the enzyme action of the product.
4. Mix the product with warm water in a small mixing cup or beaker. Most enzyme treatments have the consistency and thickness of mayonnaise when mixed with warm water. Stir the preparation until the treatment is smooth and free of powder lumps.
5. Apply the enzyme to the face with a soft mask brush. Stay clear of the eye area and other sensitive areas unless otherwise directed by manufacturer's instructions.
6. Many companies recommend steaming during the application of the treatment and during treatment setting time. The steam helps keep the treatment warm and also helps to keep the preparation from drying out on the surface. It is important to keep the preparation moist. If enzymes are allowed to dry on the face they can be irritating to the skin and are also hard to remove. Allow the treatment to set for about eight minutes. Remove with tepid, damp sponges or a damp, soft, facial cloth. Be careful

to remove the enzyme treatment thoroughly. It is easy to leave remnants of the peeling, particularly around the perimeter of the face, such as under the chin, on the jawline, and in front of the ears. This leftover enzyme can be irritating if not removed after the appropriate amount of time.

7. Brushing is not necessary when using an enzyme treatment. In fact, it can be irritating. Do not use the brush during an enzyme treatment.

8. Because of the follicle dilation caused by the enzyme, desincrustation using galvanic current is usually not necessary. It can also be irritating to thin, sensitive, or dry skins when combined with enzyme treatment. Excessively oily skin, acne-prone skin, and thick, oily skin with multiple comedones may benefit from galvanic desincrustation after an enzyme treatment. Use your best judgment and remember, when in doubt, don't!

9. Proceed with extraction in a normal manner. You will probably find that you do not have to use nearly as much pressure during extraction. This will appeal to the client as well, because treatment is more comfortable.

10. Apply a toner to lower the pH of the skin immediately after extraction. It is important to lower the pH after the enzyme treatment.

11. Proceed with the rest of treatment as normal. You should not massage the skin before applying the enzyme. This may increase irritation potential. Any facial waxing should be done toward the end of the treatment session, not before the enzyme is applied. The waxing procedure will also physically remove dead cells. It is best to perform waxing after the enzyme is removed, or, on sensitive skin, suggest that the client make a separate appointment for a different day.

12. You may find that you do not need to use as aggressive a mask as usual after an enzyme treatment. Some masks also remove dead cell buildup. On dry or thin skins, apply a gel mask, a cream mask, or simply apply a thick layer of hydrating fluid as a mask. These types of masks are nonhardening and are easier to remove from sensitive or thin skins.

Most skin-care salons charge an additional fee for enzyme treatments. You may want to allow the client to try the enzyme treatment once at no charge so that the client can see the nice results.

ALPHAHYDROXY AND GLYCOLIC PEELING TREATMENTS

Before reading this section, review the section on alphahydroxy acid in Chapter 17, The New Science of Aging Skin Treatment. Glycolic acid is available in a variety of strengths for salon use. The typical concentration of glycolic acid used in salon treatment is between 15 and 30 percent. Higher strengths are usually used only by dermatologists. It is strongly suggested that you not experiment with higher percentages of glycolic acid!

The Cosmetic Ingredient Review of the Cosmetics, Toiletries, and Fragrance Association has issued a recommendation that licensed estheticians use alphahydroxy acid salon exfoliation products that do not exceed 30 percent concentration and have a pH of 3.0 or above. Higher concentrations or lower pH can cause irritation.

Before administering alphahydroxy acid exfoliation, the client should have been using an 8 to 10 percent concentration gel, lotion, or cream at home for at least two weeks. Home use of the AHA before AHA exfoliation should be mandatory because it helps acclimate the skin for higher strength salon products. Failure to use AHA at home as described may result in increased discomfort during the procedure and increased chances of redness and irritation after the exfoliation treatment.

The standard treatment consists of a ten-minute application of 30 percent, pH 3.0 gel. This is administered twice a week for three weeks for a client beginning AHA treatments. Maintenance treatments are usually twice a month, but vary with client needs, budgets, and sensitivity levels. It is very important to pay attention to manufacturers' instructions, which may vary from product to product.

Alphahydroxy exfoliation works by dissolving surface binding lipids that hold the cells of the corneum together. AHA treatments can be used to help the same conditions listed for enzyme exfoliation but will also improve hyperpigmentation, fine lines and wrinkles, and surface roughness. Continual use refines pore appearance and helps achieve even texture and coloration.

Mild glycolic treatment may be influenced by the cleansing procedure that takes place before extraction. The cleansing procedure determines how much surface oil is removed before applying the glycolic peeling treatment. The following is a typical procedure for glycolic treatment, but read the instructions of the particular product you are using and follow them.

Procedure for Glycolic Exfoliation

1. Cleanse the skin with a mild cleansing milk, removing makeup.
2. Apply a compress to the eyes to avoid accidentally spilling the solution into the eyes.
3. Set a timer for ten minutes, or the length of time suggested by the manufacturer. Apply the glycolic acid gel with two cotton swabs held together. Begin with the forehead, and apply the gel using small, circular motions with the cotton swabs. Proceed to other areas in a precise clockwise pattern. It is important to follow a precise pattern to ensure even application of the gel.

The glycolic treatment is allowed to stay on the skin for the prescribed amount of time, as recommended by the manufacturer. A typical time for a low-strength solution is ten minutes. After ten minutes remove the gel from the face with cool, wet, gauze pads. Rinse the face well with the wet gauze. You may follow this with a cool spray of plain water in an atomizer and another cleanup with wet gauze. Finish by applying a sunscreen moisturizer (Plate 42).

This treatment is normally performed twice a week for the first three weeks. The pretreatment before application of the glycolic acid gel can influence the strength of the treatment. The strength of the cleansing products used will determine the amount of surface oils and corneum cells removed before application of the gel.

You should, during the first treatment, cleanse with a very mild cleansing milk. If the first treatment does not produce any redness or irritation, the second treatment may be preceded by a slightly stronger milk cleanser. For the third visit, again assuming there is no irritation, you may add a mild toner to complete the cleansing. The fourth treatment may be strengthened by using a slightly stronger milk cleanser with a slightly stronger toner. The cleansers and toners used should never be extremely strong or alcoholic.

It is strongly recommended that a minimum of six treatments be given before assessing the results. Results will not be particularly dramatic after one treatment. It takes several applications of 30 percent alphahydroxy acid, over several weeks, to see appreciable results in many cases (Plates 39a, 39b).

After the initial treatment, you may decide to repeat the treatment weekly, biweekly, or monthly, depending on the results. You should reassess the condition of the skin after the first few applications to determine a further treatment course.

Precautions to Take When Administering Glycolic Peelings

1. Always make sure the skin has been pretreated with lower strength alphahydroxy acid at home for at least two weeks before administering salon-strength treatment. Failure to do this may cause irritation. For instructions on home care AHA treatment, see Chapter 17, The New Science of Aging Skin Treatment.

2. Do not use the alphahydroxy acid treatment if the client is currently using prescription tretinoin (Retin-A or Renova®), adapalene (Differin®), or azelaic acid (Azelex®), or other prescription peeling agents. Treatment with any of these drugs should be discontinued for several weeks before using salon alphahydroxy exfoliation treatments.

3. Do not use glycolic or alphahydroxy acid on Accutane® patients.

4. Do not administer AHA treatments if the client is under a dermatologist's care for any skin disorders, without first obtaining approval from the dermatologist.

5. Be careful to use eyepads, and avoid getting the alphahydroxy acid close to the eyes.

6. Do not use the peeling gel on a male client immediately after he has shaved. It is best to wait several hours after shaving to apply glycolic salon treatment.

7. Check with the client before each successive treatment to make sure the client has not experienced any irritation from the previous treatment. If irritation developed after the previous treatment, do not add precleansing steps as discussed earlier. Avoid any area that is peeling, red, or irritated, or wait a few days before resuming treatment.

8. Do not administer AHA treatments to any skin that is already irritated. This includes rosacea flares, seborrheic dermatitis, eczema, windburned or sunburned skin, or skin that is irritated from a previous treatment of any type. Never double-exfoliate skin, or use other keratolytics at the same time, chemical or mechanical, especially microdermabrasion.

You should not combine professional alphahydroxy acid application with other salon facial treatments when first beginning AHA treatment. After the initial series of AHA salon applications, you may administer glycolic treatment during facial treatments, depending on the client. As always, check manufacturer's instructions for instruction regarding combining AHA treatment with other types of salon skin-care treatments.

The skin should never be exfoliated before AHA application. Avoid pretreatment with any technique or product that is stimulating, heating, or irritating.

AHA treatment with low-strength gel can be administered indefinitely on a weekly, biweekly, or monthly basis, depending on the client and the skin type.

Using AHA Treatment for Acne

The procedure is essentially the same as we have just discussed. You may notice an apparent increase in comedones and blackheads during the first few treatments. Because AHA is an exfoliating treatment, it uncovers closed comedones and loosens open comedones while exfoliating the dead-cell layer on the surface of the skin, which can be fairly heavy on oily, problem skin. You should explain the possibility to the client that the skin may seem to get worse before it gets better. Continued treatment, along with alternating extraction treatments on different days, will help loosen the acne impactions (Plates 40a, 40b).

Treatment for Hyperpigmented Skin

Again, the treatment method is essentially the same. The client should, as always, be pretreated at home for several weeks before starting salon treatment. The client should use home care products that include a melanin suppressant such as hydroquinone, kojic acid, magnesium ascorbyl phosphate, arbutin, asafetida extract, or a combination of these agents. There are premixed solutions available that include combinations of the above with alphahydroxy acids. The theory here is to remove already stained corneum cells while suppressing melanin production in the melanocytes. Needless to say, hyperpigmented clients should wear a daily broad-spectrum sunscreen of SPF-15 or 30, and should avoid sun exposure completely. Infrared rays, which are not blocked by sunscreen products, cause heat in the skin, resulting in melanin production (Plates 41a, 41b).

Stronger Glycolic Peeling

Stronger solutions are available for salon use, but with added strength comes added risk. Thirty-percent solutions are available for salon use, but they should be used conservatively and should never be left on the skin for more than two minutes. The amount of time glycolic acid is allowed to contact the skin is directly related to the strength and depth of the treatment. Do not experiment! Stick to manufacturer's directions at all times!

Medical AHA Treatment

Dermatologists and plastic surgeons may use glycolic acid solutions in concentrations of 50 to 70 percent. These are medical grade strengths and should never be used by estheticians unless they are working under the direct supervision of a dermatologist or plastic surgeon. High strengths are used to treat deeper wrinkles, solar lentigines, and actinic keratoses.

STRONGER PEELING TREATMENTS

The treatments we have been discussing using 20 to 30 percent alphahydroxy acid are generally very safe and helpful for cosmetic effects. This level of alphahydroxy acid is acceptable for almost all skin types and produces a good cosmetic effect with a very low amount of potential irritation. One company calls their treatment "rapid exfoliation," indicating that it is actually a "high-tech exfoliator," rather than a "chemical peel."

The stronger peels are of three types and three levels.

Surgical phenol peeling is a deep peeling procedure that should only be administered by a dermatologist or a plastic surgeon. This procedure involves applying a very strong solution of a very strong chemical called phenol. Phenol peeling must be administered in a doctor's office or surgical unit. Phenol, in large amounts, can be absorbed into the bloodstream and rarely can cause heart fluctuations. The heart is monitored during this procedure to ensure safety. The phenol peel penetrates to the aged, severely wrinkled skin, and can also be used to treat skin growths such as repeated instances of skin cancers and actinic keratoses (Plates 43a, 43b). It may produce hypopigmentation of the skin and a ruddy surface to the face (Plates 44a, 44b). For further information on phenol peeling, please read Chapter 19, Treating the Plastic Surgery Patient.

Laser resurfacing is a surgical technique of using a laser to reduce wrinkles and skin texture imperfections. This will be discussed in depth in Chapter 19.

Medium depth peels include 50 to 70 percent glycolic acid applications and 40 to 50 percent trichloracetic acid, better known to the medical community as TCA. TCA at this strength penetrates to the layer of the dermis, and again is a procedure that should only be administered by a dermatologist or a plastic surgeon. Combinations of TCA and glycolic acid are sometimes used by doctors to treat deeper wrinkles.

TCA does not have the potential for absorption into the bloodstream like high concentrations of phenol. Lighter peelings can be given with TCA at concentrations of 15 to 35 percent, but they do not have the dramatic results of the deeper phenol peels. Some doctors will use repeated treatments with these smaller concentrations of TCA. TCA in general also does not have as great a potential for scarring as phenol peeling.

Some companies sell low-percentage TCA to estheticians. It is the opinion of this author that TCA belongs in the hands of dermatologists and plastic surgeons only. TCA is too unpredictable, and is beyond the scope of esthetic exfoliation.

Superficial peeling is the deepest type of chemical peeling performed by estheticians. Superficial peelings, unlike deep and medium medical peelings, only remove cells from the stratum corneum. The most frequently used type of chemical is known as Jessner's Solution, which is a mixture of salicylic acid, resorcinol, lactic acid, and ethanol. Some superficial peeling formulas also contain a small amount of phenol, usually 2 percent, and sometimes sulfur. Although Jessner's Solution is a liquid, some cream forms of peels are similar and produce similar effects on the skin.

One of the latest exfoliation treatments available to the esthetician is 20 percent salicylic acid in a special vehicle called a Microsponge®. With proper training, this liquid exfoliation treatment is a safe and effective procedure.

These superficial chemical peels are helpful for treating small, superficial wrinkles, dark spots, and other forms of hyperpigmentation, melasma, and acne-prone skin.

The superficial peel evens the surface skin pigment, smoothes the appearance of the skin, and dries the surface of acne and problem skin. Like AHA, superficial peeling

Surgical phenol peeling is a very deep peeling procedure performed by a plastic surgeon or dermatologist. The peel affects the dermis and has considerable risks.

Medium depth peels are performed by dermatologists or plastic surgeons. These trichloracetic acid (TCA) peels affect the dermis, but not as deeply as phenol.

Superficial peeling effects the epidermis and is performed by estheticians or physicians. These peels include alpha and beta hydroxy acids, Jessner's solution, and resorcinol peeling treatments.

may also increase the amount of surface acne lesions, because it loosens impactions and causes them to move toward the surface. In other words, it may cause acne to get worse before it gets better.

Candidates for Salon Superficial Peelings

Clients who have sun-damaged skin, hyperpigmented skin, or other forms of melasma are the best candidates for superficial peeling. Technically, most adult clients can benefit from these peelings, because most adults do have some form of fine wrinkling or hyperpigmentation.

There are, of course, many other alternatives for treating these cosmetic problems. Glycolic acid, hydroquinone solutions, or a combination can be very effective for many forms of hyperpigmentation. Low-strength AHA peelings are also another alternative. Most estheticians will attempt to treat these cosmetic conditions with more conservative treatments, such as the ones listed above before resorting to superficial chemical peeling.

Make sure that your client has started on home care before administering superficial chemical peeling. This pretreatment will ensure that the client's skin is in better shape before using chemical peelings. Many estheticians insist that a client have facial treatments for a period of time before administering a chemical peel. This is not a bad idea because it allows you to learn about the client, the client's skin, and the client's needs before using peelings.

Many clients will call the salon specifically asking about chemical peels. Information given out over the phone should be minimal, because you have not seen the client's skin. Ask the client to make an appointment for a consultation before you issue an opinion about her skin. Many clients have cosmetic problems that can be treated by other simpler methods than chemical peels. Some clients are not using proper home care. Good home care and salon care may make the difference they need and establish a good, healthy program for their skin for a lifetime. Chemical peeling should not be looked at as a "band-aid" or a "magic bullet" for skin problems. The client needs to continually take care of the skin at home on a regular basis.

Other forms of lighter peelings such as enzyme or AHA may be sufficient for treating the client's problem.

Chemical peeling is probably the most drastic and dramatic treatment administered by an esthetician. There are some disadvantages to superficial peeling. These include discomfort, temporary discolorations, a small risk of allergic reaction, a bad appearance to the skin during the actual procedure, and a possibility of hyperpigmentation. All of these disadvantages should be explained to the client long before the procedure is administered. When the client agrees to have the superficial chemical peel, the client should be required to sign a release saying that the client has been informed of all the possible side effects and discomfort that may be associated with chemical peeling. Clients should also be shown pictures of what clients look like during the peel so that they know how they might look.

These few paragraphs are not meant to discourage the use of chemical peelings. They are meant to clarify that clients do not always fully understand chemical peeling or for what conditions it is intended. Clients who are not familiar with good skin care and do not use a regular skin-care program will generally not have as good or as long-lasting results as clients who have regular salon treatments and are good about home care.

You should also get to know a client's personality. Chemical peeling is uncomfortable, and during the procedure the skin looks terrible. A client who is nervous or who becomes hysterical easily should not have chemical peelings. You will save yourself a world of trouble by getting to know your client well before performing chemical peeling.

Other clients who should not have chemical peeling are:

1. Clients who are pregnant or are lactating.
2. Clients who have a history of heart problems.
3. Clients who have a history of medical problems. These clients should have written permission from their physician. Examples of these conditions include, but are not limited to, eczema, lupus, seborrhea, rosacea, psoriasis, bacterial skin infections, mental disorders, extremely sensitive or hyperallergic skin, and other systemic problems. Take a thorough health history, and refer the client to a medical doctor if you have any questions.
4. Clients who have a history of fever blisters or herpes simplex, which can be stimulated by chemical peeling. Clients should discuss this with a physician.
5. Clients using Accutane® or other dermatological drugs.
6. Clients using retinoic acid (Retin-A), which should be discontinued about three months before superficial peeling is administered.
7. Clients who have extremely thin telangiectatic or couperose skin.

THE PRE-PEEL CONSULTATION

At least a week before the peeling is scheduled, you should have a consultation appointment with the client. Explain to the client what normally happens, step-by-step. Make sure the client understands the discomfort and how the client will look during the procedure. Explain that the client should not have any sun exposure for eight weeks after peeling and must use a broad-spectrum sunscreen at all times. Clients who are being treated for hyperpigmentation should always be especially careful about sun exposure.

Show the client pictures of what a normal peel looks like during the process. Take pictures of the client's skin before and after the procedure. This will allow you to show the client the improvement in the skin's appearance.

Have the client sign a release saying that the client has been fully informed about the possible disadvantages of peeling and the actual procedure that takes place. It is very important to be honest with the client.

Superficial peeling will not:

• Remove deep wrinkles.
• Remove scarring or acne pocks.

- Repair severe sun damage to any appreciable degree.
- Cause a lifting effect on the skin.

    Superficial peeling will:

- Improve the skin's texture.
- Even the coloring.
- Help lighten hyperpigmentation.
- Improve fine lines and rough textures.

THE SUPERFICIAL PEELING PROCEDURE

Several different procedures are used for superficial salon chemical peeling, which will vary according to the manufacturer. The following are two examples of typical procedures for liquid and cream peelings. These are meant to serve only as examples. *Always follow the manufacturer's direction for the preparation that you are using.*

Liquid Peeling

The liquid type of peeling solution is normally Jessner's Solution. Another is a 20 percent solution of salicylic acid. Again, you should follow any specific directions furnished by the manufacturer. You should also have complete hands-on training on the treatment before attempting the procedure in the salon! The solution is applied with cotton swabs to the face. The following procedure is typical:

1. Complete all the pre-peel consultation procedures discussed.
2. Remove the client's makeup thoroughly with a cleansing milk.
3. Apply a "prep" lotion furnished by the manufacturer. This solution is usually acetone, which removes excess oils and surface dead cells.
4. Turn on a small fan and place it so it blows gently on the client's face. Do not turn the fan to high speed, because this may blow the liquid. Some companies do not recommend using a fan at all for this reason. Some fans are small enough for clients to hold them in their hands.
5. Put on a pair of latex gloves. Paint the liquid solution onto the face using two cotton swabs held closely together. Begin with the forehead and apply the solution in small, gentle, circular motions. Do not apply pressure with the swabs. Proceed from the forehead down the cheek and around the face. It is very important that the application be as even as possible. Do not apply the solution to the lips, ears, or upper lids. Lower lids may be treated, but it is strongly suggested to stay within ⅛-inch of the lower lid edge. Again, this depends on the manufacturer's recommendations. The client should keep the eyes shut during the procedure.
6. Allow this coat to "dry" for two minutes. If you notice any white areas forming on the face, this is known as **frosting**. Frosting occurs when the peel is complete. Some clients will frost after one coat, and some after two or three coats of solution. If frosting does not occur after the first coat, repeat the application procedure, and wait for

Frosting describes a white appearance of the skin that appears after applying a strong exfoliation or peeling substance.

another four minutes. Occasionally, areas of the face will frost when other areas will not. If this happens, reapply the solution to the unfrosted areas only.

7. Apply the solution at 4-minute intervals until frosting occurs. Most clients will only require one to three coats.

The solution remains on the face, and the client should stay in the salon for about an hour.

A strong burning sensation will be felt when application starts. The intensity of the burning sensation will vary with the client. This is the reason for the fan, which helps cool the sensation. After about 15 minutes, this burning sensation will stop, and the skin feels numb and slightly tingly (Plate 45, Plates 46a-f).

The Cream Peel

The preparation procedure is the same as for the liquid peel. No prep solution is used with the cream peel.

1. With gloved hands apply the cream peel to the forehead, cheeks, nose, chin, neck, and finish with a very light application to the lower lids using a cotton swab. Apply evenly. The face will begin to burn and sting. Again, this sensation can be lessened by the use of a fan and usually subsides after 15 to 20 minutes.

2. You do not have to watch for frosting with this treatment. It will happen automatically. There is no need for a second application until the next day. This thick treatment stays on the face for 1½ hours. After this time the cream is gently removed with a tongue depressor and then cleansed well with cool, wet, cotton compresses.

3. After removing the treatment, apply the thick moisturizing cream furnished in the peeling kit. The client will continue to apply this emollient cream to the face at home. The skin should be well lubricated with the emollient at all times.

4. On the second day, the same procedure is repeated in the salon with this cream peel. The client continues to keep the skin moist with the emollient cream.

Although these procedures sound fairly simple, you must be thoroughly trained and experienced to perform them correctly. You must have hands-on training to perform chemical peeling. Do not think you are qualified simply from reading this chapter or a manufacturer's handbook. You should observe several peeling procedures before attempting to perform peeling!

AFTER THE TREATMENT

Immediately after treatment the skin often looks slightly red and flushed. There is often little change in the first day. On the second day of either peel, the skin will become tan-looking, sometimes splotchy.

On the third day the skin becomes very dark and often splotchy and will feel very tight and dry. Peeling will begin around the mouth and chin first, then the cheeks, then the eyes. The neck and forehead are the last to peel. The skill will peel usually from the third through the sixth or seventh day. Occasionally, the peeling will continue for several more days. The client should be warned not to pull on the loose skin. This can cause infection and possible hyperpigmentation. It is best for the client to visit the salon daily for a quick check, and the esthetician can gently peel off areas that are ready.

Clients should not wash the face at all during the peeling procedure. They may use moisturizer, depending on the manufacturer's instructions. Cool water may be applied, but not cleanser.

Granular scrubs and other keratolyic preparations should be discontinued for at least the first two weeks after peeling. These include glycolic acid, benzoyl peroxide, sulfur, resorcinol, Retin-A, salicylic acid, lactic acid, or any other peeling or exfoliating agent.

The skin should be completely protected with a daily sunscreen for at least eight weeks after peeling. Direct sun exposure must be avoided.

REACTIONS TO PEELING

Rarely, a client will have an allergic reaction to a chemical peeling. The symptoms may include severe itching, swelling, severe redness, and stinging. Refer this client to a dermatologist who is familiar with your services, particularly your peeling procedures. Normally, a steroid cream is prescribed, which quickly alleviates the problem.

Dark skin types sometimes have a tendency to hyperpigment after a peel. Many estheticians will not administer chemical peeling to darker or black skins. If the client pulls off skin that is not ready, splotchy hyperpigmentation can occur. Normally this fades within a few weeks, as long as the skin is protected with a sunscreen. Sometimes you may need to treat the skin with a mild bleaching cream, if the hyperpigmentation does not decrease within two or three weeks after peeling.

Your proficiency in chemical peeling will increase as you perform more and more peelings. This is why it so important that you thoroughly train with someone accomplished in the practice of superficial peeling and observe the actual peeling that takes place during the six or seven days after the procedure is performed. With this training you can become proficient at superficial chemical peeling.

Topics for Discussion

1. Discuss the difference between mechanical and chemical peeling.
2. What is the difference between "peeling" and "exfoliating"?
3. What are some skin conditions that can benefit from enzyme peeling?
4. What are the differences between deep, medium, and superficial peels?
5. Discuss the consultation procedures for superficial chemical peeling.
6. What conditions will not be improved with salon superficial peeling?
7. Discuss the procedures and possible problems associated with salon chemical peeling. Why is it so important to receive hands-on training?

Chapter 19

Treating the Plastic Surgery Patient

Objectives

More and more frequently, clients are having plastic surgery performed. In this chapter we will discuss the many types of plastic surgery procedures used, and common problems of the plastic surgery patient. We will also discuss treatments for preparing the patient for plastic surgery, counseling the plastic surgery patient for referral, and how to treat cosmetic side effects of plastic surgery.

Management of postoperative skin-care and makeup needs by a licensed esthetician (skin-care specialist) can be beneficial to both the surgeon and the patient. An esthetician who is well-trained and experienced in clinical pre- and postoperative care can help the postoperative patient by providing services in proper skin care, moisturization, control and mitigation of erythema and milia, camouflage makeup instruction for coverage of bruising, post-laser erythema, and contouring techniques for diminishing the look of swelling, not to mention providing health education and emotional support. The esthetician can be the patient's "lifeline," managing problems that may not be pathological, but are of great concern to the patient.

CONCERNS OF THE PATIENT

Patients are frequently referred to the esthetician and arrive at the esthetician's clinic or salon very concerned about their immediate appearance. Rarely are these problems pathological, but are usually purely cosmetic and self-limiting. However, they are of immediate concern to the patient who needs cosmetic help, relief of discomfort, and reassurance to make it through the postoperative period.

Psychological Needs

The esthetician can play a significant role as a health educator and psychological support for the patient. An ear that understands the immediate concerns of the patient is sincerely appreciated by the patient. The esthetician should be well-versed and experienced in postoperative procedures in order to answer basic questions regarding cosmetic prognosis.

Proper Esthetician Training

It is vitally important that the esthetician be adequately trained to assist in managing postoperative cosmetic surgery patients. This means that the esthetician should have hands-on experience with actual patients under the supervision of a cosmetic surgeon, dermatologist, or a very experienced postoperative trained esthetician. Estheticians should take all the classes and seminars they can on postoperative procedures and post-laser esthetic treatment.

PLASTIC SURGERY

Years ago plastic surgery was considered by many to be a sign of vanity and reserved only for the rich and famous. Now plastic surgery is performed daily in every major American city. It is no longer considered unacceptable for people to want to look better. There are two basic types of plastic surgery—*cosmetic* surgery and *reconstructive* surgery.

Cosmetic surgery generally refers to surgical procedures used for cosmetic purposes only.

Cosmetic surgery generally refers to surgical procedures used for cosmetic purposes only. These procedures include eyelid, face, and forehead lifts, dermabrasion, chemical peelings, liposuction, laser resurfacing, collagen injections, and other procedures. Body cosmetic surgery includes body sculpting contour surgery, body liposuction, tummy tucks, and breast augmentation or reduction.

Reconstructive surgery generally refers to surgical procedure techniques used to correct noncosmetic abnormalities such as skin cancer removal, surgery needed due to accidental injury, and other physical deformities.

Reconstructive surgery generally refers to surgical techniques used to correct noncosmetic abnormalities such as skin cancer removal, surgery needed due to accidental injury, and other physical deformities. These surgical procedures are often medically necessary, and in some cases, such as melanoma, can be treatment for serious, life-threatening diseases.

For the purposes of this discussion, we will primarily discuss facial cosmetic surgery, although we will briefly discuss reconstructive surgery.

TYPES OF SURGEONS

Several different types of physicians perform plastic, reconstructive, and cosmetic surgery. All of these doctors receive four years of medical school training, followed by an internship and residency that takes four or more years to complete. These various specialists are then board certified by their particular specialty associations.

General plastic surgeons perform all types of plastic, reconstructive and cosmetic surgery. They often also perform hand surgery. They perform surgery on all areas of the face and body. They are board certified by the American Board of Plastic Surgery, which is associated with the American Society of Plastic and Reconstructive Surgeons (ASPRS). These doctors generally limit their practices to plastic surgery.

Facial plastic surgeons specialize in plastic surgery of the face, head, and neck. They generally do not perform body surgery. They are usually trained in otolaryngology, the specialty area of medicine that treats diseases of the ears, nose, and throat, and surgery of the head and neck. Their professional association is called the American Academy of Facial Plastic and Reconstructive Surgeons. They may perform facial cosmetic or reconstructive surgery, but may also perform surgery on the sinuses, ears, nose, and throat.

Ophthalmic surgeons are medical doctors who treat eye diseases and perform eye surgery. They perform eyelid surgery, or reconstructive surgery involving the eyes.

Dermatological surgeons are dermatologists who also perform plastic or cosmetic surgery.

You should always work with surgeons who are board certified in their specialty areas.

> **General plastic surgeons** perform all types of plastic, reconstructive, and cosmetic surgery.

> **Facial plastic surgeons** specialize in plastic surgery of the face, head, and neck.

> **Ophthalmic surgeons** are medical doctors who treat eye diseases and perform eye surgery.

> **Dermatological surgeons** are dermatologists who also perform plastic or cosmetic surgery.

COMMON TYPES OF COSMETIC SURGERY

We will first discuss the various types of facial cosmetic surgery procedures. We will break these procedures into several subjects: symptoms of need for plastic surgery, discussion of the actual surgical procedure, suggestions for pre- and post-care treatment (salon treatment and home care recommendations for before and after surgery), makeup needs of the postoperative patient, and long-term needs of the patient.

*Warning: Do **not** perform services on any postoperative patient until the patient has been released and approved for esthetic treatment by the attending cosmetic surgeon or dermatologist! Treating a patient before or without the surgeon's approval, or without proper training is dangerous and a tremendous legal risk.*

Rhytidectomy

Rhytidectomy is the medical term for a face-lift.

> **Rhytidectomy** is the medical term for a face-lift.

Presurgical Facial Characteristics
These characteristics include sagging skin with marked lack of elasticity, folds of skin in the jawline and neck area, jowls in the cheek and jawline area, and general lack of skin tone.

Surgical Procedure

Incisions are made in front of, or inside, the ears, following around the back of the ears, and into the hairline in the back of the head. After the incision is made, the face is literally "pulled up," and excess skin is clipped away. In some cases, the underlying muscle structure may also be surgically altered, or excess fat may be removed. In some cases a small incision may have to be made under the chin. After the excess skin is removed, the skin is reconnected in the areas of the incisions and sewn together with materials called **sutures** (often called "stitches" by laypeople). In some cases surgical staples are used instead of suture material (Plates 47a–d).

After surgery the face is very swollen and bruised. The head is wrapped in gauze dressing to provide support for the surgical area. The patient is instructed to keep the head elevated for several days, even when sleeping, to provide gravity for draining fluids. Skin discolorations, mainly due to bruising, are typical after surgery and may last for weeks. Some patients notice numbness in certain areas, particularly in front of the ears.

The sutures and dressings are removed a few days after surgery by the plastic surgeon. Most patients are pleasantly surprised by how little pain is associated with rhytidectomy, but any pain can be managed with medication. The skin may feel very tight at first, but generally feels better after a few weeks when the facial swelling has subsided.

Pretreatment for the Lift Patient

The same pretreatment procedures are followed for blepharoplasty, rhytidectomy, and forehead lift. Ideally, treatment should begin at least three months before surgery. Treatments should be administered weekly or biweekly for a minimum of six treatments. The purpose of these treatments is to thoroughly cleanse the skin, to improve circulation through massage and electrical treatment, and to have the skin in the best condition before surgery. Skin that is in prime condition before surgery will most often look better after surgery, and the good condition will aid healing.

Before starting the treatment program, you should talk to the client extensively about plans for the surgery, including the dates of the surgery. Plan your treatment schedule around the date of the actual surgery. You should explain all the benefits of skin treatment in general, as well as how important it is for the patient to take perfect care of the skin before and after the surgery, as well as emphasizing the need for ongoing care after the surgery is completed. You should give the client realistic expectations of what you will accomplish, and the differences between what the surgeon and the esthetician will do to improve the appearance of the skin and face.

1. To begin treatment, thoroughly cleanse the face.
2. Thoroughly examine the face under a magnifying lamp, making notes of all problems, especially conditions that will not be improved by plastic surgery, such as comedones, milia, fine wrinkles, hyperpigmentation, rough, dehydrated areas, etc. Type the skin and write up a detailed analysis as you would for any new client.

Sutures are materials used in reconnecting areas of surgical incisions.

Regardless of the surgery, you should treat the skin as you always would for the analyzed condition. Design treatment based on the examination. Client home care will also be directly related to the analysis, as always.

3. Begin the procedure by using the steamer on the skin for eight to ten minutes. During the steam you may apply an exfoliating treatment if necessary. Scrub creams are frequently helpful, provided the skin is suitable for scrubs. Brushing may be used over a layer of hydrating fluid. Using hydrating fluid during steam can greatly help to soften a rough-textured surface. If the skin is oily, apply a desincrustant pre-mask to the skin to help soften comedones and sebaceous filaments. Enzyme exfoliation may also be helpful to this type of skin.

4. After steaming, proceed with galvanic desincrustation (assuming there are no contraindications) to all areas with comedones, sebaceous filaments, or other impactions. Oil-dry (alipidic), poreless areas of the skin should not be treated with galvanic desincrustation.

5. Begin extraction of any impacted areas. Be thorough, but do not perform more than ten minutes of extraction in one visit.

6. After extraction, apply a toner with an antiseptic.

7. Apply a lightweight, noncomedogenic hydrating fluid to the face and begin a thorough massage appropriate for the skin type. Oily skin should not be excessively massaged, nor should areas that are still clogged. A good facial massage will be excellent for improving the circulation before surgery.

8. Apply more hydrating fluid and apply high frequency to the skin with the mushroom electrode for two to three minutes.

9. Apply a mask appropriate for the skin type. You may need to use more than one mask, such as a cleansing clay mask for the oily areas and a soft-setting gel or cream mask for dry areas. After the setting time has passed, remove the mask and apply a moisturizer with sunscreen.

Home Pre-care

The main difference between this home care procedure and that of a regular client is that the client must be very diligent about performing home care daily. Not enough emphasis can be placed on good routine home care. You should mention that home care may need to be altered after surgery depending on the case and the surgeon's wishes.

Bruising and Vitamin K

Vitamin K is a fat-soluble vitamin necessary for proper clotting of the blood. Topical vitamin K creams are now available. These are used to treat bruising of all types on all body areas, telangiectasias and distended capillaries, and are also used as a presurgical treatment to help prevent and reduce bruising from plastic surgery. These creams are available to the esthetician to sell and recommend to their clients.

For two weeks before facial surgery, the vitamin K cream should be applied daily or twice daily to all areas that will be affected by bruising during surgery. This includes surrounding areas as well as areas where incisions will be made. After surgery and with the surgeon's approval, vitamin K can continue to be used in areas of bruising, but should not be used on incisions until they are completely healed and approved for use by the surgeon.

Postsurgical Skin Care

Immediate post-care for the patient will be handled by the surgeon. The client should check with the surgeon to see when regular home care can resume.

After the client has been given the approval by the surgeon to continue home care, the client should be instructed to be extremely gentle with the skin, being careful not pull on the skin or apply significant pressure to the suture areas. Light massage at home, always using a hydrating fluid, will help dissipate bruising. Instruct your client how to perform light effleurage and tapotement (piano massage) to the face nightly.

Post-care Salon Treatment

Never begin treatment of a postsurgical client without the approval of a plastic surgeon. After you have established a good working relationship with a plastic surgeon, you should sit down and discuss both of your expectations for post-care of the patients he or she sends you. The plastic surgeon may establish a general set of rules for administering postsurgical treatment to patients. You will both be fully informed of each others' procedures and precautions. The patient should not have treatment while sutures are still in the skin, unless otherwise directed by the surgeon. Be extremely gentle with all facial procedures. The client may still be sensitive from the surgery, and you do not want to pull on the suture areas or apply firm pressure, especially immediately after surgery. Generally, salon treatment can resume about two to three weeks after surgery.

The main objectives of post-care are to help improve the circulation, reduce swelling, and help dissipate any discolorations from bruising. Long-term goals of postsurgical treatment are to improve the texture and appearance of the surface of the skin, putting the "icing on the cake" by routinely providing care to improve the surface appearance.

Assuming the patient has approval from the surgeon, the following is a typical postsurgical treatment:

1. Apply liquid cleanser to the face with gloved hands, using very gentle application movements. Use very soft facial cloths, sponges, or cotton pads to remove the cleanser, being careful not to pull on the skin too much.
2. Apply a light hydrating fluid to the skin and allow it to be steamed for about eight minutes. Cool steam is a good choice if the client has redness present.
3. Remove the hydrating fluid and examine the skin under a magnifying lamp. Check for bruised areas and look carefully at the suture areas. In general, suture areas should be avoided during treatment.
4. If there is a lot of surface flaking, apply a diluted nondrying exfoliator, such as honey and almond scrub, and gently massage, removing the scrub with the same careful technique. Avoid using brushing or suction immediately after surgery. Wait about three months before using these techniques after rhytidectomy.

5. Any extraction should be very minimal. In general, unless there are large open comedones, extraction should be avoided at this particular time.

6. Apply a lightweight hydrating fluid and begin a thorough but gentle massage, using light effluerage and tapotement. Avoid petrissage, rolling, friction, or any rough type of massage. Plenty of hydrating fluid should be used to keep the skin slippery during the massage, which helps to avoid excessive pulling. Concentrate on the eyes and neck, using gentle, circular effleurage movements.

7. Apply more hydrating fluid and apply high frequency with the mushroom electrode set at a very low intensity. Move around the face in small, gentle, circular movements for about three to four minutes.

8. Apply a nonsetting, nonstimulating mask, or apply a thick coat of hydrating fluid. It is very important that whatever you put on the face be easy to remove. Setting masks and thicker creams may be more difficult to remove, causing you to pull on the face more than normal.

9. After the mask has processed for ten minutes, wet it well using a spray of cool toner to help loosen it for removal. Remove the mask gently using soft facial cloths, sponges, or cotton pads. Apply a moisturizer-protectant appropriate for the skin type with sunscreen.

10. Although it is best to avoid makeup immediately after treatment, this may be impossible for the plastic surgery patient. Be understanding and help her with makeup after treatment. Do not start any "new" treatments on the client immediately after surgery. There is a rare possibility of allergic reaction, particularly with new products that the client has not tried. Do not recommend new products for home use at this point. Wait until the healing process is further along to start any new procedures.

Makeup Needs

The postsurgical rhytidectomy patient will likely experience extensive bruising. Many patients who undergo extensive presurgical skin care at home and in the salon seem to have less bruising, and any bruising seems to dissipate faster.

Bruises are the main problem immediately after surgery. As soon as the surgeon approves, the esthetician may help the client with camouflage makeup for the bruising. You should make available to the client a heavy coverage camouflage makeup to help conceal the bruises. The bruising usually occurs under the eyes, on the lids, in a half-moon pattern on the upper cheeks, in front of the ears, and sometimes along the jawline and neck.

Prepare the skin in the normal manner. Yellow toner may help conceal purple bruises. You may wish to apply a layer of amber or yellow toner before applying the coverage.

Apply the coverage makeup with dabbing movements using a latex makeup sponge. Blend in the edges with the client's normal foundation. As the patient heals, bruises will start to change color as the blood is absorbed by the body. Bruising also tends to shift with gravity; that is, bruises that start on the jawline may slowly seem to move down the neck and decollete, and occasionally onto the chest. During this time there may be variation in color, ranging from normal black-purple bruising to yellow or green. Apply the proper color toner to help neutralize the colors.

After the bruising has totally subsided and the suture lines have healed completely, have a second makeup lesson with the client and teach her to cover the incision scars. Work with her hairstylist to establish a good hairstyle that will help conceal the scars from the incisions. This is particularly necessary in front of the ears. Occasionally, a plastic surgery patient will experience a small amount of hair loss in the surgical area, and sometimes hair areas from above the ears end up in back of the ears. Again, the skills of a good hairstylist are very important.

Within a few months of surgery, after all swelling has subsided, the client should have a new makeup lesson, teaching her how to best complement her new look, emphasizing the new contours that the surgeon has created.

Long-Term Needs

The main long-term need is great skin care! Clients will often be interested in new products and treatments to improve the look created by the surgery. Most patients are very interested in protecting their "investment" by taking good care of their skin.

Blepharoplasty

Blepharoplasty is the surgical procedure for "lifting" the eyes and removing excess skin from the eye area.

Blepharoplasty is the surgical procedure for "lifting" the eyes and removing excess skin from the eye area.

Presurgical Facial Characteristics

These characteristics include puffiness, bags under the eyes, and drooping or flapping upper lids. Sometimes the drooping of the upper lids is so dramatic that it actually interferes with the patient's vision.

Surgical Procedure

The patient is anesthetized or sedated. Incisions are made in the normal fold of the upper lid, and excess skin is trimmed away. The suture line is made in the actual fold of the lid, rendering it practically invisible when it heals.

Lower lids are corrected by making an incision in the lower lash line. The fat pocket in a "bag" is removed, and, again, the excess skin is trimmed away and sutured along the lower lash line. Newer procedures now often allow the lower lid to be corrected from the inside of the lid, completely eliminating outside incisions.

The brows are lifted by making an incision in the lower part of the browline. Excess skin and fat is removed from this area as well. More and more patients are having a **forehead lift** at the same time as their eyes are corrected. Much of the sagging of the upper lid may be attributed to elastosis in the forehead. In a forehead lift, an incision is made about an inch back into the hairline. The excess skin is removed from the hairline incision, simultaneously lifting the brow area. This procedure is becoming more and more popular. Forehead lifts may be a problem in persons with extremely high fore-

Forehead lift is a surgical procedure that helps to correct elastosis of the forehead and lift the brows.

heads or in men who have receding hairlines or male pattern baldness, because the scars will not be concealable (Plates 48a–d).

Pretreatment
The same basic procedure is followed as is already outlined in the pretreatment section for rhytidectomy.

Home Pre-care
Use the same procedures as for rhytidectomy patients.

Postsurgical Skin Care
Follow the same post-treatment recommendations for post-rhytidectomy patients. Mild massage of the lids, after they have healed and with the surgeon's approval, may help to dissipate discoloration from bruising and swelling. Makeup needs will be the same.

A patient may occasionally choose to have only a forehead and eye lift, without a general face lift. Although this is sometimes appropriate, particularly in young individuals who only have eyelid drooping and puffiness, in most cases, general face lifting is also necessary. Most plastic surgeons will encourage these clients to proceed with face lifting at the same time as the corrective procedure for the eyes.

Rhinoplasty

Rhinoplasty is the term for surgically altering the nose. Commonly called a "nose job," many clients of many different ages request this procedure. In an older individual, a rhinoplasty may make the entire face look younger, particularly if the nose is "drooping."

Presurgical Facial Characteristics
This will vary in the rhinoplasty procedure. The nose may be crooked, too long, too short, upturned, or drooping. In many cases rhinoplasty is medically necessary to correct internal blockages of the breathing passages caused by chronic sinus problems or a deviated septum (Plates 49a–d).

Surgical Procedure
An incision is made inside the nostrils. The bones of the nose are reshaped using special surgical tools. The nose is then "redraped" over the new bone structure. Occasionally, excess skin and cartilage is removed, and any internal problem affecting breathing is corrected. After surgery a splint is placed on the nose, which is removed after a few days. The nose will be quite swollen immediately after the surgery. Swelling may last for weeks after surgery, and results cannot be assessed until the swelling has completely subsided.

Pretreatment
In the salon, the follicles of the nose should be cleaned routinely before surgery. It is advisable for the client to have about six weekly or biweekly treatments, concentrating

on deep cleansing as well as general skin care. The same procedure should be followed as for rhytidectomy, outlined earlier in this chapter. If the general skin of the face is in excellent shape, the skin in general will be in better condition for healing.

Home Pre-care

Again, the procedure is the same used for rhytidectomy patients. You may recommend that the client apply a deep cleansing mask to the nose, especially clients with extremely oily skin, with many clogged follicles on the nose.

Postsurgical Skin Care

You must be extremely careful with treatment of the nose for several months after surgery. Remember, the bones have been reshaped, and no pressure should be applied. This is particularly important regarding extraction. Essentially, no extraction on the nose or on surrounding tissue should take place for several months after surgery.

In lieu of extraction, you may use enzyme treatment on the nose to help remove excess cell buildup. Comedones on the nose may be increased after surgery due to trauma, surgical dressings, and because cleaning the nose may be uncomfortable for the client. Use of enzyme peelings or desincrustant pre-masks on the nose will help to soften pore accumulations.

If this is followed by clay-based deep cleansing masks, improvement may be obtained without extraction on the nose area. The tissue around the nose and upper cheeks should be treated in the same manner. Use "wet" treatments—do not apply treatments that need to be rubbed or lifted off. Stick to fluid type treatments that can be easily removed. Clay-based masks should be thoroughly moistened before removal. After the clay mask dries, spray it with a cold spray of diluted toner to loosen and wet it before removal.

You may notice that the client is uncomfortable, even during massage and basic cleansing. Be very gentle when cleansing the nose area, and avoid any movements that pull upward on the nose.

Avoid the use of brushing or suction on the nose area. Galvanic desincrustation can be beneficial, but be careful with the amount of pressure used.

Makeup Needs

Because of swelling, clients may need help with contouring makeup to minimize the appearance of swelling, particularly during the first few weeks after surgery. Bruising of the eyes and cheeks may occur. Use the same procedures outlined earlier in this chapter to help the client cover these areas.

Long-Term Needs

After several months have passed, you may proceed with extraction, being very careful and gentle. The client may need frequent treatments to help with clogged pores, especially while extraction is being avoided.

Dermabrasion

Dermabrasion is the technique of reducing acne scarring, scar tissue and, in some cases, wrinkles.

Dermabrasion is the technique of reducing acne scarring, scar tissue, and in some cases, wrinkles.

Presurgical Facial Characteristics

These characteristics are acne scarring, "icepick" scarring, "pock" marks from acne, hypertrophic (raised) scarring, and wrinkles in limited areas, such as around the mouth.

Surgical Procedure

The patient is anesthetized or sedated. The surgeon uses a rotating attachment, similar to an esthetician's electric brush, except the attachment is an abrasive steel instrument. The skin is literally "sanded," and the tissue is "planed" to a low level, helping to smooth out imperfections.

Generally, only areas that are affected by the scarring are treated. Although the treatment sounds painful, most patients are surprised at how little pain is involved (Plate 50).

Pretreatment

This procedure probably requires the most intensive pre- and postoperative salon treatment. Many dermabrasion patients are present or former acne sufferers, who often still have very oily, problem skin. If the acne has been or is cystic, the client should be seen by a dermatologist for treatment. It is vitally important to be sure that acne is not recurring before performing surgery. If the surgery is performed while cysts are still developing, the patient may risk more scarring after surgery.

Assuming the client has finished any dermatological treatment, treat the client as you would any acne or oily skinned client, using deep cleansing treatments routinely in the salon before the surgery. Frequent treatment, weekly or biweekly, before surgery is usually necessary. Follow the treatment program outlined in Chapter 12, Acne and the Esthetician. The ultimate goal is to have the skin completely clear, oiliness under control, and as clean as possible before surgery.

Home Pre-care

Again, follow the procedures outlined in Chapters 12 and 13. The client should use completely noncomedogenic products at home. Keratolytics such as salicylic acid, resorcinol, sulfur, glycolic acid, and benzoyl peroxide are useful before surgery. Because of the nature of the dermabrasion procedure, keratolytics must be discontinued after the surgery, until otherwise prescribed by the plastic surgeon or dermatologist.

Postsurgical Skin Care

During the dermabrasion procedure, the skin is traumatized, and this often results in multiple milia development. Sometimes dozens and dozens of milia appear after a dermabrasion. After the surgeon has approved your treatment of the skin, you may begin treatment of the milia. There is also a lot of redness usually present. Normally, treatment in the salon may resume three to four weeks after surgery. The following is a suggested treatment for post-dermabrasion clients with multiple milia:

1. Cleanse the face thoroughly with cleansing milk.
2. Steam the face with lukewarm steam over a layer of desincrustant pre-mask or solution. Do not use brushing, enzymes, or suction on the skin at this time.
3. Using a sterile lancet, begin extraction of the milia, which are usually very soft and easily removed. Do not perform this procedure unless you have been thoroughly trained in extraction of milia! Only extract for a few minutes, and discontinue immediately if redness seems to worsen. The skin is still erythemic from the surgery. You must be very careful not to traumatize the skin.
4. After extraction, spray the skin with an antiseptic toner solution.
5. Apply cold compresses to the extracted area. Allow to sit for 15 to 20 minutes.
6. Do not apply tightening or abrasive masks to freshly dermabraded skin. The skin has already been exfoliated through the surgical procedure.
7. After compresses have set on the face for 15 to 20 minutes, remove them and apply a noncomedogenic moisturizer-protectant sunscreen.

Treatment for the milia may take several weeks. The client should visit for treatment either weekly or biweekly.

Postsurgical Home Care

Advise the client to use a rinseable cleanser, a mild toner, a protectant sunscreen, and a night hydrating fluid. Remember, you are still dealing with oily skin, but this oily skin has been severely exfoliated! Avoid the use of any keratolytic or peeling agents for at least the first eight or ten weeks, depending on the surgeon's recommendations. All home care should still be completely noncomedogenic, as it should be for any oily skin. You should explain the differences in home care to the client before the surgical procedure so that the client can anticipate and understand the need for the change of products.

Makeup Needs

The client will need help in concealing the redness caused by surgery. Using a green-colored toner and beige-based makeup is helpful in concealing the redness in the areas treated. The client's normal makeup can be blended into the outer nontreated areas. Remember to keep all makeup products noncomedogenic!

Long-Term Needs

After the initial post-treatment is completed, the milia have subsided, and the redness has diminished, the client generally has much smoother skin. The client should have a makeup lesson to learn to best complement the change in skin texture. The skin normally still has oily tendencies, and treatment should be adapted to the current conditions of the skin four to six months after surgery. At this time it may be appropriate to return to the keratolytic treatments previously used.

Chemical Peeling

We have already discussed surgical chemical peeling in Chapter 18. Here we will discuss only phenol-type peeling treatments administered by plastic surgeons or dermatologists.

Presurgical Facial Characteristics

These characteristics include multiple deep wrinkles and superficial lines in the areas to be treated. Treatment may be isolated to one or two areas, such as around the mouth. Many clients will often seek information about chemical peeling for acne scarring, but dermabrasion is the most commonly used procedure for acne scarring. Chemical peeling can also be used for medicinal purposes to treat recurring skin cancers and pre-cancers.

Surgical Procedure

After sedating the patient, the plastic surgeon paints the affected areas of the face with a phenol solution. The patient is closely monitored. The face may or may not be taped with adhesive-like tape strips. The tape, if used, is removed within a few days of the procedure. The skin looks very red and scabbed at this point. Patient discomfort is common and is controlled by prescribed medication. The doctor will often recommend a special ointment to keep the skin lubricated at this point.

Pretreatment

Salon pretreatment should begin about twelve weeks before the treatment. Treatment every two weeks is typical. Several layers of skin are actually "burned off" during phenol peeling. The main reason for treatment is to have the skin in the best shape possible before surgery. Postoperative care, and particularly makeup, is often more important in the phenol peeling patient.

Home Pre-care

Designed for the sun-damaged, but sensitive skin.

Postsurgical Skin Care

Extensive redness is typical for several weeks after chemical phenol peeling. Treatment should not begin in the salon until approved by the surgeon, usually about three weeks after surgery. All keratolytic and exfoliating treatments should be completely avoided, unless otherwise recommended by the surgeon.

Use an extremely gentle, soothing treatment. Avoid the use of any scrubs, peels, or stimulating treatment. Cool aloe compresses are often used as a mask. The primary purpose of esthetic treatment for postoperative peel patients is to help with redness. Effleurage and very light tapotement are the only massage movements that should be used. Masks should be gels or liquid hydrating treatments that do not tighten and can be easily removed. Milia may form during healing, similarly to dermabrasion but usually not as severe. Patients who have received chemical peeling often need more emotional support than other plastic surgery patients. The skin may be red for weeks after surgery, and hypopigmentation is sometimes a side effect. The skin may appear grainy, and pores may appear larger than before surgery. The client will need esthetic help to minimize these problems with proper skin care or makeup.

See the upcoming section on treatment for post-laser patients for step-by-step treatment instructions.

Post-Home Care

The client, with the surgeon's approval, should use very mild cleansers, usually milks or liquid rinseable cleansers followed by a mild, nonalcoholic toner. Sunscreen must be used. Skin often no longer tans after a chemical peel, making routine use of sunscreen a must. Hydrating products that are fragrance-free are the best bet.

Creams with soothing ingredients such as dipotassium glycyrrhizinate, green tea extract, or bisabolol help minimize redness. The client, again, should avoid scrubs or any sort of peeling or exfoliating products!

Home care for post-chemical peel patients is similar to that for post-laser patients. See the upcoming section on post-laser home care for more information.

Makeup Needs

Plastic surgeons frequently refer chemical peel patients for makeup lessons to help conceal the redness after a chemical peel and to help the patient conceal any lines of demarcation that may be present as a result of the peel treatment. Application of a green-colored toner after proper skin preparation will help neutralize redness. Then apply a liquid foundation, carefully matching the patient's neck color. In some cases cream makeup may provide better coverage, but liquid generally looks more natural if it is feasible to cover with a liquid. Teach the client to carefully blend in any lines of demarcation, such as darker areas that have not been treated by the chemical peel. Makeup designs that focus attention on the eyes may help draw attention away from other treated areas of the face.

Long-Term Needs

Besides good general skin care, the chemical peel patient will need help with the aforementioned possible side effects of the peel.

Phenol peeling is most often recommended for seriously sun-damaged, wrinkled, and leathery skin. Although the peel procedure does seem to tighten the face, it is not a substitute for face-lift. The phenol peel is often reserved for patients who need serious help because of severe wrinkling and rough textures from sun damage. The possible side effects of phenol peelings must be considered acceptable risks for this sun-damaged skin.

ESTHETIC MANAGEMENT OF THE POST-LASER PATIENT

The following information is condensed from an article written by the author for *Les Nouvelles Esthetiques—American Edition*. The author wishes to thank Les Nouvelles Esthetiques for its cooperation in reprinting this information.

Make sure all products used in this treatment are designed for use on post-laser patients. After receiving approval from the surgeon to treat the post-laser patient, gently cleanse the skin using a nonfragranced, emulsion cleanser with cool wet cotton pads.

Place the client under cool steam. This uses a special vapor machine that operates from ultrasonic vibration.

Apply a hyaluronic serum with antioxidants. This will soothe and improve hydration. Make sure that the serum is designed for use on laser patients. It should NOT have a low pH!

Apply a nonfragranced hydrating fluid with lipids to reinforce the barrier function. Massage very gently with slow effleurage movements and light tapotement.

Unfold a 4 x 4 (16 ply) gauze pad across the face.

Apply cold "globes" to the face in gentle symmetrical stroking movements.

Slowly move the globes around the face. Apply more hydrating fluid after removing the gauze.

Apply a cooling, non-drying, non-setting gel mask with chamomile, matricaria, licorice, or bisabolol.

Apply cool wet cotton compresses to remove the gel mask. Be careful not to pull on the face.

Apply concentrated fragrance-free lipid serum to any lasered area, such as the eyes and around the mouth.

(All Post-Laser Treatment Photos Courtesy Mark Lees Skin Care, Inc.)

Figure 19–1 Post-laser treatment

Laser Surgical Procedures

Plastic surgery, like many other fields, is benefiting from advanced technology. The best current example is the popularity of lasers for skin resurfacing. Lasers are basically very concentrated stream forms of polarized light. In laser resurfacing, the laser is used to retexturize the surface of the skin, literally vaporizing layers of skin. This helps to literally "plane down" wrinkles and, if "full-face" laser is performed, does have a slight firming effect on the face.

Lasers can be used for surface lines and wrinkles and minor scarring. For shallow imperfections, lasers are good alternatives to surgical chemical peeling, because the penetration level is easier to control. The depth of the procedure is controlled by how many "passes" the patient has, basically how many times the surgeon passes across particular areas of the face.

There are two types of lasers currently being used for resurfacing: carbon dioxide (CO_2) and erbium. The CO_2 laser is generally stronger and is a better choice for deeper wrinkles and more severe sun damage. CO_2 cannot be used on the neck, however, because the skin on the neck is not as thick as facial skin. The erbium laser is primarily used for a "refreshening" procedure, in younger clients or clients with less severe wrinkling. The two types of laser are used in combination by some surgeons. Some surgeons also use a laser at the same time as when performing another procedure such as rhytidectomy or face-lift. Lasers can also be used on particular areas such as around the mouth and eyes. Patients can experience many cosmetic side effects during recovery from laser surgery. The esthetician can play a significant role in the management and control of these esthetic side effects.

Pretreatment

The surgeon will generally meet with the patient several weeks before the surgery. Medical pre-care varies from doctor to doctor, but generally consists of use of either Retin-A or an alphahydroxy acid home care product coupled with a melanin suppressant such as a 4 percent hydroquinone preparation.

PROCEDURES FOR THE ESTHETICIAN

Before Surgery

The esthetician should meet with the client and establish a plan of treatment. This may vary slightly with the particular individual needs of the patient and the procedures being performed. For example, laser resurfacing may accompany a blepharoplasty, or a partial resurfacing may be performed with a face-lift. Some patients will elect to only have their perioral or periocular regions resurfaced.

Typically, the esthetician should perform at least one deep cleansing procedure, carefully removing impactions, comedones, or milia. Some patients will require more than one session for cleansing, again depending on individual needs.

A series of treatments performed weekly for six weeks before surgery can be very helpful in optimizing the health of the skin. This should consist primarily of light exfoliation using 30 percent alphahydroxy acid, which will help remove dead cell buildup and dislodge clogged follicles.

The mission of pre-care is to have the skin in top shape before the resurfacing, theorizing that skin that is in excellent condition will heal better and have fewer potential complications than skin that is in poor condition.

On the last visit before the resurfacing, the esthetician should consult with the client and instruct her in her step-by-step postoperative home care program, making sure that the client has all the products she needs. A camouflage makeup shade should be chosen and the client should have very basic instructions on how to use this product. As previously mentioned, a more involved makeup lesson should be performed 2 to 3 weeks after the resurfacing to individualize the technique for the particular case.

After Surgery

Laser Patient Referral

The plastic or dermatological surgeon generally refers patients after any sutures are removed, usually around 11 to 12 days post-laser, and after the skin is sufficiently re-epithelialized and no longer raw, to reduce any risks of infection or poor healing. *It is only with the surgeon's approval that the esthetician should proceed with esthetic treatment.*

The esthetician will evaluate the individual case for skin type, age of the patient, amount of redness, dryness, discomfort, and areas of treatment. A good esthetician should also be trained to recognize conditions such as infection that should be referred back to the surgeon (Case Studies—Plates 51a–f).

Hyperpigmentation

Hyperpigmentation is a problem for some patients following laser resurfacing. Generally, the lighter the skin of the patient, the less the hyperpigmentation problem or risk. Laser is not a good alternative for any patient who experiences hyperpigmentation easily.

Pre-care use of a prescribed 4 percent hydroquinone preparation helps reduce the likelihood of pigment problems after the procedure. Postoperative hyperpigmentation may also be avoided by the proper use of a broad-spectrum SPF-15 or higher daily-use sunscreen, which will be used routinely after the skin has healed. Management of any severe postoperative hyperpigmentation should be referred back to the surgeon.

Redness

Redness or erythema is typical of many resurfacing procedures, particularly laser resurfacing. This is one of the biggest, if not the biggest, concern of post-laser surgery patients, and a side effect that the esthetician can help alleviate. Patients are anxious to get back to work and their normal lifestyle without appearing red and drawing attention to their situation.

Redness is easily covered with camouflage makeup for the short term, but in laser and chemical resurfacing patients, this redness can last for weeks, and in some cases, for months. Patients are very interested in reducing the redness, not just covering it up.

The use of lipid-based products, antioxidant complexes, and effective hydrators can help reestablish the barrier function of the epidermis and minimize postoperative redness.

Dryness

The surgeon often prescribes an antibiotic ointment for the first few days after the laser procedure. Sometimes the surgeon will use a dressing such as Flexan® to protect the face.

After the dressing is removed, the surgeon will often recommend a heavy, occlusive, emollient, petrolatum-type product. This is to protect the skin with a barrier while the skin is reestablishing the epidermal tissue and the natural barrier function. Although these products definitely serve their purpose and are temporarily necessary, heavy, occlusive ointments are very sticky and oily and are not user-friendly. They cannot be used with makeup and are uncomfortable.

Dryness of the skin, particularly during the transitional period from the post-resurfacing patient's use of a heavier, occlusive emollient, and the return to a daily use moisturizer, can be aesthetically displeasing as well as uncomfortable for the patient. Patients frequently complain of tightness and discomfort, as well as unsightly flaking that can accentuate skin wrinkles or imperfections and add to difficulty in makeup application. Foundations tend to clump in areas of extreme dryness, adding to the patient's cosmetic problems, even with camouflage coverage makeups. This can actually draw attention to the area, rather than detract from it.

Dehydration

Because the surface layers have basically been removed, the skin must re-epithelialize to reestablish the various layers of the epidermis. While the skin is re-epithelializing, it has a very poor barrier function, which results in dehydration, sensitivity, and erythema. The skin feels and looks very dehydrated during this period. With the doctor's approval at the appropriate time after the procedure, the esthetician can help to properly hydrate the skin, reducing the feeling of tightness, and easing the rough texture of severely dehydrated skin.

Ingredients to Help Restore Barrier Function

The substance between the epidermal cells is referred to as the interstitial fluid, intercellular matrix, or cement. This substance is a complex mixture of lipids such as ceramides, sphingolipids and glycosphingolipids, phospholipids, cholesterol, and fatty acids, with hydrating water-binders called natural moisture factors (NMFs) such as sodium PCA. These combined ingredients in the proper proportions, can help "patch the mortar between the bricks" in the intercellular matrix, which is essentially absent after laser resurfacing. This helps to reestablish the protective barrier function that keeps skin protected and well-hydrated, and will significantly reduce redness following surgery. The use of products and serums based in lipid replacement ingredients, coupled with hydrating ingredients such as sodium hyaluronate, glycerin, or sodium PCA can help mimic the natural barrier function, resulting in better hydrated, smoother, and more comfortable skin. The serums are often in a silicone base. These products can be lighter weight and much more user-friendly than cumbersome, heavy ointments.

Because freshly resurfaced skin tends to be much more sensitive and reactive than normal skin, it is very important that all products used on post-laser patients be fragrance-free to avoid sensitizing the skin. It is also very important that the products have been properly tested by an independent laboratory for irritancy.

Treatment Methods

Use of in-office facial treatments can help minimize redness. These treatments involve the use of fragrance-free lightweight hydrating fluids using functional ingredients such as the aforementioned sphingolipids, glycosphingolipids, cholesterol, and phospholipids, along with hydrating ingredients such as glycerin, sodium PCA, and sodium hyaluronate. Light and gentle facial massage with a hydrating fluid, and the use of cold therapy or compresses, along with proper products can help reduce redness in a fairly short period of time. If you are certified in Manual Lymph Drainage, this may be appropriate for post-laser patients. Soothing, nonhardening gel or cream mask treatments are implemented to increase moisturization and help remove dry, dead skin flakes gently. This treatment modality also reduces the appearance of dryness, tightness, and flaking, and helps achieve the appearance of skin smoothness.

Proper home care instruction of the patient should comprise the use of a very mild, fragrance-free, low- or nonsurfactant (one that does not foam much) cleanser, because stronger surfactant cleansers can further irritate and add to the dryness. Use of a well-formulated antioxidant serum may also help soothe the redness and dehydration. Some vitamin preparations may not be appropriate, especially if they sting when applied, or increase redness after application.

Routine use of a good hydrator with a concentrated lipid serum eases dehydration and flaking as well as decreasing redness.

This combination of treatment products will also serve as a good pre-makeup treatment, allowing for smoother application of color cosmetics.

Sun Protection

Obviously, post-laser patients should have absolutely no direct sun exposure. They should do everything they can to protect their skin from the sun, and it doesn't hurt to remind them that sun is probably the reason they needed the laser in the first place!

Because of the irritancy potential of many absorbing sunscreen ingredients, sunscreen application is usually not advised for the first 18 to 21 days after laser surgery. If any sunscreen is used during this time, it should be a reflecting screen, such as one with micronized zinc oxide or titanium dioxide as an active ingredient.

After the epidermis is reestablished, about 18 to 21 days, the client should be instructed to use a broad-spectrum sunscreen SPF-15 or above on a DAILY basis. This should be a routine part of their daily care for the rest of their lives. The easiest way to do this is to find a wearable facial moisturizer with a built-in SPF-15 sunscreen or block. Make sure the client understands that a little dab of sunscreen is probably not enough. Instruct the client to apply several dots to the face and neck and massage it in, allowing a few minutes for it to absorb before applying makeup. Don't forget your hands and arms, too—another very vulnerable spot for sun damage and sun-induced aging!

Milia Formation

Milia frequently develop during healing of resurfacing procedures. Estheticians are a great help in removing these unsightly cosmetic lesions, which are of much concern to the patient.

Freshly lasered skin is *very* fragile and delicate. Do not extract milia unless you have extensive experience in performing milia extraction, and have the approval of the referring surgeon.

Return to Normal Routine

The client can return to the normal skin-care routine after two to three months. This is, of course, assuming that the client had an appropriate regimen established prior to surgery. Daily use of a mild effective cleanser, broad-spectrum SPF-15 sunscreen day cream, alphahydroxy acid products appropriate for the skin type, topical antioxidants, and lipid-based hydrators are all helpful in management of the aging skin. There is mounting evidence that these few procedures do help skin look younger, and maintain the proper health of the skin.

Ongoing Care

The esthetician can help the patient with ongoing care, cosmetic and skin-care needs. Additional skin-care procedures can be added long after the skin has healed from surgery, further improving the appearance of the results of the surgery.

Makeup lessons after the immediate postoperative adjustment period can teach the patient how to best accentuate her new look and detract from any imperfections. The well-trained esthetician can further advise the patient on sun protection, and keep the patient abreast of new developments in skin-care, makeup, and plastic surgery techniques that might be appropriate for the patient.

General skin-care instruction and help in selecting the right program for the client is a very important service, both for the short and long term. The licensed esthetician plays a very important role in management of postoperative cosmetic surgical side effects, health education skin-care instruction, and support for the patient's psyche as the patient returns to normal lifestyle.

OTHER SURGICAL PROCEDURES

Liposuction is the term for surgical removal of fat deposits. The procedure uses a vacuum-like instrument that suctions away fat from areas such as the chin or the cheeks. Liposuction is often also used on the body, such as the hips and thighs. A small incision is made in the skin, and the instrument is inserted into the subcutaneous fat layer, where treatment is administered. Bruising is the main side effect of this procedure. Chin or cheek liposuction is often performed at the same time as a face-lift.

There are no specific additional pre- or postoperative salon procedures for facial liposuction, except as already outlined for face-lift surgery. Treatment of the incision areas should be avoided, and harsh massage should be avoided. Treatment, as always, should not begin until the surgeon approves.

Liposuction is the term for surgical removal of fat deposits.

Collagen injections are procedures performed by a plastic surgeon and involve injecting collagen into depression scars or wrinkles to reduce the appearance of the lesion.

Salon Treatment for Post-Laser Patients

Before any salon procedure, you must have a direct referral and approval for treatment from the plastic surgeon! Do NOT treat the client without the surgeon's approval!

1. Have the client complete a health history form, carefully checking for previous allergies, sensitivities, and other contraindications for treatment.

2. Seat the client and carefully examine her skin, *without cleansing first*. There is a chance that the client is not yet ready for treatment, and you must thoroughly examine and check for areas that are still healing. Normally, surgeons will refer the post-laser client around 11 to 12 days after the procedure. Clients should be ready if they have the surgeon's referral. Carefully observe and record areas of redness (erythema), rawness, dryness, dehydration, flaking, and milia. Should you notice any pus or strange-looking lesions, refer the patient back to the surgeon, or call the surgeon for advice.

3. If everything appears normal for postoperative condition, gently cleanse the skin with cool predampened cotton pads with a very gentle cleanser. After cleansing, apply a *nonfragranced* hydrating fluid that contains lipids and hydrating agents such as glycerin, hyaluronic acid, or sodium PCA. The skin should be slightly damp before application.

4. Place the client under (not hot) vapor. Cool steam is preferable. If warm vapor is used, focus it at least 18 inches away from the client's face. The point is to gently moisten the face, not to warm or stimulate it. Vapor should be administered for about five to eight minutes.

5. Gently wipe down the face again with fresh cool cotton pads. Apply more hydrating fluid and gently massage the face in long, gentle effleurage strokes. Do not use any stimulating massage movements. Gentle tapotement (piano movements) is appropriate.

6. Apply more hydrating fluid to ensure the skin is very moist and lubricated. Apply high frequency with the mushroom electrode at a low setting. Use circular movements for about two to three minutes. Stop immediately if the face reddens or if the client complains of discomfort.

7. Once again, apply hydration fluid over the face. Unfold a 4 × 4 gauze square and place across the face. Apply the cryoglobes in gentle circles across the face for about five to seven passes.

8. Apply more hydrating fluid, and then apply a cool wet cotton compress in three strips across the face. Allow this compress to stay on for five to ten minutes.

9. Gently remove any excess fluid with fresh cotton pads. Apply several drops of lipid serum over the entire face.

10. Depending on the redness level, you may apply makeup. However, if the skin is extremely red now or prior to treatment, or if this is the first treatment, it is often best not to apply makeup immediately after treatment. In many cases, it is better to deal with skin care on the first day and makeup instruction the next day.

Collagen injections are almost always an in-office procedure. Bovine (cow) collagen is injected into the dermis through an **intradermal** injection. The wrinkle depression in the dermis is "inflated" with the collagen, immediately reducing the appearance of the wrinkle. Collagen injections are frequently used for treatment of nasolabial wrinkling, eyelines, and small depressions, pocks, and hypotrophic scars (Plates 52a, 52b).

Intradermal means inside the dermis, which is where collagen and other filler material may be injected to fill out hypotrophic scars, wrinkles, or pock marks.

Treatment should be avoided in the freshly treated area. The area may appear "lumpy" for up to several weeks after the injection. The body will slowly absorb the collagen, so collagen injections need to be repeated for best results, usually every few months.

Collagen injections are often the first procedure sought by clients for minor wrinkles and other small imperfections. They are a good treatment for spot wrinkles, but are not a substitute for a face-lift. Collagen injections appeal to clients because they are nonsurgical, but often the client needs other surgery in addition to collagen to "polish" the results of surgery.

Implants are used to improve the cheeks and chin. These are small "sacks" of silicone or saline (saltwater solution) that are implanted in the chin and cheek areas to improve low cheekbone appearance or receding chins. Avoid treating the area immediately after surgery, following the surgeon's recommendations. Implants are often performed at the same time as a face-lift.

Implants are used to improve the cheeks and chin.

Gortex® is a synthetic material that has been developed as a filler that is more permanent than collagen. This can be used in lipline or nasolabial injections.

Permanent eyeliner or **makeup** is often performed by plastic surgeons, but in some states is legal for estheticians to perform. The procedure involves a "tattooing" type process that implants small amounts of pigment in the skin. The procedure is often used to create a permanent eyeline or lipline, but can also be used in the cheek area, and occasionally to help correct dark, flat lesions, such as small, red macules. Courses available through many schools teach permanent makeup. Check with your instructor regarding the laws in your state affecting permanent makeup.

Permanent eyeliner or **makeup** means "tattooing" a permanent eyeline or lipline. It can also be used in the cheek area, and occasionally to help correct dark, flat lesions, such as small, red macules.

Reconstructive surgery, as previously discussed, is used to help correct skin scars and abnormalities that are caused by accidents, disease, or congenital (birth) defects.

These procedures vary greatly, due to the many differences in the problems being treated. Plastic surgeons often remove facial skin cancers, using their skills to best conceal the demarcations from these treatments.

Home Care for Post-Laser Patients

The first 11 to 12 days are directly supervised by the surgeon.

- Days 1 to 5—Antibiotic ointment
- Days 5 to 12—Occlusive (petrolatum) applied routinely
- Days 11 to 30—Gentle cleanser, soothing antioxidant serum, hydrating fluid, lipid serum
- Day 30—Return to normal routine as advised by the esthetician or surgeon

Sunscreen is usually not used until day 18 or until erythema is reduced. Sunscreens can be irritating or sensitizing to freshly lasered skin. Sun exposure must be totally avoided.

These are general guidelines and may vary with the patient or the surgeon.

Often there is no time for pretreatment of these areas. The patient normally sees the esthetician after the surgery has occurred. Often seeking makeup help, the patient is frequently referred by the surgeon for help with concealing scars from the surgery. Sometimes several operations may have to take place to help revise scars from accidents or skin cancer. Makeup help may be required for coverage during and between these operations.

We will not discuss the correction of these types of scars here. The esthetician should take specialty courses in paramedical camouflage makeup in order to help these patients.

REFERRALS

The plastic surgery candidate will often first seek counseling from the esthetician. Carefully evaluate the client's concerns, and then refer the client to a plastic surgeon. Because plastic cosmetic surgery is an elective procedure, the client will often want to think about the possibility of surgery for some time before proceeding.

You should have brochures available from your referring surgeon that briefly describe the various types of surgery. Plastic surgeons will gladly furnish these at no charge to you once you have established a working relationship. It is best to have relationships with several surgeons. Suggest to the client that they have consultations with at least two different surgeons, to make sure they feel comfortable with the doctor and to see pictures of the doctor's work. Secondly, referring a client to more than one doctor can reduce any liability you might encounter if, by chance, a client has a bad experience with the surgeon.

You should have a working understanding with the plastic surgeon of each other's procedures and needs. Prepare a pre- and postsurgical brochure discussing esthetic procedures and how they help plastic surgery patients. Work with your plastic surgeon on this brochure, so that both of you are involved and are knowledgeable about typical procedures. When in doubt about treating a cosmetic or plastic surgery patient, always consult the doctor!

Many workshops and classes are available on paramedical makeup and working with plastic surgeons. You should take these courses to best prepare yourself for working with a plastic surgeon.

Topics for Discussion

1. What is the difference between cosmetic and reconstructive surgery?
2. What are the various types of physicians who perform plastic surgery?
3. What are some general postoperative skin-care procedures that should be avoided?
4. Why is it important for the plastic surgery patient to have presurgical skin-care treatments?
5. What should the esthetician do when there is a question about a treatment procedure for a plastic surgery patient?

6. Discuss preparing a brochure about esthetic treatment for a plastic surgery patient. Why is it important for both the esthetician and the plastic surgeon to be involved in preparing such a brochure?

7. Discuss the use of surgical lasers for resurfacing. What concerns of the laser patient must be handled by the esthetician?

Chapter 20

Recognize and Refer Medical Conditions

Objectives

The esthetician should be trained to recognize common medical conditions and diseases of the skin and refer them to the proper medical authority—in most cases the dermatologist.

This chapter is designed to illustrate and briefly discuss some of the medical conditions that the esthetician may observe in routine practice. Although not all of these conditions are life-threatening, many skin conditions need to be referred to the dermatologist for proper medical treatment.

The esthetician will often have clients who come to the salon for treatment of what they may think is a cosmetic disorder, but is actually a dermatological condition. The esthetician should never diagnose a medical condition, but should be able to recognize conditions that require medical treatment. The esthetician should be well educated about the different types of common skin diseases and conditions and should be able to discuss conditions with the dermatologist. The esthetician should also be familiar with the cosmetic effects of certain skin disorders and know how they can help with cosmetic symptoms that the client may need to conceal.

This chapter will teach you about medical conditions that need medical referral. You should always refer any condition that you do not understand or that is obviously not just a minor cosmetic problem.

Before discussing the medical conditions in this chapter, it is important to discuss common medical terminology—specifically dermatological terminology. The medical community has very precise descriptions for symptoms of the skin. Using these specific terms, dermatologists can very accurately describe lesions and therefore diagnose illnesses more efficiently. (The author wishes to thank Rube Pardo, M.D., Ph.D., and the Department of Dermatology at the University of Miami, for their assistance in preparing this section on dermatological terminology.)

PRIMARY AND SECONDARY LESIONS

A **lesion** is any mark on the skin that is not a normal part of the skin. It does not necessarily mean that the skin is diseased. A freckle is a lesion; so is a wrinkle. However, lesions can also be symptoms of disease, such as melanoma, shingles, or measles. **Primary lesions** of the skin are lesions that are in the early stages of development.

Secondary lesions are lesions that primary lesions eventually become.

Macules are flat (nonelevated) marks on the skin in which there is only a change in the normal color of the skin. Again, a freckle can be an example of a macule, and the flat red mark left after a pimple has healed is also a macule. It is simply a descriptive term meaning that this is a flat area with a change in the normal color of the skin. The adjective used to describe a lesion is macular. Large macules, larger than 1 centimeter, are called **patches**. **Papules** are raised areas on the skin that are generally smaller than 1 centimeter. **Plaques** are papules that are larger than 1 centimeter.

Nodules are raised lesions that are larger and deep in the skin. A nodule looks like a lump, but the skin can be moved over the lesion. Very large nodules are called **tumors**.

A **pustule** is a lesion that is filled with pus, which we have previously discussed in Chapter 12, Acne and the Esthetician. Extremely deep infections with pockets of pus are called **abscesses**.

Vesicle is the medical term for blisters. They contain body fluids. A **bulba** is a large vesicle. A vesicle or bulba that has ruptured so that the fluid is exposed to the surface of the skin is said to be weeping or oozing.

A **wheal** is a hive. Wheals are caused by a concentration of the fluid in the tissue. Wheals are reabsorbed into the bloodstream via the lymphatic system.

Erosion refers to a shallow depression in the skin. Scratches on the skin are called **excoriations**, which we have already discussed in Chapter 12, Acne and the Esthetician. Deep erosions are called **ulcers**, in which part of the dermis has been lost.

Diseased skin often has remnants of body fluids, pus, or blood caked to a lesion. This is described as **crust**.

Scales are patches of dry, dehydrated skin without crust.

Erythema refers to any area of redness associated with a lesion. Bruises are known as **hematomas**. **Purpura** are hemorrhages of the blood vessels.

Lesion is any mark on the skin that is not a normal part of the skin.

Primary lesions are lesions that are in the early stages of development.

Secondary lesions are lesions that primary lesions eventually become.

Macules are flat (nonelevated) marks on the skin in which there is only a change in the normal color of the skin.

Patches are large macules that are larger than 1 centimeter.

Papules are raised areas on the skin that are generally smaller than 1 centimeter.

Plaques are papules that are larger than 1 centimeter.

Nodules are raised lesions that are larger and deeper in the skin. A nodule looks like a lump, but the skin can be moved over the lesion.

Tumors are very large nodules.

Pustule is a clump of white blood cells that have formed and risen to the surface of the skin.

Abscesses are extremely deep infections with pockets of pus.

Vesicle is the medical term for blisters.

Bulba is a large vesicle.

Atrophy means wasting away. Skin that has thinned from age or chronic sun exposure is said to have atrophied. **Hypertrophy** is thickening of a tissue. Hypertrophic scars are raised scars, due to thickening of a tissue. **Atrophic scars** are depressed scars, such as acne pocks, caused by loss of tissue.

A number of terms are used to described the shapes of certain lesions. A **linear** lesion is a line-like lesion. A ring-shaped lesion is called **annular**. Lesions that have a snake-like pattern are called **sepiginous**. **Geographic** lesions look like a map. **Target**, or **iris**, lesions have a center with a round surrounding area, such as a pustule.

Keratosis is a general term meaning a thickening of a stratum corneum, such as seborrheic keratosis, described in Chapter 16, Sun and Sun Damage.

Eczematization refers to a combination of symptoms, including erythema, weeping, crusting, and present vesicles.

A **nevus** is a mole. More than one mole are described as nevi. **Lentigines** are freckles. Dyschromias are skin color abnormalities. **Hyperpigmentation** refers to any condition that has more than the normal amount of melanin. **Hypopigmentation** refers to any area with less than the normal amount of pigment.

ACNE

We have already thoroughly discussed acne in Chapter 13. Severe acne requires medical attention. Grade 4 acne is severe inflammatory acne with cystic lesions. Cysts should always be referred to the dermatologist. The medical treatment for cysts includes injections with steroids, which help to shrink the lesion. Some cysts may be lanced by the dermatologist and drained. Both topical and oral antibiotics may be used to help control inflammatory acne conditions. Common topical preparations may include the antibiotics erythromycin (trade name A/T/S®) or clindamycin (trade name Cleocin T®). These preparations are available only by prescription and are liquid roll-ons that are applied to the skin either daily or twice daily. The doctor may suggest that the client not use certain cosmetic products that will increase irritation. Frequently, dermatologists will prescribe prescription keratolytic products such as prescription-strength benzoyl peroxide treatments, retinoic acid (Retin-A), adapalene (Differin®), azelaic acid (Azelex®), or other peeling and sloughing agents. These products are discussed in detail in Chapter 13.

Other acne-related medical conditions include *acne rosacea, perioral dermatitis,* and *seborrheic dermatitis,* which are all also discussed in previous chapters.

COMMON INFECTIONS OF THE SKIN

Infections of the skin may be grouped into three types: bacterial, fungal, and viral.

Common Bacterial Infections

Impetigo is a skin infection that is commonly seen on the face, particularly in the lower part of the face, but it can occur anywhere. This disease is characterized by large, open,

---

Wheal is a raised red lesion associated with sensitivity or allergy. Wheals are also called hives.

Erosion refers to a shallow depression in the skin.

Excoriations are scratches on the skin.

Ulcers are deep erosions in which part of the dermis has been lost.

Crust is caked body fluids, pus, or blood remnants left from diseased skin.

Scales are patches of dry, dehydrated skin without crust.

Erythema refers to any area of redness associated with a lesion.

Hematomas are bruises.

Purpura are hemorrhages of the blood vessels.

Atrophy means wasting away.

Hypertrophy is thickening of a tissue.

Atrophic scars are depressed scars such as acne pocks, caused by loss of tissue.

Linear lesion is a line-like lesion.

Annular lesion is a ring-shaped lesion.

Sepiginous lesion is a lesion that has a snake-like pattern.

Geographic lesion looks like a map.

Target, or **iris**, lesion has a center with a round surrounding area, such as a pustule.

Keratosis is a general term meaning thickening of the stratum corneum, such as seborrheic keratosis.

Eczematization refers to a combination of symptoms, including erythema, weeping, crusting, and present vesicles.

Nevus is a mole.

Lentigines are freckles.

Hyperpigmentation refers to any condition that has more than a normal amount of melanin.

Hypopigmentation refers to any area with less than the normal amount of pigment.

Impetigo is a skin infection that is characterized by large, open, weeping lesions.

Folliculitis is a bacterial infection of the hair follicle.

Pseudofolliculitis is caused by irritation from shaving. Ingrown hairs are the main cause of pseudofolliculitis.

Furuncle is a severe infection of the hair follicle. It is also known as a boil.

Carbuncles are large boils that often result in abscesses.

Septicemia, also known as blood poisoning, occurs when a bacterial infection enters the bloodstream.

Cellulitis is a deep infection of the dermis caused by streptococcus.

Erysipelas, also known as St. Anthony's Fire, is a severe form of bacterial cellulitis.

Mycoses are fungal infections.

Tinea veriscolor is what many refer to as sun "spots" or sun "fungus." These white splotches are a fungal condition.

Tinea pedis is commonly known as athlete's foot, which is a fungal infection of the skin on the foot.

Tinea corporis is better known as ringworm.

Candidas are yeast infections.

Herpes refers to a group of viruses.

weeping lesions. They look like large sores, similar to acne, except that impetigo lesions weep and appear damp. The lesions can range in size. Impetigo is frequently seen in children and is extremely contagious. Impetigo is caused by staphylococcus bacteria. The disease is treated by the use of antibiotics (Plate 53).

Folliculitis is a bacterial infection of the hair follicle. The infection results in irritation and is characterized by multiple pinpoint irritations around the pore openings (Plate 54). **Pseudofolliculitis** is caused by irritation from shaving. It also appears as irritated follicles but is not usually infected. Ingrown hairs are the main cause of pseudofolliculitis, seen frequently in the beard area of male clients, especially the neck.

A more severe infection of the hair follicle is called a **furuncle**, also known as a boil. Large boils often result in abscesses and are referred to as **carbuncles**. Folliculitis, furuncles, and carbuncles are treated with antibiotics. If a furuncle or carbuncle bursts on the inside of the lesion, the bacteria may enter the bloodstream, causing **septicemia**, also known as blood poisoning. Septicemia is characterized by a red erythemic line running from the source of primary infection. Septicemia is extremely serious, and should be treated immediately by a physician. **Cellulitis** is a deep infection of the dermis, caused by streptococcus (Plate 55). A severe form of cellulitis is called **erysipelas**, also known as St. Anthony's Fire. Again, this is extremely serious and should be seen immediately by a physician.

Fungal Skin Infections

There are a number of fungal infections of the skin. Fungal infections are called **mycoses**.

Tinea veriscolor is sometimes called *sun fungus.* It is often seen on the backs and chests of persons who are tan. Tinea veriscolor inhibits the production of melanin in the skin, which results in its appearance as white patches. It is not actually directly related to sun exposure, but is often seen on tanned persons, because the skin will not tan in the areas where tinea veriscolor is active. The disease is easily treated with the use of antifungal prescription medications.

Tinea pedis is commonly known as *athlete's foot,* which is a fungal infection of the skin on the foot. The disease is characterized by severe itching and scaling, particularly on the sole of the foot. Again, tinea pedis is easily treated by the use of antifungal prescription medications.

Tinea corporis is better known by the public as ringworm. It can occur on any area of the body and presents itself as a ring-like lesion (Plate 56).

Candidas are yeast infections. They can cause a variety of skin infections. Oral thrush, seen often in infants and persons with suppressed immune systems, such as AIDS patients, is a yeast infection of the mouth characterized by white patches inside the mouth.

Viral Skin Infections

Herpes refers to a group of viruses. Herpes simplex is the cause of common cold sores, which generally appear on or around the mouth and often appear as oozing red ulcers (Plate 57). They are very contagious, and should be treated by a physician. Facial treatments should be avoided for clients with active lesions. Certain facial treatments such as chemical peels have been known to cause a flareup of the herpes virus.

Herpes zoster, better known as *shingles,* is caused by the same virus that causes chickenpox. Herpes zoster is harboured by the nervous system and generally follows a pattern along the nerves in the skin. The lesions of herpes zoster look like multiple red blisters (Plate 58). Subjective symptoms may include burning, tingling, or numbness, and severe cases can result in extreme pain. Minor infections can be only a nuisance, and the disease subsides by itself. However, the infection can reoccur and in some cases causes scarring and pain due to nerve inflammation. There is no cure for herpes zoster, although there are some prescriptions helpful in controlling it. Herpes zoster is another infection that may be especially a problem in immunosuppressed individuals, such as AIDS patients.

Molloscum contagiosum is a viral infection frequently seen on the faces of children, which appears as groups of small, flesh-colored papules. They often resemble milia, but are in groups or clusters and are hard to the touch (Plate 59). They must be treated by a physician.

One of the most frequent viral lesions seen are warts. **Warts** are caused by a variety of viruses known as *papovaviruses* or *veruccae.* Wart treatment varies with the lesion, including topical acid therapy using salicylic acid or trichloroacetic acid. Other dermatologic treatments include freezing the lesions with liquid nitrogen or cautery with an electric needle. Warts are contagious, especially to the same individual, and can be spread to another area of the body easily. Warts may be seen by the esthetician on the face, feet, and hands, especially the nails, and should be referred to a dermatologist for treatment (Plate 60).

Pityriasis rosea is a patchy, red, rashlike disorder. It can occur anywhere on the body, but is frequently seen on the trunk. Groups of patches may develop. Many outbreaks resemble the pattern of a Christmas tree on the trunk. There is no real cure for pityriasis rosea, but it usually subsides after a few weeks. Itching associated with infection can be treated with topical prescription steroid creams (Plate 61).

COMMON REACTIONS, RASHES, AND IRRITATIONS

In Chapter 6 we have already discussed common allergies that the esthetician sees routinely. **Dermatitis** means inflammation of the skin. It is a descriptive term used to describe many different types of skin inflammation and irritation. Dermatitis is an irritation, rather than a disease. It is generally not caused by pathological organisms, such as infections caused by viruses, bacteria, and fungi. Many of the other terms already discussed in this chapter are used as adjectives to describe different types and patterns of dermatitis.

Contact Dermatitis

Contact dermatitis is probably the most common form of dermatitis observed by the esthetician. Contact dermatitis is an irritation caused by either an allergic reaction or irritation to something or some substance touching the skin or coming in contact with

Herpes zoster, better known as shingles, is caused by the same virus that causes chickenpox. The lesions of herpes zoster look like multiple red blisters.

Molluscum contagiosum is a viral infection frequently seen on the faces of children, which appear as groups of small, flesh-colored papules.

Warts are caused by a variety of viruses known as papovaviruses or verrucae.

Pityriasis rosea is a patchy, red, rashlike disorder.

Dermatitis is inflammation of the skin.

Contact dermatitis is an irritation caused by either an allergic reaction or irritation to something or some substance touching the skin or coming in contact with the skin's surface.

the skin's surface. Cosmetics are a frequent cause of contact dermatitis. Other frequent causes of contact dermatitis include jewelry, laundry products, clothing fabrics and dyes, plants (such as poison ivy), and other substances (Plates 62a, 62b).

There are two basic treatments for contact dermatitis. The first, of course, is to avoid contact with the offending substance. This is sometimes hard to pinpoint, because we touch so many substances on a daily basis. Often the dermatologist can tell much about the source of irritation by the location of the dermatitis. Irritation of the hands is often caused by household products. Health and personal care professionals, including estheticians, often suffer from dermatitis related to substances they touch at work.

Irritation from hand washes, disinfectants and antiseptics, and even allergies to latex gloves are frequently seen in these professionals. Estheticians also come in contact with a large number of cosmetic products, which can also be a source of irritation.

The process of eliminating the offending substance is often a matter of trial and error, eliminating one or all substances and testing by slowly adding steps of substance contact. Allergies are sometimes easier to detect. The dermatologist can often run allergy patch tests, and allergies have a tendency to be more acute, or sudden, than irritation dermatitis.

The second part of contact dermatitis treatment is to soothe and stop the inflammation. Topical steroid creams are often prescribed by the dermatologist to ease the symptoms of allergic or irritant dermatitis. These prescription creams usually work fairly quickly, assuming that the source of irritation has also been eliminated.

Dermatitis can have many characteristics visually, but is usually red (erythemic), and often itchy or burning. The term *eczema* refers to the same condition as *dermatitis*.

Atopic Dermatitis

Atopic eczema, also known as atopic dermatitis, is a chronic inflammatory condition of the skin that is hereditary and may be related to respiratory allergies or asthma.

Atopic eczema or dermatitis is a more complicated form of dermatitis. It is a more severe and chronic condition, and is associated, in most cases, with heredity. It may be affected by illness, stress, and other changes. Some patients suffer from atopic dermatitis all their lives.

Atopic eczema can be controlled with the use of prescription steroid creams and oral antihistamines. Cosmetologically, the atopic eczema patient will be more likely to have irritant reactions to cosmetics. If you have a client with atopic eczema, discuss any cosmetics with the client's doctor. In general, stick to fragrance-free, simple products—the simpler the better, and the fewer ingredients, the better. Use the same care as discussed in Chapter 6.

Occasionally, you may notice a rash following a pattern on the face that does not clear up. Rashes in a butterfly pattern across the cheeks can be a symptom of lupus erythematosus. We have already discussed lupus in Chapter 2. If you notice a recurrent rash on a client's face, you should refer the client to a physician, as you should all rashes and chronic redness (Plate 63).

Psoriasis

Psoriasis is an inflammatory disorder of the skin that is caused by the skin and epidermis "turning over" faster than it does in a normal individual. Largely hereditary, it can be chronic and last over a lifetime. The disorder is not contagious and is not related to any pathological organism. It is a disorder, not a disease (Plate 64).

Psoriasis primarily affects the skin on the body and is often symmetrical, which means it occurs simultaneously on both sides of the body in the same place. It often affects the elbows, the knees, and other extremities.

Treatments used to control psoriasis include steroid creams, antihistamines, and light therapy using controlled exposures of UVA. Some new oral drugs are also being used to treat chronic cases.

Urticaria

An outbreak of **urticaria**, or hives, is due to allergies. Urticaria often quickly fades without treatment, but the source of the allergy should be identified. Dermatologists use topical steroids, oral steroids, antihistamines, and allergy testing to treat and identify causes of urticaria.

Urticaria, or hives, is due to allergies.

Keratosis Pilaris

Keratosis pilaris is a condition in which the skin exhibits redness and irritation in patches, accompanied by a rough texture, and small pinpoint white papules that look like very small milia. Keratosis pilaris is often found on the cheeks and upper arms. It is often seen in children and teenagers, but can affect any age group. In most cases, it is a nuisance disorder. Doctors have been successful in treating keratosis pilaris with glycolic or lactic acid solutions, but it often goes away by itself.

Keratosis pilaris is a condition in which the skin exhibits redness and irritation in patches, accompanied by a rough texture, and small pinpoint white papules that look like very small milia.

Telangiectasias are enlarged or broken capillaries, often referred to as **couperose** by European estheticians. Telangiectasias are permanent and are caused by a variety of factors, including chronic sun exposure, exposure to extreme temperatures, friction, or injury to the skin. They are characteristic of rosacea, as we have discussed in previous chapters. They can also be caused or worsened by use of vasodilators, which are drugs or substances that cause dilation of the blood vessels. Included in the category of vasodilators are tobacco and alcohol. Alcoholics often have many telangiectatic vessels. Treatment ranges from freezing and electrocautery to laser and injection. Most telangiectasias are only a beauty nuisance, but clients with multiple telangiectasias should be referred to a dermatologist for treatment or evaluation.

Telangiectasias are small, red enlarged capillaries of the face and other areas of the body.

Couperose refers to diffuse redness including telangiectasias of the face and other areas of the body.

The esthetician can treat telangiectasias with vitamin K creams, which significantly help reduce their appearance. A new type of skin-care equipment, ultra-high frequency, may also be helpful in management of telangiectasias. Telangiectasias do have a tendency to reoccur, even when they are treated by the dermatologist with laser or electrodessication, the use of an electric needle to cauterize the capillaries and cut off the blood flow to the area.

GROWTHS

We have already discussed solar-induced growths of the skin. These include sebaceous hyperplasias, seborrheic keratoses, basal and squamous cell carcinomas, solar lentigenes, and melanoma. Solar-induced skin growths are seen frequently by estheticians.

Skin tags are very small, threadlike growths. They are benign lesions, but frequently are irritated by jewelry or clothing, rubbing against them.

Xanthomas are fatty pockets found on the eyelids.

Xanthalasmas are much flatter than milia, have a yellowish appearance, are below the skin's surface, and may have irregular shape.

You should review Chapter 16, Sun and Sun Damage, and be very familiar with identifying these growths, especially cancers and pre-cancers.

Skin tags are very small, threadlike growths. They are frequently seen on the eyelids, neck, and decollete. They are benign lesions, but frequently are irritated by jewelry or clothing rubbing against them. Most people find them unattractive, and they should be removed. They are easily removed by the dermatologist using freezing, electric needle, or scissors (Plate 65).

Skin tags are largely hereditary, and have been associated with obesity, pregnancy, postmenopause, diabetes, and intestinal disorders. These medical associations are another reason that skin tags should be seen by a physician.

Xanthomas or **xanthalasmas** are fatty pockets found on the eyelids. They look like large closed comedones, and are frequently found on the upper and lower lids. They are somewhat flat and are usually oval or egg-shaped.

Xanthalasmas should be referred to a dermatologist for removal by extraction or excision. They are often associated with high cholesterol, and often the dermatologist will order tests to determine cholesterol levels.

We have only touched on the many disorders and diseases that can affect the skin. We have, however, discussed many conditions frequently observed by the practicing esthetician.

Again, this chapter should educate you, to recognize symptoms that could indicate conditions that should be referred to a dermatologist or other appropriate physician. Estheticians treat cosmetic disorders of the skin. They should never attempt to diagnose or treat a disease or medical disorder.

Always refer any suspicious rash, growth, or other abnormality to a dermatologist.

Topics for Discussion

1. What is the difference between a primary and a secondary lesion?
2. What are some common infections of the skin? What are their causes?
3. What are some common fungal infections?
4. Use your knowledge of dermatological terminology to describe a grade 3 acne condition.
5. Why should estheticians be familiar with common forms of skin disease?

Chapter

21

Medical Relations

Objectives

The esthetician and the medical doctor can beautifully complement each other's work. It is important to learn to work with doctors, especially dermatologists and plastic surgeons.

In this chapter you will learn about medical relations, and you will learn important factors in having good relationships with the medical community. We will also discuss common problems between the two professions and what you can do to make these relationships successful.

More and more estheticians routinely work with physicians, usually dermatologists and plastic surgeons. In many instances estheticians work in the offices of doctors.

This chapter will address how esthetics and medicine relate. Specifically, we will discuss how physician-esthetician relationships work and how to establish working relationships with members of the medical community.

HOW ESTHETICIANS WORK WITH PHYSICIANS

Estheticians can provide many services that complement a medical practice. For example, estheticians can provide deep cleansing facial treatments for acne patients and problem skin clients who also receive medical treatment from a dermatologist. Estheticians can help educate the patient about home care and can help recommend proper home care. They can also teach clients how to cope with the cosmetic side effects of many dermatological drugs.

The dermatologist may refer a client to an esthetician for help in choosing non-comedogenic cosmetics, or they may ask the esthetician to find a cosmetic that will work for a specific client without certain ingredients to which the patient may be allergic. Paramedical camouflage makeup cases are often referred by dermatologists.

Patient Referrals from the Esthetician

You are in a position, seeing dozens of clients a week, to send many referrals to the dermatologist for problems such as cysts, rashes, allergies, possible skin cancers, sun damage, and other skin afflictions that we have discussed in Chapter 20. So many skin diseases and abnormalities require medical care. Always refer any cases that you are not sure about!

MEDICAL TRAINING

Let us discuss the kinds of doctors you may work with and what kind of training they have.

Dermatologists are specialists in the diseases of the skin, hair, and nails. They treat diseases, whereas estheticians treat cosmetic disorders. They study for four years of college and then four years of medical school, at which time they are awarded the Medical Doctor degree (M.D.). Another type of physician is the Doctor of Osteopathy (D.O.). Osteopathic school is very similar to medical school, except that osteopathic physicians traditionally have more holistic training, with emphasis on nutrition, body alignment, and so forth. D.O.'s are basically licensed to practice just like M.D.'s.

After medical or osteopathic school, doctors generally have a year of internship and then two to four years of specialty residency in dermatology. They train under dermatologists at major hospitals or universities. After all these years of training, they take their board exam in dermatology, administered by the American Academy of Dermatology, the professional association for dermatologists. This special certification is what dermatologists refer to when they say they are board certified.

Dermatologists may also subspecialize in several fields. MOHS surgeons have further specialty training in micrographic surgery, a specialized form of surgery for hard-to-treat skin cancers. Other dermatologists may be dermatological surgeons, specializing in skin surgery, or may practice plastic surgery.

Another up-and-coming field in dermatology is **cosmetic dermatology**. This field certainly relates well to the field of esthetics. These dermatologists have specialty training in cosmetic disorders and diseases of the skin and have a good understanding of

Cosmetic dermatology is a subspecialty of dermatology treating appearance-oriented problems of the skin.

human appearance and beauty. Cosmetic dermatologists generally have a very good understanding of esthetics and the needs of the esthetic client.

Plastic surgeons have four years of college and four years of medical school, internship, and then several years of residency in plastic surgery.

Qualifications for board exams and the different types of physicians who practice plastic surgery have already been discussed in Chapter 19.

OTHER DOCTORS

Besides dermatologists and plastic surgeons, there are other types of doctors that estheticians should be acquainted with and be able to refer cases to. Generally, these physicians are M.D.'s who are board certified in their various fields of specialty.

Gynecologists specialize in treating women's reproductive and urinary systems, and often help women with hormonal disorders. Acne, unwanted hair growth, and hyperpigmentation are all symptoms that can be hormone related.

Endocrinologists specialize in treatment of diseases of the endocrine system. The glandular system, if it is diseased, can seriously affect the skin. Thyroid or adrenal disorders, for example, can affect the skin, hair, and nails. **Rheumatologists** are specialists in rheumatoid diseases, including lupus.

Internists specialize in the treatment of internal diseases, including heart problems, diabetes, and other internal afflictions. Clients who have body massage may need referral to orthopedic surgeons, neurologists, or chiropractors. Cosmetic dentists, who specialize in the treatment of cosmetic disorders of the mouth and teeth, can also help make the client look better.

Endocrinologists specialize in treatment of diseases of the endocrine system.

Rheumatologists are specialists in rheumatoid diseases, including lupus.

Internists specialize in the treatment of internal diseases, including heart problems, diabetes, and other internal afflictions.

WHAT IS "PARAMEDICAL" ESTHETICS?

There has been a great deal of controversy in the esthetics profession about the term "paramedical." This term evolved out of a need for some estheticians to clarify or legitimize what they do.

Many estheticians prefer the term "clinical," meaning that the esthetician is practicing skin care with a scientific approach. A clinical esthetician understands skin from a scientific perspective and understands how to manage the skin using results-oriented techniques. A medical esthetician may work in a dermatologist's or plastic surgeon's office, administering medical-related treatments under the doctor's supervision. This may include administering higher strength glycolic peels, or helping with immediate postoperative care for surgical patients.

YOUR FIRST CONTACT WITH A PHYSICIAN

You must establish contact with a physician in order to have a working relationship. Many doctors are not familiar with estheticians or their training. This is why it is so important to have a complete résumé listing all your credentials. You should also list any specialty you have and any additional degrees you may hold. List only academic training. In other words, do not list particular product training that you may have had, unless it includes training in a specialized area, such as acne, clinical camouflage, comedogenicity, etc. If you hold a special certification such as a CIDESCO or BABTEC diploma (see Chapter 22, The Scientific Approach), make sure you list it here, along with a short explanation of the certificate, because the doctor may not be familiar with esthetic board certifications. Specifically list if you have real clinical training or advanced training in the sciences.

Make sure you list all the positions you have held, any professional affiliations, such as membership in esthetic organizations, and special awards. Make sure your résumé looks very professional. It may be beneficial to contact a résumé service organization to help you write it.

WHAT DOCTORS LIKE . . . AND DON'T

Doctors have very serious, scientific training. They generally do not have much training in artistic fields and are not always well-acquainted with special techniques in the esthetics field. Be specific about what kind of special training you have had. Doctors are trained in the scientific method—make sure you read Chapter 22. This will help you better understand why doctors are sometimes skeptical about estheticians.

Sometimes it may seem that doctors do not care much about esthetics. Often a doctor is more concerned about a patient's medical condition than about a cosmetic problem. Medical concerns outweigh cosmetic concerns. In other words, a physical reaction is more important than how something looks. If a patient has skin cancer, for example, getting rid of the cancer outweighs how the skin will look after medical treatment. Ideally, of course, both factors will be taken into consideration, but the patient's life and medical condition are always first!

Doctors in general are impressed with estheticians who have a good working knowledge of dermatology and how the human body functions in general. It helps to have additional training in other medically related fields. Estheticians who are also nurses, for example, often do very well working with dermatologists. If you have a good background in a science-related field, it will help you greatly when communicating with physicians. Doctors also appreciate it when an esthetician takes a scientific approach to cosmetic treatment. Examples of this are practicing clinically, using sterile techniques, using time-tested methods, and respecting when a client needs dermatological care, rather than esthetic care.

The biggest dislike of dermatologists, and doctors in general, is unscientific, "miraculous" approaches to beauty. If you make exaggerated claims or always tout the latest "miracle" treatment, you will not get much respect from the medical community. "Natural" treatments also raise medical eyebrows. There are advantages and disadvantages to using "natural" products. As one prominent dermatologist said, "Tuberculosis is natural, and so are scorpions!" For more information on why "natural" is not always best, read Chapter 6.

The bottom line is that most doctors are honest with patients and expect the same from you. They know that neither of you can perform miracles. Be honest with your medical colleagues. Admit when you don't understand something. And don't act as if you are the dermatologist's equal. You are in entirely different, related fields.

WHAT TO LOOK FOR IN A RELATIONSHIP WITH A DOCTOR

Just as doctors expect certain standards from estheticians, you should expect the same standards from the doctors with whom you work.

Unfortunately, managed care has caused financial uproar for some physicians, who find it more lucrative to work in a cash business like skin care. There have been instances when doctors who are not even specially trained in dermatology or any other skin-related form of medical science suddenly open cosmetic or skin-care clinics. Many of these doctors are looking to make money without accepting insurance.

Unfortunately, there are also some doctors who are more interested in money than in good and fair treatment of patients, and see the opportunity to make a lot of money in skin care. These types of doctors have created a lot of resentment among many esthetic skin-care professionals.

It is important to look for a doctor who is board certified or board eligible in his/her specialty. It is equally important to associate with an established specialist who has a good reputation and who treats estheticians like licensed professionals, not like subservient flunkies.

If you work as a medical esthetician in a doctor's office, make sure you are paid similarly as you would be if you were in private practice. There are doctors who are wonderful, caring people, who care about their patients and want the very best care. These are the doctors you want to work with.

One of the best scenarios is to find a board-certified dermatologist or plastic surgeon who wants a *referral* relationship, rather than have the esthetician in the office. This allows the esthetician to accept doctor referrals while still working independently. The esthetician can feel comfortable referring patients, knowing that the doctor does not have an in-house esthetician who might assume skin-care treatments for the referred patient.

THE INTERVIEW

Call and make an appointment with the dermatologist to talk. Tell the receptionist who you are and briefly explain why you would like to talk to the dermatologist. If the receptionist is hesitant about making the appointment, leave a message for the doctor to call you. If the doctor returns your call, ask for an appointment to come by and talk.

Remember, not all doctors understand what estheticians do. Briefly explain what services you perform and your particular specialties. Bring your résumé. You may want to bring a good book with you to show what kind of education you have had.

Ask if the doctor has any particular specialties, and suggest working with you. Relax and get to know the doctor as a person. You will often find you have more in common than you think.

Ask the dermatologist for any patient brochures distributed in the office. Familiarize yourself with these brochures and any other patient education materials the doctor uses routinely. This will acquaint you with the doctor's techniques and may also give you an idea of how you could fit into the practice.

Invite the doctor to visit your salon. Offer a free treatment, and after the treatment offer some free samples of products. Do everything just as you normally would. Tell the doctor that you will act as if he or she were any other client. This way the doctor will see how you really work. Most dermatologists are actually very impressed with a good facial treatment. You might also offer a free treatment to the doctor's nurse or assistant. They often are involved with patient education in the office!

After you get to know the doctor you may ask if you may observe some procedures. Spending a day with a dermatologist is a truly enlightening experience! You will see cases you never see in the salon, and you will leave with a better understanding of medicine in general.

Don't forget that the interview is also a great opportunity for you to see how you feel about the doctor with whom you are meeting. Is he or she friendly and warm? Does he/she have a holistic approach to medicine? Does he/she already have a working understanding of esthetics? All of these factors will help indicate a successful medical referral situation.

DOCTORS' CONCERNS

Allergies

Have a good understanding of how allergies develop and how irritation occurs. Dermatologists see a lot of allergic reactions and a lot of contact dermatitis. Be knowledgeable about common cosmetic ingredient allergies and patch testing. Ask the doctor to help you understand the method of allergy testing.

Comedogenic Cosmetics

This is an area where you can really win a dermatologist over. If you have a good understanding of comedogenicity and acne, you can provide an excellent service to the dermatologist, helping patients find noncomedogenic, nonacnegenic cosmetics and skin-care products.

Rosacea and Sensitive Skin

Many patients are diagnosed with rosacea, and many people have sensitive skin. Having a good knowledge of rosacea management and sensitive skin is very helpful to dermatologists.

Sun Damage

Dermatologists are impressed if you have a good knowledge of skin cancer and sun damage. They will be equally unimpressed if you offer tanning sessions in your salon!

Electrolysis

Here is another excellent service for esthetic referral. Dermatologists see a lot of cases of unwanted hair that may be a result of another medical condition. Electrolysis is generally very well accepted by dermatologists and doctors in general.

Paramedical Makeup

Doctors very often refer patients for help with camouflage and corrective makeup. It is important for you to be well versed in corrective makeup techniques and clinical camouflage makeup. Doctors will frequently refer patients with scars or birthmarks, accident victims, post-skin-cancer treatment patients, and patients with disfigurements for help with makeup. Do not be discouraged if this is all they refer at first. Eventually, one of those patients will have skin-care treatments and will return to the doctor with glowing results and comments!

Extraction

Dermatologists often refer patients for treatment of comedones. They are often already treating the patients with other prescription drugs. Knowing how to treat these patients will help you prove yourself to the doctor. Discuss your extraction techniques with the doctor and set up a list of rules for various types of patients.

Tretinoin/Retinoid Acid

Tretinoin (Retin-A, Renova®, azelaic acid (Azelex®), adapalene (Differin®), and other prescription topical drugs are often prescribed by dermatologists. These and other topical drugs can have side effects on the skin, and often make the skin more sensitive to some cleansers, cosmetics, and other skin-care products. You should be familiar with management of clients being treated with other drugs that can affect the skin, what ingredients and products should be avoided, and which are unacceptable treatments for sensitive skin. Helping clients find suitable products while being treated with these drugs is an important part of a clinical skin-care practice.

Accutane® patients are another group of patients who need help with extra gentle skin care. See Chapter 12 and Chapter 17 for further information.

Seborrhea and Other Inflammations

The doctor will be interested in how you deal with the patient who has a history of seborrheic dermatitis or other types of dermatitis.

Perhaps you are lucky enough to have attended a school that has a lecturing dermatologist on staff. This type of learning experience is an extremely valuable preparation for working with a dermatologist. Try to take continuing education classes with dermatologists or take classes that address some of the pertinent topics we have discussed as being important issues to them. Read all that you can, obtaining brochures and purchasing dermatology textbooks to study on your own. There are several condensed versions of these types of texts, and a variety of good books are available, written in easy-to-understand language, that discuss common dermatological problems.

Some pharmaceutical companies are progressive enough to offer training to allied health professionals, including estheticians. Many of these programs are new, and more will, no doubt, be offered in the future. Many of the esthetician's journals offer regular interviews with medical experts and frequently contain articles about the subjects we have discussed. Taking a course in medical terminology is also a good idea so you will better understand medical language.

HOW TO REFER A CLIENT

When you notice that a client has a problem that needs referral, tell the client to call your referring dermatologist for an appointment. Send the dermatologist a referral slip telling about your client, why you are referring the client, and what services you have been performing to help the client. Make arrangements with the dermatologist to have him or her send you a reply referral letter letting you know what their diagnosis was and what treatment they have prescribed. In this letter they will tell you what should be done in the salon as a follow-up. Occasionally, a dermatologist will tell a client not to have esthetic services for a period of time. This should be explained in the doctor's letter, as well as the reason for this recommendation. Sometimes, particularly if the patient has minor skin surgery, or has recurrent dermatitis, or has a communicable disease, it is necessary to discontinue esthetic treatment.

SOME COMMON PROBLEMS

Many estheticians have discussed problems they often have in their relationships with dermatologists. Many of these are caused by miscommunication between the doctor and the esthetician. This is why it is so important to have an open line of communication with the dermatologist. We will discuss some of the most common complaints estheticians have about dermatologists and the common problems dermatologists have with estheticians.

Why Do Dermatologists Only Recommend Certain Product Lines?

Just as you are educated about certain product lines, dermatologists receive training about certain products. Drug companies sponsor product knowledge classes and workshops, just as cosmetic companies do. So it is only natural that the doctor recommend familiar products. An esthetician would not recommend unfamiliar products either.

Doctors recommend what is widely available to their patients. They also recommend products they know their patients can afford. Dermatologists are particular about many allergy-causing, comedogenic, or irritancy-inducing chemicals used in cosmetics. Therefore, it is important that you have products available that meet these standards. You should try to have available moderately priced, noncomedogenic, hypoallergenic cosmetics that are as frangrance-free as possible. Dermatologists are concerned about allergies, and fragrances frequently cause allergies. This does not mean that this type of product is all you should carry, but you certainly should have a specialty line available for this type of client. Furnish information to dermatologists about your products, and furnish them with some sample products to try themselves.

Why Do Dermatologists Always Recommend Soap and Water?

Soap and water are readily available to most patients in all income groups. Soaps that dermatologists recommend rarely cause allergy problems. Soaps are more rinseable than many cleansing milks, an important factor in treating skin problems. Talk to the dermatologist about recommending rinseable "soapless" soaps, which have the same rinseability as soap, but without the residues and possible higher pH. Again, you should have this type of product available, and it should be fragrance-free.

When I Send a Client to a Dermatologist, the Client Doesn't Come Back to the Salon!

This could result from different situations. First, get the doctor to agree to send you a referral letter letting you know about the client's progress, if esthetic treatment should be discontinued, and, most importantly, why.

Occasionally, a client will find that the visit to the dermatologist solves the problem and simply elects not to return to the salon at that time.

Occasionally, you will discover that you are working with an "esthetician-basher"! The best way to deal with this kind of doctor is to find another doctor whom you can work with!

Again, you may want to choose to refer to a doctor who does not have an in-house esthetician, rather than to a doctor who does. You may risk losing a client to the doctor's esthetician.

Dermatologists' Problems with Estheticians

Here are some common complaints dermatologists have about estheticians.

The Esthetician Is Not Scientific

To fully understand this, please read Chapter 22, The Scientific Approach. Many products on the market were developed based on anecdotal evidence, which is not scientifically sound. If you use and recommend products with exaggerated claims, or that have no scientific basis, this is a problem for many dermatologists. The solution to this problem is to carry products that are as scientific as possible and that do not make unbelievable claims.

The Esthetician Uses Products That Are Too Heavy or Comedogenic

Both of these are "no-nos" with dermatologists. As previously discussed, carry a good line of lightweight, fragrance-free, noncomedogenic cosmetics.

Patients Complain That the Esthetician Is "Hard-Sell"

An esthetician should never take a "hard-sell" approach, no matter what kind of client you are dealing with. Carefully evaluate each client's individual needs, as well as lifestyle, budget, and skin-care needs. You should let the doctor know the range of what your products cost so they can brief their patients.

Some patients simply cannot afford esthetic services. Medical doctors see patients with serious medical problems, many of whom may not be able to afford esthetic services. Try your best to help these patients find an affordable product that they can use at home, even if they don't visit regularly for services.

WORKING WITH THE PLASTIC SURGEON

Plastic surgeons are generally easier to work with than dermatologists. Cosmetic surgeons have clients who can afford elective cosmetic surgery. These clients can usually also afford esthetic services and more upscale products.

Because plastic surgery is often elective, plastic surgeons are more interested in esthetics, due to the artistic aspects of their specialty. They are interested in having their patients look as good as possible. Esthetic services "put the icing on the cake" by accentuating their work. Good skin care and proper makeup really enhance a good cosmetic surgery procedure. As previously discussed in Chapter 19, you should establish a relationship with a plastic surgeon and have an understanding with the surgeon about treatment procedures so that you both know what to expect from one another.

The bottom line is that good communication and a healthy respect for each other's professions is the key to a successful working medical relationship.

Topics for Discussion

1. What are some services that you can provide to the dermatology patient?
2. What type of conditions might you refer to the dermatologist?
3. Discuss a physician's training.
4. Discuss scheduling a first-time meeting with a dermatologist.
5. What are common communication problems between estheticians and dermatologists?
6. Discuss some ways to improve relations between the esthetics and medical communities.
7. Discuss how to choose the right doctor to whom you can refer clients.

The Scientific
Approach

Objectives

Improving your education is a vital part of professional growth. Setting standards and learning to evaluate new developments is an essential part of any profession.

In this chapter we will discuss the need to be scientific in your approach to the practice of esthetics and the many educational opportunities that are available for advancement in the profession of esthetics.

Esthetics, like other health-related fields, is not an exact science. Too many factors are involved to determine the exact cause of a skin problem or to suggest an exact solution to a skin problem. So many factors are involved in any treatment involving the human body, whether the treatment is esthetic or medical. Therefore, estheticians can only give a "best guess" opinion about skin conditions and what they recommend to help.

We can, however, make an educated guess, taking the time to learn as much as we can about the human body in general and the skin in particular.

THE SCIENTIFIC METHOD

Scientific method refers to the experimental technique of developing a hypothesis, or idea, based on available information. The hypothesis is tested, interpreted, and results are published.

The **scientific method** refers to the experimental technique of developing a hypothesis, or idea, based on available information. After the hypothesis is established, the method involves testing the idea and interpreting and publishing the results of the experiment. Let's look at an example. Years ago, doctors observed that certain keratolytic agents helped to peel the skin. They knew that many forms of acne were essentially caused by dead cells building up and clogging the follicles. It made sense that a keratolytic agent applied to the skin of acne patients would help loosen and remove dead cell buildup, opening the follicle and therefore increasing the oxygen content of the follicle canal. They also knew that acne bacteria could not survive in the presence of oxygen. They assembled a group of acne sufferers and experimentally applied keratolytic agents routinely to the skin of these patients. They tried to control the patients' other habits. In other words, if some of these patients were using special soaps, or vigorously scrubbing the skin, this could affect the results of the study. Factors that can affect an experiment are called *variables*. If there are too many variables in a study, it is hard to determine what causes changes that occur in an experiment.

Control group is the group in an experiment that does not change behavior.

In order to see if other factors caused changes besides the keratolytic agents, these scientists assembled a **control group**, a group of acne patients who did everything the same as the experimental group but did not apply the keratolytic. Instead they were given a product that looked the same as the keratolytic product but that did not actually contain the keratolytic. Such a product is called a *placebo*. Scientists observed that the group of acne patients who used the product with the keratolytic experienced marked improvement in their acne, whereas the group who applied the product without keratolytic had no improvement.

This method of research showed that keratolytics can help acne patients. The scientists carefully observed the number of acne lesions present on all of the patients' faces before and after the experiment. They carefully calculated the percentage of decrease in acne lesions of the group using the keratolytic and compared it to the control group. Then they applied specially designed mathematical formulas to measure the differences they observed. Using this type of mathematical calculation is called **statistics**. If there is a measurable difference in factors before and after the experiment, as there was in the group using the keratolytic, the results are said to be statistically significant. The scientists then published the results of their study, and the theory of using keratolytics to help acne eventually became standard practice.

Statistics are precise mathematical measurements of changes in an experiment.

This is a very simplified example, but it illustrates the scientific method. Other factors can influence a study. The number of subjects (patients) studied is an important factor. If too few people are studied, the study will not be significant. If the study does not take place over a long enough period of time, the study will not be significant. Research like this takes a lot of time and money. Drugs may be tested for years and years before being released. Side effects and possible dangers of using the drug must also be studied. If a drug helps a certain condition, but at the same time hurts another area of the body, it often cannot be practically used. Cosmetics generally have less research performed on them than drugs. The main reason for this is money. It is very expensive to perform complicated research studies. Also, as we learned in Chapter 11, if a cosmetic manufacturer makes a claim that it affects anything but appearance, it is considered a drug and is subject to governmental regulations that require much more research. This is why doctors often consider the need for cosmetic treatment to be questionable. Cosmetics are generally not tested nearly as extensively as drugs and therefore are not as scientifically sound as pharmaceuticals, according to many scientists.

Research on cosmetics is often performed on the ingredients rather than the product itself. The active agent is tested in the laboratory to determine its benefits, and then it is mixed with a usable vehicle, such as a cream or lotion. More and more cosmetic companies are testing their products and measuring improvement in the subjects' appearance.

If a product contains ingredients that are thought to be beneficial for the skin, this theory is called *anecdotal*. Anecdotal evidence is based on observation and theory, but the theory has not been thoroughly scientifically tested, as we discussed earlier. This doesn't mean that the product has no beneficial cosmetic effects; it simply means that the results and use are based on anecdotal, rather than scientific, findings.

An example of anecdotal information is the use of plant extracts and essential oils. There has been some scientific research in the use of these extracts, but not enough to establish scientifically significant findings for all of the many extracts that are used in cosmetics. Pharmaceutical companies frequently use chemicals that are actually extracted from plants, but the chemicals are isolated and pure, rather than using the entire extract, as many cosmetic companies do.

This brings up the subject of "natural" versus "synthetic." Natural cosmetics are regarded by some estheticians as superior to "chemicals." But plant extracts are nothing more than a group of different chemicals, because all materials on earth are made of chemicals! This is the main, and justified, argument against "natural" products. As we discussed in Chapter 6, if a person experiences an allergic reaction to salicylic acid, it is easy to determine that the person is allergic because salicylic acid is used as an isolated chemical. But if a client has an allergic reaction to a product containing sweet birch extract, a plant source for salicylic acid, it is hard to determine if the client had a reaction to salicylic acid or to one of the many other chemicals that comprise sweet birch extract.

This example is why dermatologists are often skeptical about the use of plant extracts and essential oils in cosmetic products. In general it is accepted that the fewer and more isolated ingredients that are used in cosmetics, the less potential there is for allergic reaction.

EVALUATING PRODUCTS

When you talk to a manufacturer about a new product or line of products, you should try to establish how scientific the research has been on the products. Ask many questions. Has the product been evaluated as thoroughly as possible? Do their claims sound believable? Or are they using "puffing" descriptions? **Puffing** refers to using complicated descriptions of the products to describe their effects on the skin. Some companies have excellent products and still use "puffing" because they are attempting to avoid

Puffing is a term used to describe the way some companies make their products sound better than they are.

making drug claims. If a company claims that a product has an effect on the functioning of the body, it is making drug claims.

What is the company's approach to skin care? Are formulations based on current research and do they use techniques that have been time tested? What are their developer's credentials? If they make claims for hypoallergenicity or noncomedogenicity, how are the products tested?

You must have a sound background to be able to ask good questions and evaluate a product. How do you prepare so you know what questions to ask? There are many things you can do to improve your scientific approach to skin care.

Go Back to School

Take some courses in chemistry, biology, and other sciences at your local community college or university. Start with beginning level classes. Many estheticians go back to school for additional classes and even degrees! A college degree in a related field such as health, chemistry, nutrition, or biological sciences is very helpful in the practice of esthetics. Many very successful estheticians have degrees in other related fields. You don't have to give up your practice to expand your education. More and more colleges offer night or weekend classes for working people. Some major universities now offer special two- to five-day classes in cosmetic sciences. One of these is the University of California at Los Angeles. For further information on this program, contact UCLA Extension.

Read Your Journals

You should subscribe to every journal in the beauty business. Contacts for magazines are listed in the bibliography section of this book.

These journals contain a wealth of information, including information about the many products available to estheticians. Many excellent estheticians write for these journals, describing their good and bad experiences. There is so much you can learn each month from reading these magazines.

Buy Any Book You Can About Skin

Visit your bookstore every month and purchase any new books about skin or health. Visit your college bookstore and purchase beginning level textbooks in anatomy, chemistry, biology, and other subjects related to esthetics.

An extremely important learning source is trade shows! You will meet and learn from some of the top estheticians, dermatologists, chemists, and researchers in the industry!

Stay for the whole show, and attend all the classes you can. You will learn a lot from your fellow attendees. The fellowship and learning experience has no price and is an extremely valuable learning tool. But you won't meet them if you don't go to the shows!

While at the shows, talk to the exhibitors and speakers and see from whom you feel you can learn the most. Ask if they offer additional training or classes. Make arrangements to attend classes offered by these specialists. Get on their mailing lists so you can receive a calendar of upcoming events or speaking engagements.

Three types of classes are generally offered at trade shows.

General education is taught at a "main stage" routinely throughout the convention. This is included in your admission fee. Usually held in a large ballroom, speakers discuss their specialties, or there are panel discussions. These lectures are usually less than an hour each.

Manufacturer education is offered in private classrooms. This is where the manufacturers teach you about their products. Obviously, manufacturers want you to buy their products after the classes. This is an excellent opportunity to evaluate new products. Remember, these lectures are usually commercial, but they are still a great way to learn more about your profession.

Workshops and seminars are often offered after the main convention. These are usually referred to as post-classes. Post-classes usually carry a separate fee and allow you to spend two or more hours with an accomplished speaker. If you read journal articles that you like or find helpful, the authors of these articles may be featured at trade show post-classes. The education in these classes is often called generic, meaning that it is not commercially product oriented. Spending this kind of time with a top esthetician is by far the best learning experience you can have.

Regional Seminars

Most skin-care companies have educational programs available, both product classes and general advanced esthetics classes. These classes often last a day or more and are offered frequently. Of course, this involves traveling to the city where the seminar is held, but you will usually find it very worthwhile.

Clinical Skin Care

As we have discussed previously, clinical skin care is a results-oriented program approach to esthetics. This combines a thorough assessment of the particular client's needs and a step-by-step plan of action, based on scientific treatment methods, and individualized home care, based on performance ingredients.

The profession is taking a turn toward clinical approaches, and although there will always be a need for relaxation therapy facial treatments, many estheticians are interested in offering clinical care, which is for many estheticians more challenging and rewarding.

Advanced Schools and Training

Basic skin-care training, in general, does not offer enough hours or the specialized instruction necessary for advanced clinical skin care. It is up to the individual esthetician to decide what type of practice he/she wishes to pursue. It is often necessary to look for schools or programs that offer advanced specialty classes.

Fortunately, more of these specialty programs are now emerging. These programs offer one- to five-day intensive learning sessions, often with well-known skin-care experts. To find more about these types of graduate programs, look for information in skin-care journals.

Join Your Professional Associations

The National Cosmetology Association (NCA) is the United States affiliate of CIDESCO International, the oldest and best-established esthetics organization in the world. CIDESCO helps to set standards for the industry and administers the CIDESCO International Examination, a board certification exam for estheticians. In many countries, estheticians attend schools that have been accredited by CIDESCO and are eligible to take the exam upon graduation. There are now several CIDESCO accredited schools in the United States. For graduates of schools that are not accredited, CIDESCO offers the "Three Year Exam." This means that if you have graduated from a licensed esthetics school, have practiced as a licensed esthetician for three years and complete a special intensive training program through CIDESCO, you may take the exam. The exam is difficult, and you should plan on several months of preparation for the test. If you pass the test, which is both written and practical, you are awarded the CIDESCO International Diploma. Estheticians who pass the exam are called CIDESCO Diplomats. The CIDESCO diploma is accepted as the highest earned title in the world for estheticians.

The NCA also offers other examinations. The NCA offers programs on the national and state level. The Esthetics America committee is a group of accomplished estheticians who have passed the Esthetics America exam, a national level test that is administered by the NCA. There are also state-level examinations that must be passed to qualify for the national exam. For further information on NCA programs, contact NCA, P.O. Box 809169, Chicago, IL 60611-9169, or in the United States call 1-800-527-1683. The American Aestheticians Education Association, P.O. Box 117896, Carrollton, TX 75011-7896, 1-800-985-2232, is an organization dedicated to providing specialized advanced education in many areas to estheticians. They have several events each year with well-known speakers and faculty.

The Esthetics Manufacturers and Distributors Alliance (EMDA) of the American Beauty Association, 401 N. Michigan Ave., Chicago, IL 60611, 1-312-245-1595, is a professional organization for skin-care manufacturers and wholesale distributors. They offer educational programs, legislative support, and help with issues of safety and standards for the esthetics profession.

Probably the biggest function of the professional organizations is serving as legislative watchdog for the profession. This helps prevent deregulation and helps ensure safety and standards for public health. Most professional organizations also offer special seminars, conventions and congresses, magazine subscriptions and journals, special insurance programs, and many other benefits.

Strive to obtain the highest credentials you can. There are three special secrets to being a great esthetician. You must receive the best education possible. You have to communicate well with people, and you have to, most of all, love your profession!

Topics for Discussion

1. Describe the scientific method.
2. What does *statistically significant* mean?
3. What kind of factors can affect a study?
4. What is the difference between scientific and anecdotal evidence?
5. Discuss how to evaluate products.
6. Why is it important to read and subscribe to esthetic journals?

Bibliography and Recommended Readings

Bark, J. (1989). Retin-A and other youth miracles. Rocklin, CA: Prima.

Bevan, J. (1979). The Simon and Schuster handbook of anatomy and physiology. New York: Simon and Schuster.

Boyd, A. (1998). The skin sourcebook. Los Angeles: Lowell House.

Brinker, N., & Chihal, J. (1997). 1000 questions about women's health. Arlington, TX: Summit.

Chase, D. (1989). The new medically based no-nonsense beauty book. New York: W.W. Norton.

Chihal, J., & London, S. (1999). Menopause: Clinical concepts. Durant, OK: EMIS Medical.

Desowitz, R. (1987). The thorn in the starfish. New York: W.W. Norton.

Dwyer, J. (1990). The body at war. New York: Mentor Books.

Fitzpatrick, T., Johnson, R., Wolff, K., Polano, M., & Suurmond, D. (1997). Color atlas and synopsis of clinical dermatology. New York: McGraw-Hill.

Flandermeyer, K. (1979). Clear skin. Boston: Little, Brown.

Fulton, J. (1984). Dr. Fulton's step-by-step program for clearing acne. New York: Barnes & Noble Books.

Gerson, J. (1999). Standard textbook for professional estheticians. Albany, NY: Milady.

Goodman, T., & Young, S. (1988). Smart face. New York: Prentice-Hall.

Gray, H. (1995). Gray's anatomy. Philadelphia: Running Press.

Haberman, F., & Fortino, D. (1983). Your skin. New York: Berkley.

Jovanovic, L., & Levert, S. (1993). A woman doctor's guide to menopause. New York: Hyperion.

Jovanovic, L., & Subak-Sharpe, G. (1987). Hormones—the woman's answer book. New York: Fawcett Columbine.

Kaiser, J. (1999). Healing HIV. Mill Valley, CA: HealthFirst Press.

Lowe, N., & Sellar, P. (1999). Skin secrets. London: Collins & Brown.

Otto, J., & Towle, A. (1993). Modern biology. New York: Holt, Rinehart & Winston.

Pugliese, P. (1991). Advanced professional skin care. Bernville, PA: APSC.

Schoon, D. (1994). HIV/AIDS & Hepatitis. Albany, NY: Milady.

Scott, A., & Fong, E. (1998). Body structures & functions. Albany, NY: Delmar.

Steigleder, G., & Maibach, H. (1984). Pocket atlas of dermatology. New York: Thieme.

Stoll, D. (1994). A woman's skin. New Brunswick, NJ: Rutgers University Press.

Teaff, N., & Wiley, K. (1996). Perimenopause—preparing for the change. Rocklin, CA: Prima.

Turkington, C., & Dover, J. (1996). Skin deep. New York: Facts on File.

Warshofsky, F. (1999). Stealing time. New York: TV Books.

Winter, R. (1999). A consumer's dictionary of cosmetic ingredients. New York: Three Rivers Press.

Wolfe, D. (1988). Introduction to college chemistry. New York: McGraw-Hill.

PERIODICALS

American Spa
East One Park Ave.
New York, NY 10016
(212) 951-6600

Cosmetic Dermatology
26 Main St.
Chatham, NJ 07928-2402
800-976-4040

Dayspa
7628 Densmore Ave.
Van Nuys, CA 91406-2042
(818) 782-7328

Dermascope Magazine
2611 Beltline Rd., Suite 140
Sunnyvale, TX 75182
(972) 226-2309

Les Nouvelles Esthetiques—American Edition
3929 Ponce de Leon
Coral Gables, FL 33134
800-471-0229

Progressive Clinical Insights (PCI)
720 Central Park Blvd.
Daytona Beach, FL 32127-7555
(904) 304-1600

Skin, Inc.
362 South Schmale Rd.
Carol Stream, IL 60188-2787
(630) 653-2155

Index

eyelid dermatitis and, 90
factors influencing, 92
fragrances and, 85–86
irritations and, 82–83
nail products and, 88
noncosmetic products and, 89
preservatives and, 86–87
sensitive skin and, 75–76
sudden reactions, 92–94
sunscreen and, 87–88
testing for irritation, 84–85
see also Dermatitis

Alphahydroxy acids (AHAs), a family of naturally occurring acids, 132
acne and, 181
contraindications of, 134
peeling treatments with, 269–72
photoaging skin and, 256–59
skin-care products with, 155–56, 157–58
strengths and effectiveness of, 133
vehicles and other ingredients with, 133–34

Amino (prefix), refers to compounds that have an amino acid group attached, 106

Amino acids, proteins that help break down simple sugars, fats, and parts of proteins, 3, 104

Amphoteric surfactants, may have either a positive or a negative ionic charge. They are frequently used in facial lotions and creams, 110

Ampoules, 151–54

Anaerobic, bacteria that do not need oxygen to grow and survive, 169

Androgens, male hormones, 59, 172

Anecdotal, means that an ingredient is supposed to provide certain benefits to the skin, but they have not yet been substantiated, or proven, by scientific means, 125

Anhydrous products, treatment products that do not contain water, 164

Animal testing, 166

Anionic surfactants, are strong cleansers and are frequently used in household products, 109

Annular lesion, a ring-shaped lesion, 305

Anorexia, and hormones, 73

Antibiotics, drugs that are made from extracts obtained from living organisms that fight bacterial infections, 25

Antibody, a protein that helps to neutralize foreign organisms entering the body, 17, 18

Antigen, refers to a foreign substance recognized by the immune system as an invader, 17, 18

Antihistamines, drugs that are produced to combat the formation of histamines, 76

Antimicrobials, 116–17

Antioxidants, topical free radical scavengers that help neutralize free radicals before they can attach themselves to cell membranes, eventually destroying the cell. They are added to cosmetic formulas to prevent oxidation, 118, 135
photoaging skin and, 259

Antiseptic washes, 52

Antiseptics, a weaker form of disinfectant. They are usually mild enough to use on the skin, 46
commonly used, 50

Apocrine glands, are present in the groin area and armpits. They produce a thicker form of sweat and are responsible for producing the substance that, when in contact with bacteria, produces body odor, 8, 56, 57

Aqueous, water-based, as in an aqueous solution, 106

Arbutin, a melanin suppressant, 233

Ascorbic acid is an acid form of vitamin C, an antioxidant; necessary for collagen production, 136

Aseptic procedure, the term scientists use to describe proper handling techniques of sterilized and disinfected equipment, 46
disposable materials and, 46–47
nondisposable items and, 47–49

Astringents, have a tightening effect on the skin or pore appearance, 127
acne and, 181

Atopic dermatitis, 308

Atopic eczema, also known as atopic dermatitis, a chronic inflammatory condition of the skin that is hereditary and may be related to respiratory allergies or asthma, 308

Atrophic scars, depressed scars, such as acne pocks, caused by loss of tissue, 305

Atrophy, means wasting away, 305

Autoimmune diseases, 27

Autoimmunity, a condition in which the immune system cannot distinguish the difference between antigens and its own body cells, 27

Azelaic acid, a form of acid, also known as Azelex, a topical prescription drug used for acne treatment, 185, 233

Azelex, 185

AZT, 33

Azulene, a hydrocarbon derived from the chamomile flower, 78, 127

B cells, also called B lymphocytes, make antibodies that are proteins that help to prevent further infection or reoccurrence, 18